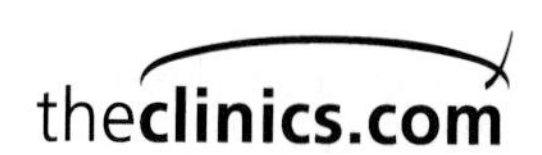

CARDIOLOGY CLINICS

Cardiovascular Magnetic Resonance Imaging

GUEST EDITOR
Raymond J. Kim, MD

CONSULTING EDITOR
Michael H. Crawford, MD

February 2007 • Volume 25 • Number 1

SAUNDERS
An Imprint of Elsevier, Inc.
PHILADELPHIA LONDON TORONTO MONTREAL SYDNEY TOKYO

W.B. SAUNDERS COMPANY
A Division of Elsevier Inc.

Elsevier Inc. • 1600 John F. Kennedy Blvd., Suite 1800 • Philadelphia, Pennsylvania 19103-2899

http://www.theclinics.com

CARDIOLOGY CLINICS
February 2007
Editor: Karen Sorensen

Volume 25, Number 1
ISSN 0733-8651
ISBN-13: 978-1-4160-4281-5
ISBN-10: 1-4160-4281-4

Cardiology Clinics (ISSN 0733-8651) is published quarterly by Elsevier Inc., 360 Park Avenue South, New York, NY 10010-1710. Months of issue are February, May, August, and November. Business and editorial Offices: 1600 John F. Kennedy Blvd., Suite 1800, Philadelphia, PA 19103-2899. Customer Service Office: 6277 Sea Harbor Drive, Orlando, FL 32887-4800. Periodicals postage paid at New York, NY, and additional mailing offices. Subscription prices are $198.00 per year for US individuals, $302.00 per year for US institutions, $99.00 per year for US students and residents, $242.00 per year for Canadian individuals, $367.00 per year for Canadian institutions, $264.00 per year for international individuals, $367.00 per year for international institutions and $132.00 per year for Canadian and foreign students/residents. To receive student/resident rate, orders must be accompanied by name of affiliated institution, data of term, and the *signature* of program/residency coordinator on institution letterhead. Orders will be billed at individual rate until proof of status is received. Foreign air speed delivery is included in all *Clinics* subscription prices. All prices are subject to change without notice. POSTMASTER: Send address changes to *Cardiology Clinics*, Elsevier Periodicals Customer Service, 6277 Sea Harbor Drive, Orlando, FL 32887-4800. **Customer Service: 1-800-654-2452 (US). From outside of the US, call 1-407-345-1000.**

Cardiology Clinics is also published in Spanish by McGraw-Hill Interamericana Editores S. A., P.O. Box 5-237, 06500, Mexico D. F., Mexico; in Portuguese by Reichmann and Alfonso Editores Rio de Janeiro, Brazil; and in Greek by Dimitrios P. Lagos, 8 Pondon Street, GR115-28 Ilissia, Greece.

Cardiology Clinics is covered in *Index Medicus, Excerpta Medica, The Cumulative Index to Nursing and Allied Health Literature* (INAHL).

Printed in the United States of America.

CONSULTING EDITOR

MICHAEL H. CRAWFORD, MD, Professor of Medicine, Lucie Stern Chair in Cardiology, University of California San Francisco; and Chief of Clinical Cardiology, University of California, San Francisco Medical Center, San Francisco, California

GUEST EDITOR

RAYMOND J. KIM, MD, Associate Professor, Cardiology Division; Director, Duke Cardiovascular Magnetic Resonance Center, Duke University Health Systems, Durham, North Carolina

CONTRIBUTORS

GREGORY B. ANG, MD, Fellow in Cardiology, Cardiology Division, Duke University Medical Center, Durham, North Carolina

EVAN APPELBAUM, MD, Harvard-Thorndike Laboratory of the Department of Medicine (Cardiovascular Division), Beth Israel Deaconess Medical Center and Harvard Medical School, Boston, Massachusetts

BARBRA BROWN, NP, Nashville Cardiovascular MRI Institute, The Heart Group, PLLC, Brentwood, Nashville, Tennessee

JAMES C. CARR, MD, Assistant Professor of Radiology, Department of Radiology, Northwestern University Medical School and Northwestern Memorial Hospital, Chicago, Illinois

ANNA LISA CROWLEY, MD, Duke Cardiovascular Magnetic Resonance Center, Duke University Health Systems, Durham, North Carolina

PETER G. DANIAS, MD, PhD, Department of Medicine, St. Elizabeth's Hospital and Tufts University Medical School, Boston Massachusetts

CHRISTOPHER J. FRANÇOIS, MD, Cardiovascular Imaging Fellow, Department of Radiology, Northwestern University, Feinberg School of Medicine, Chicago, Illinois

JOHN D. GRIZZARD, MD, Assistant Professor, Department of Radiology, Virginia Commonwealth University Medical Center, Richmond, Virginia

THOMAS H. HAUSER, MD, Harvard-Thorndike Laboratory of the Department of Medicine (Cardiovascular Division), Beth Israel Deaconess Medical Center and Harvard Medical School, Boston, Massachusetts

W. GREGORY HUNDLEY, MD, FACC, FAHA, Department of Internal Medicine, and Department of Radiology, Wake Forest University School of Medicine, Bowman Gray Campus, Medical Center Boulevard, Winston-Salem, North Carolina

ROBERT M. JUDD, PhD, Associate Professor, Department of Medicine and Radiology, Greenberg Division of Cardiology, Weill Medical College of Cornell University, New York, New York

HAN W. KIM, MD, Duke Cardiovascular Magnetic Resonance Center, Duke University Health Systems, Durham, North Carolina

RAYMOND J. KIM, MD, Associate Professor, Cardiology Division; Director, Duke Cardiovascular Magnetic Resonance Center, Duke University Health Systems, Durham, North Carolina

IGOR KLEM, MD, Faculty, Greenberg Division of Cardiology, Weill Medical College of Cornell University, New York, New York

WARREN J. MANNING, MD, Harvard-Thorndike Laboratory of the Departments of Medicine (Cardiovascular Division) and Radiology, Beth Israel Deaconess Medical Center and Harvard Medical School, Boston, Massachusetts

REZA NEZAFAT, PhD, Harvard-Thorndike Laboratory of the Department of Medicine (Cardiovascular Division), Beth Israel Deaconess Medical Center and Harvard Medical School, Boston, Massachusetts

MANESH R. PATEL, MD, Assistant Professor, Department of Medicine, Division of Cardiology, Duke University Medical Center, Durham, North Carolina

ANDREW J. POWELL, MD, Department of Cardiology, Children's Hospital Boston; Associate Professor of Pediatrics, Harvard Medical School, Boston, Massachusetts

DIPAN J. SHAH, MD, Nashville Cardiovascular MRI Institute, The Heart Group, PLLC, Brentwood, Nashville, Tennessee

ANNE MARIE VALENTE, MD, Boston Adult Congenital Heart Service, Department of Cardiology, Children's Hospital Boston; Instructor in Pediatrics and Internal Medicine, Harvard Medical School, Brigham and Women's Hospital, Boston, Massachusetts

THOMAS F. WALSH, MD, Department of Internal Medicine, Wake Forest University School of Medicine, Winston-Salem, North Carolina

JONATHAN W. WEINSAFT, MD, Assistant Professor, Department of Medicine, Greenberg Division of Cardiology, Weill Medical College of Cornell University, New York, New York

JAMES A. WHITE, MD, Assistant Professor, Department of Medicine, Division of Cardiology, University of Western Ontario; and Director of Cardiovascular MRI Clinics Research, London Health Sciences Centre & Lawson Health Research Institute, London, Ontario, Canada

SUSAN B. YEON, MD, JD, Harvard-Thorndike Laboratory of the Department of Medicine (Cardiovascular Division), Beth Israel Deaconess Medical Center and Harvard Medical School, Boston, Massachusetts

CONTENTS

FORTHCOMING ISSUES

May 2007

3D Echocardiography
Edward A. Gill, MD, Nevin Nanda, MD,
and Roberto Lang, MD, *Guest Editors*

August 2007

The Athletes Heart 2007:
At Border Between Physiology and Pathology
Antonio Pelliccia, MD, *Guest Editor*

November 2007

Heart Failure
James B. Young, MD,
and Jagat Narula, MD, *Guest Editors*

RECENT ISSUES

November 2006

Adult Congenital Heart Disease
Gary D. Webb, MD, *Guest Editor*

August 2006

Advanced 12-Lead Electrocardiography
S. Serge Barold, MD, *Guest Editor*

May 2006

Interventional Cardiology
Samin K. Sharma, MD, *Guest Editor*

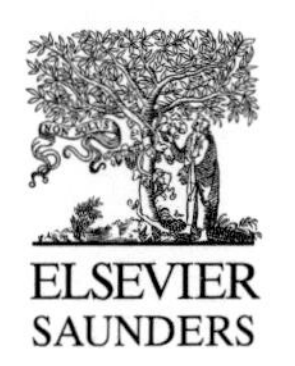
ELSEVIER
SAUNDERS

Cardiol Clin 25 (2007) ix

CARDIOLOGY
CLINICS

Foreword

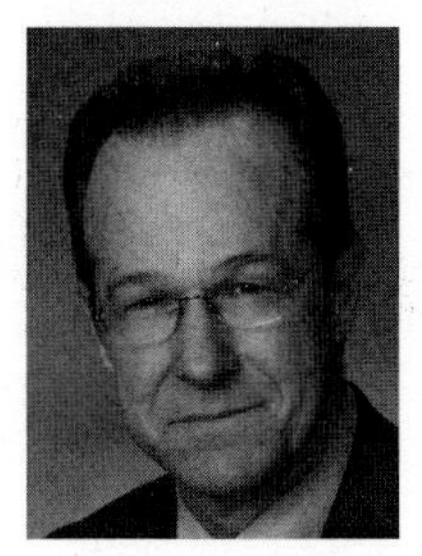

Michael H. Crawford, MD
Consulting Editor

Cardiac MRI has been around for about 25 years. I remember when it first arrived it seemed to have tremendous potential, but after a decade of limited utility, many of us became disenchanted. At the same time CT scanning seemed to be making great strides in cardiovascular imaging, so MRI languished. Now MRI seems to be making a comeback, or more precisely, becoming more clinically useful. MRI always has been viewed as superior for left ventricular mass and volume measurements, differentiating myocardial masses, and diagnosing aortic dissection. Now it is making strides in detecting myocardial ischemia and viability, diagnosing congenital and valvular heart disease, and imaging peripheral and coronary arteries.

Dr. Raymond Kim, who leads the Duke University cardiac MRI team, has assembled a group of international experts to cover the current clinical utility of cardiac MRI. Advances in the field finally seem to be fulfilling the promises made 25 years ago, as are described in the articles in this issue. Thus, it is time to get reacquainted with cardiac MRI and all its possible uses. This issue of *Cardiology Clinics* meets that need.

Michael H. Crawford, MD
Division of Cardiology
Department of Medicine
University of California, San Francisco Medical Center, 505 Parnassus Avenue, Box 0124
San Francisco, CA 94143-0124, USA

E-mail address: crawfordm@medicine.ucsf.edu

doi:10.1016/j.ccl.2007.03.002

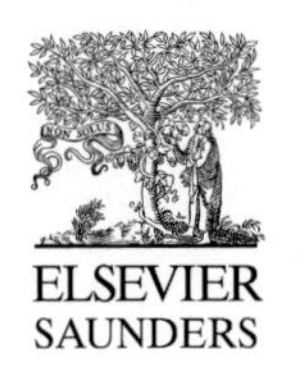

ELSEVIER
SAUNDERS

Cardiol Clin 25 (2007) xi

CARDIOLOGY
CLINICS

Preface

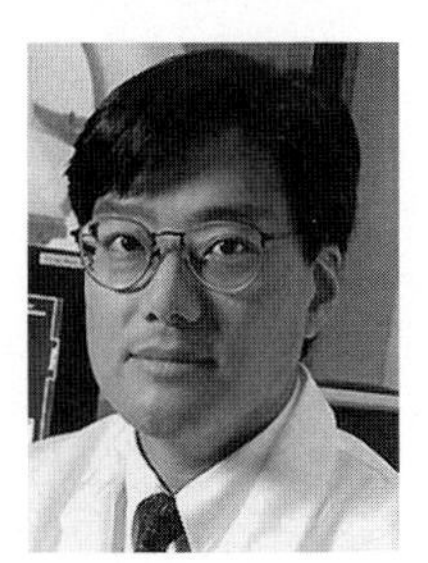

Raymond J. Kim, MD
Guest Editor

I am delighted to serve as the Guest Editor for this issue of *Cardiology Clinics*. This is a timely issue, because cardiovascular magnetic resonance (CMR) recently has made great strides into the clinical arena. Although the modality long has been recognized as a reference standard for cardiac volumes and morphology, only 5 to 6 years ago, CMR was primarily a research tool. It was known as a hot, cutting-edge modality, but, truth be told, scans for clinical purposes were rare and primarily for boutique disorders such as arrhythmogenic right ventricular cardiomyopathy and cardiac neoplasms. In contrast, CMR is considered now a competitive first-line test for bread-and-butter indications such as the evaluation of ischemic heart disease and heart failure.

The reasons for this shift are myriad, and include the rapid development of stress perfusion CMR and the burgeoning applications for delayed-enhancement imaging. In accord with its growing clinical importance, the articles in this issue—all by international experts with vast expertise in clinical CMR—focus less on topics that have only research value and more on issues directly relevant to patient care.

The contributors have performed admirably in providing a succinct yet thorough review of the topics. I hope that readers will find this issue to be of practical value, and worthy of adding to their collection of well-thumbed clinical resources. Enjoy.

Raymond J. Kim, MD
Duke Cardiovascular Magnetic Resonance Center
Duke University Medical Center
Box 3934, Durham, NC 27710, USA

E-mail address: raymond.kim@duke.edu

0733-8651/07/$ - see front matter © 2007 Published by Elsevier Inc.
doi:10.1016/j.ccl.2007.03.001

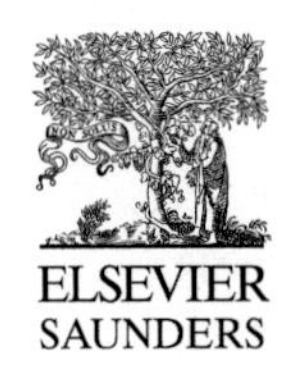
ELSEVIER
SAUNDERS

Cardiol Clin 25 (2007) 1–13

CARDIOLOGY
CLINICS

A Clinical Cardiovascular Magnetic Resonance Service: Operational Considerations and the Basic Examination

Han W. Kim, MD*, Anna Lisa Crowley, MD, Raymond J. Kim, MD

Duke Cardiovascular Magnetic Resonance Center, Duke University Medical Center, Box 3934, Durham, NC 27710, USA

In the last decade, cardiovascular magnetic resonance (CMR) has emerged as an important clinical technique that can be used to evaluate a broad range of cardiovascular pathologies. Technical advances have expanded CMR from primarily a tomographic imaging modality that provided static images of morphology to one that is dynamic, allowing the rapid, high-resolution imaging of ventricular function, valvular motion, and myocardial perfusion. In addition, CMR is now considered the "gold standard" for the assessment of regional and global systolic function, myocardial infarction and viability, and congenital heart disease. At specialized centers, CMR has become a clinical workhorse for the evaluation of ischemic heart disease and for heart failure and cardiomyopathies. Despite this versatility, general acceptance of CMR in cardiovascular medicine has progressed slowly. Although multifactorial, this slow acceptance is primarily due to two reasons. First, referring physicians remain unfamiliar with the wide variety of CMR examinations that are available for routine clinical use, and second, clinical expertise in the practice of CMR is scarce and currently limited to a handful of centers. The expanding availability of CMR education will likely alleviate these bottlenecks. The most recent training guidelines of the American College of the Cardiology (ACC) and the American College of Radiology include (ACR) CMR as an integral component of basic cardiology and radiology training [1,2]. The purpose of this article is to provide a basic understanding of important operational considerations when starting a CMR service and to describe a conceptual framework of the components of a CMR examination.

Operational considerations

MRI scanner and CMR facility

It is important to recognize that an MRI scanner is not a single device but consists of multiple separate components. A schematic of these components is shown in Fig. 1. Approximately 800 square feet is required to house the components of the MRI scanner. Allocating space for a patient waiting room, changing rooms, lavatories, a patient preparation area, offices, and reading stations is also desirable. Specific guidelines for facility design have been published by the ACR [3,4]. Other considerations that are important in surveying the suitability of a site for CMR include evaluating the potential area for extrinsic electromagnetic interference and vibration (which may introduce image artifacts), ensuring an adequate power and chilled water supply, and confirming the ability of the structure to support the weight of the scanner. MRI scanner manufacturers help to assess the suitability of the allocated space before drafting a floor plan for the facility. In addition to space considerations, equipment compatible with MRI, such as a contrast power injector, drug infusion pump, and

* Corresponding author.
E-mail address: kim00050@notes.duke.edu (H.W. Kim).

0733-8651/07/$ - see front matter
doi:10.1016/j.ccl.2007.01.001

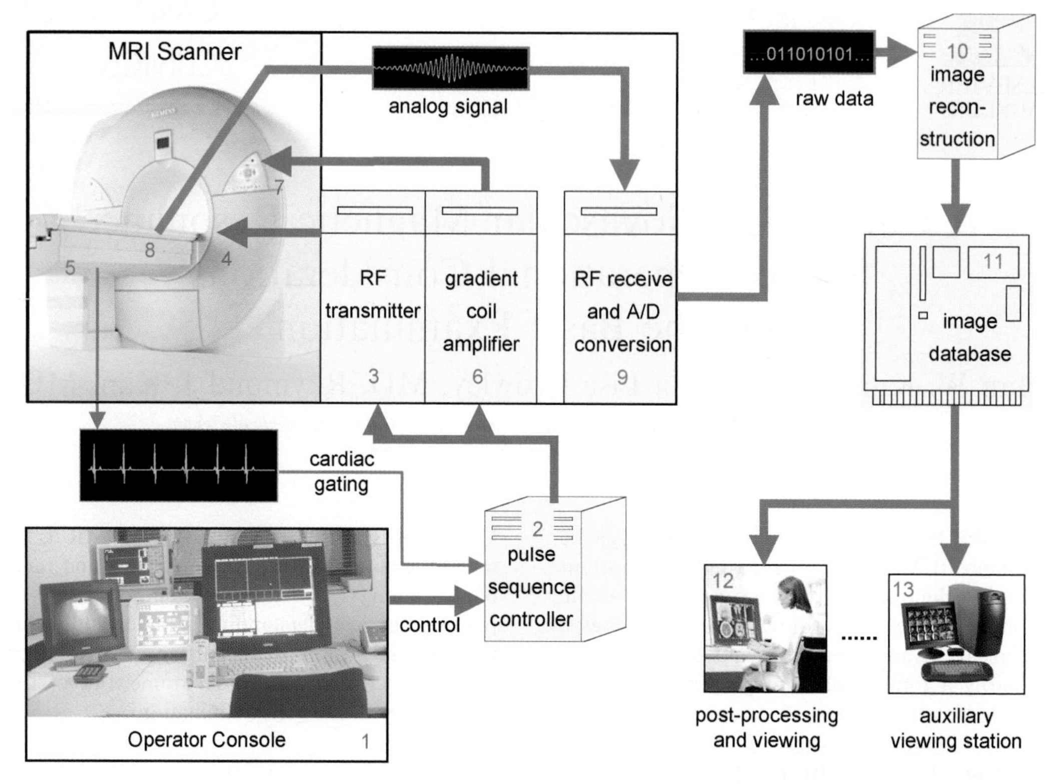

Fig. 1. Components of the MRI scanner. For a CMR study, the operator defines the type of examination and manipulates the imaging parameters from a control computer console using a graphic user interface (1). Software, known as a pulse sequence, is selected from a menu to acquire images that are appropriate for the diagnostic question. The precisely timed radiofrequency (RF) pulses, used to stimulate tissues, are generated by the pulse sequence controller (2), RF transmitter (3), and RF coil (4). For CMR, the ECG signal (5) from the patient is often used for timing. Spatial image information is encoded by the gradient coil amplifier (6) and gradient coil (7), which alter the net magnetic field, known as "B_o," of the MRI scanner. The magnetic resonance signal from the body is detected from fixed receiver coil arrays (8) that are built into the patient table and from flexible arrays that can be placed on top of the patient. These received signals, which are usually analog, are processed and digitized by an analog-digital (A/D) converter (9) and then passed to a computer dedicated to image reconstruction (10). The final images are stored in an image database or a picture archiving and communication system (11) and can undergo postprocessing at a workstation (12) and interpretation at auxiliary viewing stations (13). (*From* Kim HW, Rehwald W, White JA, et al. Magnetic resonance imaging of the heart. In: Fuster V, O'Rourke RA, editors. Hurst's the Heart. New York: McGraw-Hill Medical, in press; with permission.)

monitoring equipment, is necessary if stress testing and contrast angiography are to be performed.

Staffing

For a dedicated CMR facility, a critical number of clinical and administrative staff members are necessary to ensure efficient workflow. For a facility with one MRI scanner, the clinical staff members include the following: (1) two technologists to share the responsibilities of screening patients for MRI contraindications, obtaining brief clinical histories, scanning patients, and postprocessing; (2) one nurse to provide preprocedural instructions (eg, avoidance of caffeine), place intravenous lines, administer medications (eg, adenosine or contrast media), and monitor patients during stress testing; and (3) one or (preferably) two physicians to supervise and interpret the CMR examinations. Having a second physician available is often desirable so that uninterrupted service can be provided when one physician is away. It is important for the supervising physician to survey the clinical history before the study to ensure that the necessary examination components are performed. The supervising physician also reviews the images before the patient's exit from the scanner because the CMR examination may frequently reveal findings that were unexpected before imaging and may require additional imaging components. The administrative staff should include members whose roles pertain to scheduling, billing, and information technology.

CMR training and credentialing

Physicians

The complexity of CMR requires that physicians undergo dedicated training. The guidelines for training from the Society for Cardiovascular Magnetic Resonance are summarized in Box 1 [1,5]. Opportunities for introductory training are available from a variety of sources, including international meetings, computer-based education, and other Continuing Medical Education accredited courses. For those interested in obtaining Level 2 or 3 credentialing, short-term visiting fellowships and dedicated 1- to 2-year fellowships are offered at a number of CMR centers. It is important that physician training emphasizes hands-on operation of the scanner, including troubleshooting, rather than just image interpretation.

Technologists

Although MRI technologists may receive extensive training in body MRI, formal education in CMR is usually limited. Thus, even experienced technologists who are new to CMR require extensive education in cardiac anatomy, pathology, and the special requirements of cardiac imaging (eg, cardiac gating, stress testing, interactive pulse sequence optimization). Often, the responsibility of this training falls on the physician establishing the new CMR service. From the point of view of the technologist, CMR is different from imaging of other parts of the body in that he or she may be required to recognize cardiovascular abnormalities during the course of the examination and to modify the imaging protocol to fully investigate unexpected findings. Correspondingly, proficient technologists are comfortable with improvising imaging protocols and pulse sequence parameters. Individuals who have prior experience in cardiac diagnostic testing (eg, echocardiography, nuclear cardiology, and so forth) may be successful in transitioning into the position of CMR technologist.

Reimbursement

Current procedural terminology (CPT) codes for CMR have been existence for many years (Table 1). For cardiac examinations, the procedures are billed under one of the 75552–75555 CPT codes. Unlike other imaging modalities for which add-on codes are often used to reflect additional imaging, only a single CPT code can be used for a CMR examination, regardless of complexity. Moreover, these codes do not take into account the recent tremendous advances in CMR and current clinical capabilities. Several organizations are working toward revising these codes to differentiate between basic and more complicated examinations (eg, function only, function + viability, function + stress testing + viability). For CMR stress testing, adjunctive nonimaging codes (see Table 1) can be combined with a cardiac (7555X) CPT code.

As with any type of imaging, reimbursement policies may vary between different payers and geographic regions. In general, precertification for MRI procedures is not required by the Centers for Medicare and Medicaid Services (CMS). In addition, most states do not have *International Classification of Diseases, Ninth Revision* (*ICD-9*) restrictions for the CMR CPT codes, although *ICD-9* restrictions are commonly used for magnetic resonance angiography (MRA). Local medical review policies may be consulted to provide guidance regarding Medicare coverage determinations. Most commercial carriers employ policies that are similar to CMS guidelines; however, private carriers may use different restrictions, require precertification, or provide reimbursement only after a "medical necessity" review. In addition, CMS and most private carriers do not provide reimbursement for velocity flow mapping (CPT code 75556).

Cardiovascular MRI examination

Pulse sequences

The versatility of CMR arises from its ability to probe a vast array of biologic parameters—by way of special software programs called pulse sequences—while using the same machine. The concept that software programming changes alone can result in completely different raw data is a unique feature of MRI and allows innovations to arise not only from technical improvements in hardware but also from novel pulse sequences. This feature, however, is responsible for the increased complexity of MRI because it may not always be clear which pulse sequence or sequences should be used for a given clinical scenario (ie, to probe the correct biologic property or properties).

Box 1. Society for Cardiovascular Magnetic Resonance guidelines for physician training

Level 1: Introductory training

- One month of training incorporated into cardiovascular medicine, radiology, or nuclear medicine program

Level 2: Criteria for the practice of cardiovascular magnetic resonance

General criteria

- Board eligible or certified in cardiovascular medicine, radiology, or nuclear medicine
- Basic knowledge, clinical training, and experience in at least one other cardiovascular imaging modality
- Unrestricted medical license

Specific criteria

- At least 3 months of training with a Level 2–qualified or Level 3–qualified (preferred) mentor
  (1) Minimum of 2 months of full-time training in a CMR laboratory (at least 35 h/wk of in-laboratory training)
  (2) Up to 1 month of independent study (may consist of coursework or case studies provided on-line or by way of CD/DVD, time at major medical meetings devoted to the performance of CMR, or other relevant education training)
- At least 50 hours of CMR-related coursework
- Supervised interpretation of a minimum 150 CMR studies
  (1) At least 25 cardiac studies
  (2) At least 25 vascular studies
  (3) For at least 50 studies, the trainee must be present during the scan, ideally as the primary operator, and should perform the analyses and make the initial interpretation
- Continuing Medical Education in CMR for at least 20 hours every 2 years
- Primary interpretation of at least 100 cases every 2 years

Level 3: Advanced competency in cardiovascular MRI

General criteria

- Same as Level 2 general criteria

Specific criteria

- Minimum of 12 months in CMR with a Level 3–qualified mentor
- Supervised interpretation of a minimum 300 CMR studies
  (1) At least 50 cardiac studies
  (2) At least 50 vascular studies
  (3) For at least 100 studies, the trainee must be present during the scan, ideally as the primary operator, and should perform the analyses and make the initial interpretation
- Participation in an ongoing quality assurance or improvement program
- Continuing Medical Education in CMR for at least 40 hours every 2 years
- Primary interpretation of at least 200 cases every 2 years

In addition, for each pulse sequence, many sequence parameters need to be set correctly to achieve optimal image quality.

An individual pulse sequence is a combination of radiofrequency pulses, magnetic gradient field switches, and timed data acquisitions—all applied in a precise order—that results in accentuation or suppression of specific biologic parameters. A simple way to conceptualize pulse sequences is to consider them as consisting of two separate elements: the imaging engine and the associated modifiers [6]. The imaging engine is a required component that provides information regarding the spatial relationship of objects within the imaging field (ie, the main component that produces the image). Modifiers are optional components that can be added to the imaging engine individually or in combination to provide specific

Table 1
Current procedural terminology (CPT) codes commonly used in CMR

CPT code	Description
Cardiac	
75552	Cardiac MRI for morphology without contrast
75553	Cardiac MRI for morphology with contrast
75554	Cardiac MRI for function/complete
75555	Cardiac MRI for function/limited
75556	Cardiac MRI for velocity flow mapping
Stress testing	
93016	Stress, physician supervision
93018	Stress, interpretation and report
J0152	Adenosine stress (30 mg)
Vascular	
70547	MRI (MRA) of neck without contrast
70548	MRI (MRA) of neck with contrast
70549	MRI (MRA) of neck with and without contrast
C8909	MRI (MRA) of chest with contrast
C8910	MRI (MRA) of chest without contrast
C8911	MRI (MRA) of chest with and without contrast
C8900	MRI (MRA) of abdomen with contrast
C8901	MRI (MRA) of abdomen without contrast
C8902	MRI (MRA) of abdomen with and without contrast
72198	MRI (MRA) of pelvis with and without contrast
73225	MRI (MRA) of upper extremity with and without contrast
C8914	MRI (MRA) of lower extremity with and without contrast
C8912	MRI (MRA) of lower extremity with contrast
C8913	MRI (MRA) of lower extremity without contrast
76377	MRI reformation (three-dimensional)

Abbreviation: MRA, magnetic resonance angiography.

information regarding tissue characteristics or to speed imaging. Fig. 2 lists some of the more commonly used imaging engines and modifiers in CMR.

Components of the cardiovascular magnetic resonance examination

Given the large number of pulse sequences that can potentially be used to evaluate cardiovascular patients, it is imperative to organize and standardize the imaging protocols to improve work flow and to ensure consistency between scanner operators. Fig. 3 depicts the protocol steps, associated pulse sequences, and the timeline of a typical core examination that includes stress testing. For simplicity, the authors have divided the CMR examination components into two groups: (1) the core examination, which is performed in most CMR examinations; and (2) optional elements, which may be performed when deemed necessary to fully investigate the clinical question. At the authors' center, we have found that organizing the pulse sequences in this manner facilitates training of technologists and fellows by providing a structure to the array of possible image engines that may be made in any given examination.

Core examination

Scouting. Scouting is the first and simplest procedure to perform. For cardiac imaging, the goal of scouting is to establish the short- and long-axis views of the heart. Due to patient anatomic variation, the short- and long-axis cardiac views lie at arbitrary angles with respect to scanner coordinates and are therefore referred to as "double oblique" planes. A schematic depicting the procedure for obtaining double oblique planes is shown in Fig. 4. For extracardiac imaging such as vascular angiography, scouting is performed in traditional imaging planes (eg, axial, sagittal, and coronal) to localize the structure of interest. Scout images are usually acquired using a single-shot imaging engine (steady-state free precession [SSFP] or half Fourier single-shot turbo spin-echo [HASTE]) during free breathing.

Function/volumes. CineMRI, using a gradient-recalled echo (GRE) or SSFP imaging engine, has been shown to be highly accurate and

MRI Pulse Sequence Structure

IMAGING ENGINE

TYPE

Spin echo (SE)
- The first pulse sequence used to image the heart.
- Only a variant, turbo spin-echo (**TSE**), is used today. Used primarily to delineate morphology.

Gradient-recalled echo (GRE)
- Common work-horse sequence used for cine imaging (produces movies similar to echocardiography), dynamic perfusion imaging, vascular imaging, and delayed-enhancement imaging (**DE-MRI**), among others.

Echo-planar imaging (EPI)
- Rapid form of imaging usually combined with GRE.
- Often used for dynamic perfusion imaging.

Steady-state free precession (SSFP)
- The most recent technique. Also known as TrueFISP, FIESTA, Balanced FFE.
- The current gold standard technique for imaging ventricular morphology and function.
- Provides high signal-to-noise. Becoming a ubiquitous choice for cardiovascular imaging. Used for coronary, vascular, perfusion, and delayed-enhancement imaging, among others.

MODE

Single-shot
- Entire dataset for one image is acquired in a single continuous stream.
- Allows "real-time" or "snap-shot" imaging during free-breathing.
- Example includes half Fourier single-shot TSE (**HASTE**) for rapid morphologic imaging.

Segmented
- Dataset for one image is acquired piecemeal over several heartbeats.
- Allows imaging with high spatial resolution and high temporal resolution (a narrow window within the cardiac cycle).

EXAMPLE IMAGES

GRE

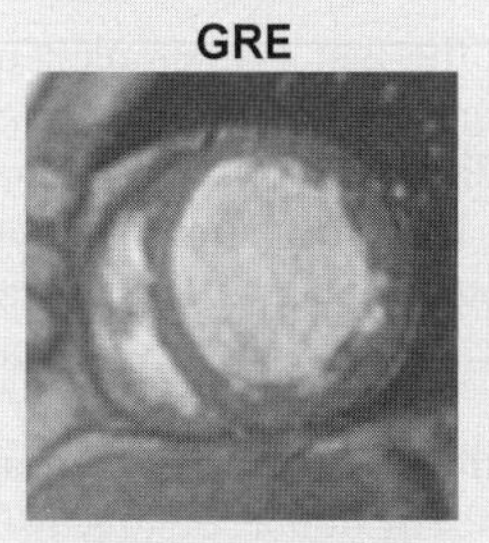

SSFP

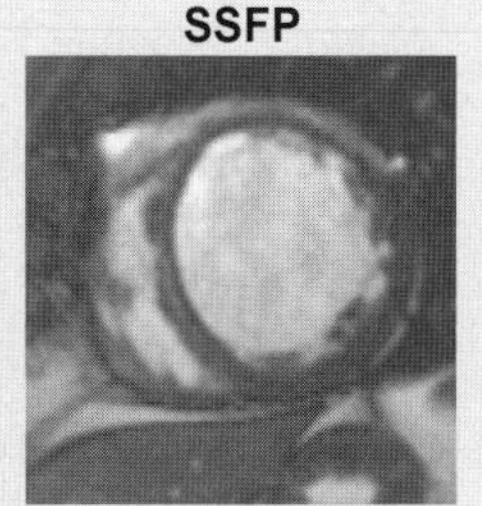

MODIFIERS

Black-blood
- Vascular structures (or cardiac chambers) with fast moving blood appear black.
- Slow flowing blood can be bright and hard to distinguish from cardiac or vascular structures (e.g. LV apex, false lumen of aortic dissection, etc).

Fat suppression
- Useful for diagnosis of cardiac and pericardial masses, right ventricular dysplasia, and to distinguish epicardial contrast hyperenhancement from fat.

Inversion prepulse
- Used to produce high levels of T1-weighting. Important component of delayed-enhancement imaging.

Saturation prepulse
- Also used for T1-weighting. Commonly used for dynamic perfusion imaging.

Tagging
- A saturation prepulse variant that labels the heart muscle with a dark grid. Useful to demonstrate intramural rotation, contraction, and strain.

Velocity-encoded
- Similar to echo doppler techniques. Used for quantification of cardiac output, shunts, and valvular dysfunction.

Parallel imaging
- Recent method used to speed imaging at the cost of signal-to-noise. Can be combined with nearly all forms of cardiovascular imaging.
- Multiple variants are in use (e.g. SENSE, SMASH, etc).

EXAMPLE IMAGES

Black-blood

Inversion prepulse

Tagging

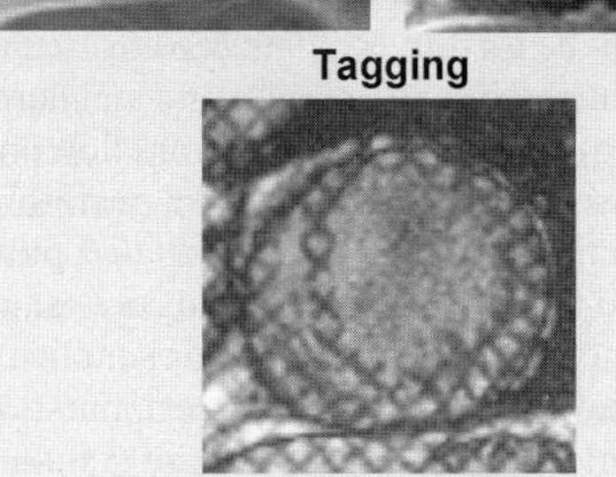

Fig. 2. MRI pulse sequence structure. The MRI pulse sequence can be considered as consisting of two separate elements: the imaging engine and modifiers. Typical images using different imaging engines and modifiers are shown at the bottom. All images are of the same short-axis spatial location. See text for further information. LV, left ventricular; SENSE, sensitivity encoding for fast MRI; SMASH, simultaneous acquisition of spatial harmonics. (*Adapted from* Shah DJ, Judd RM, Kim RJ. Technology insight: MRI of the myocardium. Nat Clin Pract Cardiovasc Med 2005;2(11):598, 599; with permission.)

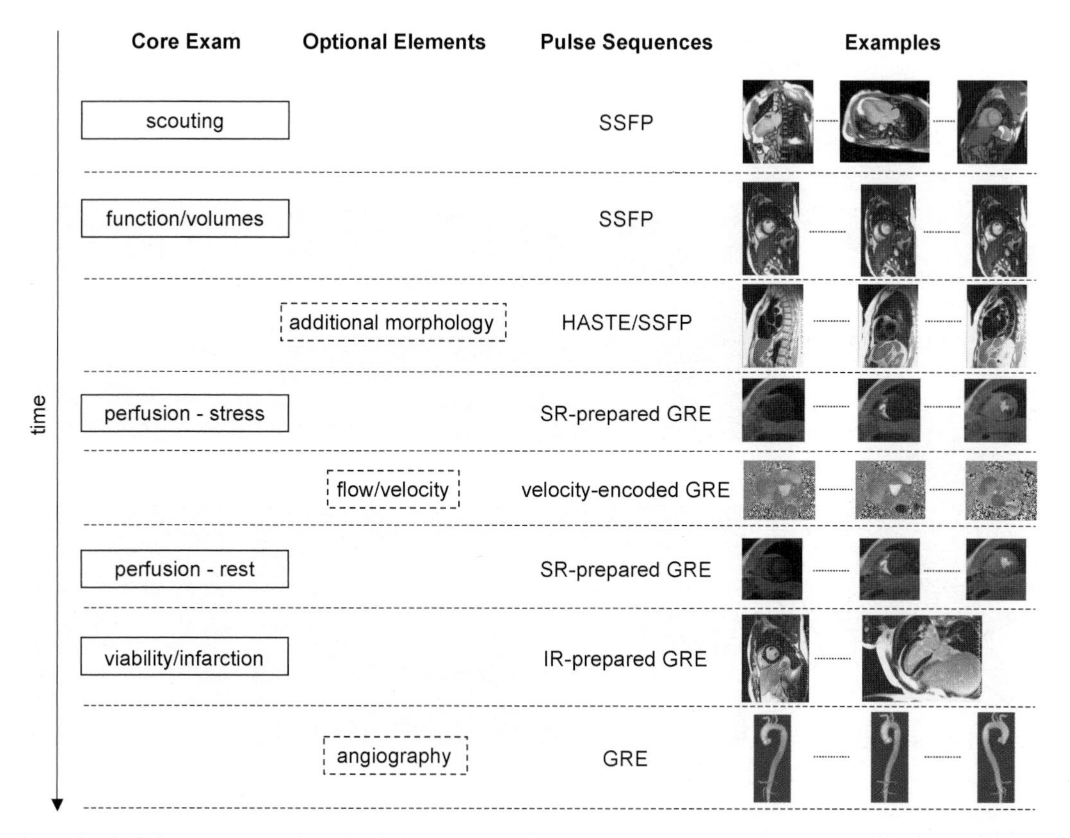

Fig. 3. Typical CMR core examination with stress testing. The protocol steps, associated pulse sequences, and timeline of a typical core cardiovascular examination that includes stress testing are depicted with example images. GRE, gradient-recalled echo; HASTE, half Fourier single-shot turbo spin echo; IR, inversion recovery; SR, saturation recovery; SSFP, steady-state free precession.

reproducible in the measurement of ejection fraction, ventricular volumes, and cardiac mass [7]. The goal of cine imaging is to capture a movie of the beating heart to visualize its contractile function. In recent years, cineMRI has become widely accepted as the gold standard for the measurement of these parameters [7]. Moreover, it is increasingly used as an end point in studies of left ventricular remodeling [8–10] and as a reference standard for other imaging techniques [11,12].

Currently, the most common imaging engine for cineMRI is SSFP. The advantages over other sequences such as GRE include intrinsically high signal-to-noise ratio and excellent blood-myocardium contrast that facilitates the identification of the endocardial border [13]. During a typical CMR examination of the heart, a short-axis stack from the mitral valve plane through the apex and two-, three-, and four-chamber long-axis views are obtained to comprehensively image all ventricular segments. In addition, valvular function (eg, qualitative assessments of regurgitation and quantitative measurements of valve stenosis by planimetry) can also be determined from cineMRI.

Perfusion at stress and rest. As a result of technical and clinical advancements, perfusion MRI is increasingly used at CMR centers for the detection of coronary artery disease [14]. The sensitivity, specificity, and diagnostic accuracy of perfusion MRI appears at least comparable, and perhaps superior, to that of nuclear single photon emission CT (SPECT). Thus, recently, the American College of Cardiology Foundation Appropriateness Criteria Working Group deemed the use of perfusion MRI as "appropriate" for evaluating chest pain syndromes in patients who have intermediate risk of coronary artery disease and for determining the physiologic significance of indeterminate coronary artery lesions [15].

The goal of perfusion MRI is the creation of a movie of the passage of contrast media (typically

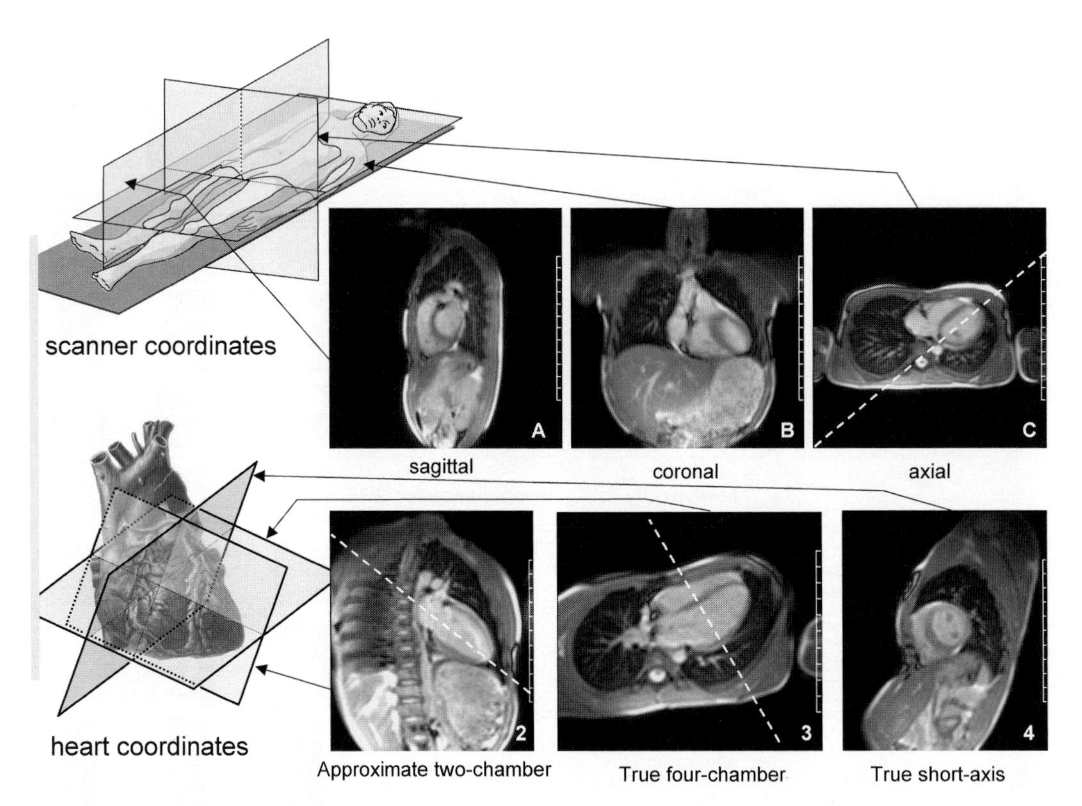

Fig. 4. Procedure for scouting. To establish the short- and long-axis planes of the heart, the following steps are followed. Step 1: images are obtained along the scanner axes (sagittal, coronal, and axial; panels 1A, 1B, and 1C, respectively). Step 2: from a pseudo–four-chamber long-axis view (usually from the axial image), one prescribes a perpendicular plane through the approximate apex, which results in an approximate two-chamber view. Step 3: another perpendicular plane is prescribed through the apex, which results in a true long-axis view (usually four-chamber). Step 4: a perpendicular plane, "bread-loafing" the heart, delivers the true short-axis plane. (*From* Kim HW, Rehwald W, White JA, et al. Magnetic resonance imaging of the heart. In: Fuster V, O'Rourke RA, editors. Hurst's the Heart. New York: McGraw-Hill Medical, in press; with permission.)

gadolinium based) during its first pass through left ventricular myocardium. Similar to SPECT, imaging is performed during pharmacologic vasodilation (usually with adenosine). Imaging under resting conditions is also performed approximately 15 minutes after stress to allow for clearance of the contrast media from the blood pool. Most clinical CMR services use gradient echo or gradient echo-echo planar-planar hybrid imaging engines with a parallel imaging modifier in single-shot mode (see Fig. 2). Four to five short-axis slices are obtained every cardiac cycle for the entire first pass of contrast transit with ECG gating.

Viability and infarction. Myocardial viability and infarction are simultaneously examined using the technique known as delayed-enhancement MRI (DE-MRI) [16–20]. In patients who have ischemic heart disease, DE-MRI is highly effective in identifying the presence, location, and extent of myocardial infarction in the acute and the chronic setting [18,20,21] and is superior to SPECT for the detection of subendocardial myocardial infarction [19]. Moreover, the technique is now considered the gold standard for identification of myocardial stunning following acute myocardial infarction [22,23] or of hibernating myocardium in chronic ischemic heart disease [24,25]. More recently, it has been used in conjunction with perfusion MRI to improve specificity and diagnostic accuracy of stress testing [26,27]. DE-MRI is also being used evaluate patients who have nonischemic cardiomyopathies including hypertrophic cardiomyopathy [6,28–30], dilated cardiomyopathy [10,31,32], and sarcoidosis [33]. The goal of DE-MRI is to create images with high contrast between abnormal myocardial tissue, which generally accumulates excess gadolinium (following intravenous administration), and normal tissue in which gadolinium concentration is low. This imaging is currently best achieved using a segmented, GRE imaging engine with an inversion recovery prepulse modifier to provide heavy T1 weighting [16–20]. A parallel imaging [34,35] modifier is also often used to shorten acquisition time. Imaging is performed approximately 5 minutes after rest perfusion imaging or 10 to 15 minutes after a one-time intravenous gadolinium dose of 0.15 to 0.20 mmol/kg if stress–rest perfusion imaging is not performed. Short- and long-axis views in the identical planes used for cineMRI are obtained during repeated 6- to 10-second breath holds. Data acquisition (readout period) is timed with the ECG in mid-diastole to minimize cardiac motion. Only every other heartbeat is used for data collection to allow for adequate recovery of longitudinal relaxation between inversion pulses (when bradycardia is present, imaging can occur every heartbeat) [36]. Recently, an ultrafast, real-time version of DE-MRI was developed that can acquire snapshot images during free breathing, although with lower special resolution and less T1 weighting [37,38]. This technique uses an SSFP imaging engine in single-shot mode with parallel imaging and provides complete left ventricular coverage in less than 30 seconds. This technique could be considered the preferred approach in patients who are more acutely ill, unable to breath hold, or have irregular heart rhythms.

Optional elements

Morphology. Cardiac and proximal vascular structures are commonly assessed by SSFP cineMRI. On occasion, additional structural/anatomic information is necessary to fully investigate a clinical question such as in the setting of congenital heart disease, cardiac masses, or patients who have aortic root dilation on initial three-chamber cineMRI. In general, a "morphology" scan consists of a series of parallel slices that "bread-loaf" the anatomic region of interest. Although any orientation may be imaged, usually axial, sagittal, or coronal planes (or all three) are chosen first.

To quickly provide substantial anatomic coverage, morphology imaging is primarily performed in single-shot mode using an SSFP or a turbo spin echo (TSE) imaging engine. The SSFP sequence is similar to that used for real-time cineMRI but has been altered to produce a stack of images that progresses through space, rather than a cine movie loop at a single location. In its native form (without additional modifiers), SSFP produces images in which blood in the cardiac chambers and vasculature appear bright; thus, it is known as a "bright-blood" technique. To first order, SSFP images are T2/T1 weighted [18]. In contrast, spin echo–based sequences such as TSE produce images in which flowing blood is dark; thus, these are known as "black-blood" techniques. Blood signal suppression may be incomplete, however, and a black-blood modifier, which consists of a double-inversion prepulse [39], is often added to improve blood nulling. A single-shot version of TSE that is commonly used in cardiovascular imaging is black-blood half-Fourier single-shot TSE (HASTE).

With SSFP or HASTE morphologic imaging, the entire thorax can be imaged in multiple orthogonal views in less than 2 minutes without breath holding. The choice between SSFP and HASTE is made depending on the clinical question and whether bright- or black-blood contrast is desired. On occasion, small structures may be obscured on SSFP imaging by bright signal from the blood. Conversely, stagnant blood flow by virtue of incomplete suppression may be mistaken as tissue on HASTE imaging. Accordingly, both techniques should be performed when images from one are inconclusive because the time cost is minimal. When higher spatial resolution is desired for certain key views, segmented cineMRI or segmented TSE can be performed during a breath hold. Black-blood sequences should be performed before gadolinium administration because shortening blood T1 impairs the suppression of blood signal. SSFP sequences can be performed before or after gadolinium administration.

Flow/velocity. Velocity-encoded cine imaging (VENC-MRI) is used to measure blood velocities and flows in arteries and veins and across valves and shunts. Also known as phase-contrast velocity mapping, the underlying principle is that signal from moving blood or tissue will undergo a phase shift relative to stationary tissue when a magnetic field gradient is applied in the direction of motion.

The goal of VENC-MRI is to produce a cine loop across the cardiac cycle, whereby on any given frame, pixel intensity is proportional to blood velocity. Generally displayed using a gray scale, white corresponds to maximum flow in one direction, black corresponds to maximum flow in the opposite direction, and midgray indicates that flow is absent. Although blood velocity can be measured in any arbitrary direction, it is usually assessed in reference to the imaging plane. Encoding velocity in the slice gradient direction allows measurement of "through-plane" velocities, and encoding in the frequency or the phase-encoded gradient directions allows "in-plane" measurement of velocity components directed vertically or horizontally within the image plane.

VENC-MRI is commonly performed using a segmented GRE imaging engine during a patient breath hold. The sequence, however, is modified to measure the effects of a magnetic field gradient on the precessing protons within flowing blood. The precise details of VENC-MRI are complex and considered more comprehensively elsewhere [40–42]; however, optimizing the maximum velocity that can be measured—which is inversely related to gradient strength (for a constant application time)—is important. Setting the maximum velocity too low leads to aliasing, whereas setting it too high leads to more noise or inaccuracy in the velocity measurement. Retrospective rather than prospective ECG gating is preferred to allow data collection throughout the entire cardiac cycle including end-diastole.

Although VENC-MRI appears analogous to Doppler echocardiography, there are important differences (Table 2). For instance, an advantage of VENC-MRI is that blood flow through an orifice is directly measured on an en-face image of the orifice with "through-plane" velocity encoding. In addition, because VENC-MRI can be performed in any arbitrary orientation, en-face flow may be directly measured across nearly any structure, even those that may be difficult to visualize by echocardiography (ie, baffles, sinus venosus atrial septal defects). With echocardiography there are two limitations. First, the blood flow profile is not directly measured but is assumed to be flat (ie, velocity in the center of the orifice is the same as near the edges) so that, hopefully, one sampling velocity would indicate average velocity. Second, the cross-sectional area of the orifice (via M-mode or two-dimensional imaging) is estimated from a diameter measurement of the orifice at a different time during the examination from when Doppler velocity is measured. Conversely, VENC-MRI has some disadvantages. Perhaps most important, VENC-MRI is not performed in real time and requires breath holding to minimize artifacts due to respiratory motion. One consequence is that it is difficult to measure changes in flow that occur with respiration.

Angiography. Contrast-enhanced MRA (CE-MRA) is performed in conjunction with morphologic imaging to fully define arterial or venous structures. CE-MRA may be added to the core examination when indicated (eg, CE-MRA of the thoracic aorta for a patient who has a dilated aortic root with aortic regurgitation) or it can be performed independently.

The goal of CE-MRA is the creation of a three-dimensional data set of a vessel or vascular bed. Gadolinium contrast media is administered as a bolus during imaging to generate high signal within the vascular structure, creating a lumenogram. The most common imaging engine for CE-MRA is three-dimensional gradient echo.

Table 2
Comparison of velocity-encoded MRI and Doppler echocardiography

Imaging characteristic	Velocity encoding	MRI Doppler echocardiography
Imaging during free breathing	Limited	Yes
Imaging during arrhythmias	Limited	Yes
Temporal resolution	~50 ms[a]	<10 ms
Peak velocity location	Yes	Location ambiguity (continuous wave Doppler)
Angle dependence	Yes, 20°	Yes, 20°
Imaging planes	Any	Echocardiographic windows
Blood flow profile	Directly measured	Flat profile assumed
Flow quantification	En face	In plane[b]

[a] The given temporal resolution is for breath-hold imaging. Temporal resolution may be significantly improved for non–breath-hold imaging, but artifacts due to respiratory motion artifact may be prominent.

[b] Conduit cross-sectional area is estimated from diameter measurement.

From Kim HW, Rehwald W, White JA, et al. Magnetic resonance imaging of the heart. In: Fuster V, O'Rourke RA, editors. Hurst's the Heart. New York: McGraw-Hill Medical, in press; with permission.

For thoracic and abdominal CE-MRA, imaging is performed during a single breath hold to minimize respiratory motion. ECG gating and imaging during diastole is necessary when imaging structures that are affected by cardiac motion or that are pulsatile (eg, aortic root). A precontrast scan is also done for off-line subtraction from the contrast-enhanced scan to eliminate background and expedite postprocessing on a workstation.

Reporting and archiving

The image reporting and archival needs of a clinical CMR service are often different from those of traditional imaging services in radiology or cardiology. At most centers, cardiac studies are interpreted using the ACC 17 segment model [43]. Reporting is significantly facilitated by the ability to simultaneously view multiple image sets. For instance, with stress testing, concurrent viewing of wall motion on cineMRI, first pass perfusionMRI at stress and rest, and viability on DE-MRI aids in distinguishing the presence of inducible myocardial ischemia from myocardial infarction or ischemia (Fig. 5). Many picturing archiving and communication systems (PACS), however, require specific customizations to display even a few series of dynamic movie loops concurrently and are not designed to display a large set of dynamic and static images at the same time. When operating a clinical service, the inability to display images in this manner can slow workflow and should be an important consideration when selecting a PACS.

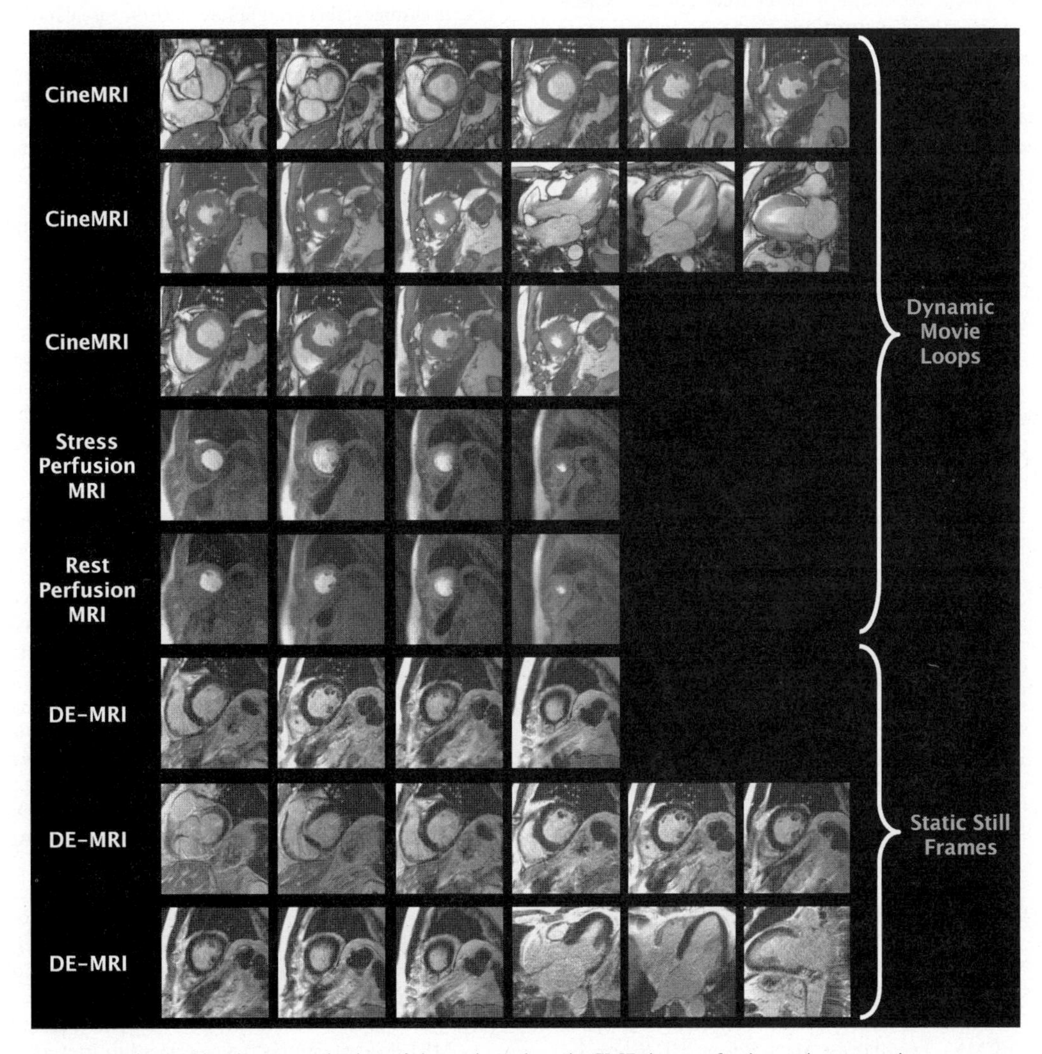

Fig. 5. Simultaneous viewing of dynamic and static CMR images for image interpretation.

A routine cardiac study can comprise 1000 images and usually requires 50 to100 megabytes of storage. Vascular studies, especially those that involve multiple stages such as a peripheral run-off examination, can be several-fold larger. At the authors' center, all studies are immediately available on-line by way of standard Web browsers. A 5.6-terabyte redundant array of independent disks (RAID) is currently used as primary storage. Another 5.6-terabyte RAID, which mirrors the original, is stored in a separate physical facility for data redundancy.

Summary

The authors' have used the model outlined in this article to build a dedicated clinical CMR service a their institution. Since its inception in 2002, the clinical volume has grown rapidly and now consists of more than 3000 billed procedures per year [14]. Of these procedures, nearly 50% of the volume is from adenosine perfusion stress testing, 25% from viability testing, and the remainder from vascular and congenital heart disease studies. This organizational structure has facilitated the growth of the authors' clinical service by standardizing imaging protocols, improving work flow, and simplifying CMR training.

References

[1] Pohost GM, Kim RJ, Kramer CM, et al. Task Force 12: training in advanced cardiovascular imaging (cardiovascular magnetic resonance [CMR]): endorsed by the Society for Cardiovascular Magnetic Resonance. J Am Coll Cardiol 2006;47(4):910–4.

[2] Woodard P, Bluemke D, Cascade P. ACR practice guideline for the performance and interpretation of cardiac magnetic resonance imaging (MRI). American College of Cardiology; 2006. Available at: http://www.acr.org/s_acr/bin.asp?TrackID=&SID=1&DID=24522&CID=546&VID=2&DOC=File.PDF. Accessed February 28, 2007.

[3] Kanal E, Borgstede JP, Barkovich AJ, et al. American College of Radiology white paper on MR safety: 2004 update and revisions. AJR Am J Roentgenol 2004;182(5):1111–4.

[4] Kanal E, Borgstede JP, Barkovich AJ, et al. American College of Radiology white paper on MR safety. AJR Am J Roentgenol 2002;178(6):1335–47.

[5] Kim RJ, de Roos A, Fleck E, et al. Guidelines for training in cardiovascular magnetic resonance (CMR). J Cardiovasc Magn Reson 2007;9(1):3–4.

[6] Shah DJ, Judd RM, Kim RJ. Technology insight: MRI of the myocardium. Nat Clin Pract Cardiovasc Med 2005;2(11):597–605.

[7] Pennell DJ, Sechtem UP, Higgins CB, et al. Clinical indications for cardiovascular magnetic resonance (CMR): consensus panel report. Eur Heart J 2004;25(21):1940–65.

[8] Bellenger NG, Davies LC, Francis JM, et al. Reduction in sample size for studies of remodeling in heart failure by the use of cardiovascular magnetic resonance. J Cardiovasc Magn Reson 2000;2(4):271–8.

[9] Osterziel KJ, Strohm O, Schuler J, et al. Randomised, double-blind, placebo-controlled trial of human recombinant growth hormone in patients with chronic heart failure due to dilated cardiomyopathy. Lancet 1998;351(9111):1233–7.

[10] Bellenger NG, Rajappan K, Rahman SL, et al. Effects of carvedilol on left ventricular remodelling in chronic stable heart failure: a cardiovascular magnetic resonance study. Heart 2004;90(7):760–4.

[11] Ioannidis JP, Trikalinos TA, Danias PG. Electrocardiogram-gated single-photon emission computed tomography versus cardiac magnetic resonance imaging for the assessment of left ventricular volumes and ejection fraction: a meta-analysis. J Am Coll Cardiol 2002;39(12):2059–68.

[12] Corsi C, Lang RM, Veronesi F, et al. Volumetric quantification of global and regional left ventricular function from real-time three-dimensional echocardiographic images. Circulation 2005;112(8):1161–70.

[13] Barkhausen J, Ruehm SG, Goyen M, et al. MR evaluation of ventricular function: true fast imaging with steady-state precession versus fast low-angle shot cine MR imaging: feasibility study. Radiology 2001;219(1):264–9.

[14] Rehwald WG, Wagner A, Albert TSE, et al. Clinical CMR imaging techniques. In: Manning WJ, Pennell DJ, editors. Cardiovascular magnetic resonance. New York: Churchill Livingstone, in press.

[15] Hendel RC, Patel MR, Kramer CM, et al. ACCF/ACR/SCCT/SCMR/ASNC/NASCI/SCAI/SIR 2006 appropriateness criteria for cardiac computed tomography and cardiac magnetic resonance imaging: a report of the American College of Cardiology Foundation Quality Strategic Directions Committee Appropriateness Criteria Working Group. J Am Coll Cardiol 2006;48(7):1475–97. Available at: http://www.acr.org/s_acr/bin.asp?TrackID=&SID=1&DID=24522&CID=546&VID=2&DOC=File.PDF. Accessed February 28, 2007.

[16] Fieno DS, Kim RJ, Chen EL, et al. Contrast-enhanced magnetic resonance imaging of myocardium at risk: distinction between reversible and irreversible injury throughout infarct healing. J Am Coll Cardiol 2000;36(6):1985–91.

[17] Kim RJ, Fieno DS, Parrish TB, et al. Relationship of MRI delayed contrast enhancement to irreversible

injury, infarct age, and contractile function. Circulation 1999;100(19):1992–2002.
[18] Simonetti OP, Kim RJ, Fieno DS, et al. An improved MR imaging technique for the visualization of myocardial infarction. Radiology 2001;218(1): 215–23.
[19] Wagner A, Mahrholdt H, Holly TA, et al. Contrast-enhanced MRI and routine single photon emission computed tomography (SPECT) perfusion imaging for detection of subendocardial myocardial infarcts: an imaging study. Lancet 2003;361(9355):374–9.
[20] Wu E, Judd RM, Vargas JD, et al. Visualisation of presence, location, and transmural extent of healed Q-wave and non-Q-wave myocardial infarction. Lancet 2001;357(9249):21–8.
[21] Ricciardi MJ, Wu E, Davidson CJ, et al. Visualization of discrete microinfarction after percutaneous coronary intervention associated with mild creatine kinase-MB elevation. Circulation 2001;103(23): 2780–3.
[22] Choi KM, Kim RJ, Gubernikoff G, et al. Transmural extent of acute myocardial infarction predicts long-term improvement in contractile function. Circulation 2001;104(10):1101–7.
[23] Gerber BL, Garot J, Bluemke DA, et al. Accuracy of contrast-enhanced magnetic resonance imaging in predicting improvement of regional myocardial function in patients after acute myocardial infarction. Circulation 2002;106(9):1083–9.
[24] Kim RJ, Wu E, Rafael A, et al. The use of contrast-enhanced magnetic resonance imaging to identify reversible myocardial dysfunction. N Engl J Med 2000;343(20):1445–53.
[25] Schvartzman PR, Srichai MB, Grimm RA, et al. Nonstress delayed-enhancement magnetic resonance imaging of the myocardium predicts improvement of function after revascularization for chronic ischemic heart disease with left ventricular dysfunction. Am Heart J 2003;146(3):535–41.
[26] Klem I, Heitner JF, Shah DJ, et al. Improved detection of coronary artery disease by stress perfusion cardiovascular magnetic resonance with the use of delayed enhancement infarction imaging. J Am Coll Cardiol 2006;47(8):1630–8.
[27] Cury RC, Cattani CA, Gabure LA, et al. Diagnostic performance of stress perfusion and delayed-enhancement MR imaging in patients with coronary artery disease. Radiology 2006;240(1):39–45.
[28] Moon JC, Mogensen J, Elliott PM, et al. Myocardial late gadolinium enhancement cardiovascular magnetic resonance in hypertrophic cardiomyopathy caused by mutations in troponin I. Heart 2005; 91(8):1036–40.
[29] Moon JC, McKenna WJ, McCrohon JA, et al. Toward clinical risk assessment in hypertrophic cardiomyopathy with gadolinium cardiovascular magnetic resonance. J Am Coll Cardiol 2003;41(9):1561–7.
[30] Choudhury L, Mahrholdt H, Wagner A, et al. Myocardial scarring in asymptomatic or mildly symptomatic patients with hypertrophic cardiomyopathy. J Am Coll Cardiol 2002;40(12):2156–64.
[31] McCrohon JA, Moon JC, Prasad SK, et al. Differentiation of heart failure related to dilated cardiomyopathy and coronary artery disease using gadolinium-enhanced cardiovascular magnetic resonance. Circulation 2003;108(1):54–9.
[32] Assomull RG, Prasad SK, Lyne J, et al. Cardiovascular magnetic resonance, fibrosis, and prognosis in dilated cardiomyopathy. J Am Coll Cardiol 2006; 48(10):1977–85.
[33] Patel M, Cawley P, Heitner JF, et al. Detection and prognostic significance of myocadial damge in patients with sarcoidosis using delayed enhancement cardiac magnetic resonance. Circulation 2006; 114(Suppl II):408.
[34] Sodickson DK, Manning WJ. Simultaneous acquisition of spatial harmonics (SMASH): fast imaging with radiofrequency coil arrays. Magn Reson Med 1997;38(4):591–603.
[35] Pruessmann KP, Weiger M, Scheidegger MB, et al. SENSE: sensitivity encoding for fast MRI. Magn Reson Med 1999;42(5):952–62.
[36] Kim RJ, Shah DJ, Judd RM. How we perform delayed enhancement imaging. J Cardiovasc Magn Reson 2003;5(3):505–14.
[37] Li W, Li BS, Polzin JA, et al. Myocardial delayed enhancement imaging using inversion recovery single-shot steady-state free precession: initial experience. J Magn Reson Imaging 2004;20(2):327–30.
[38] Sievers B, Elliott MD, Hurwitz LM, et al. Rapid detection of myocardial infarction by sub-second, free breathing delayed contrast-enhanced cardiovascular magnetic resonance. Circulation 2007;115(2): 236–44.
[39] Edelman RR, Chien D, Kim D. Fast selective black blood MR imaging. Radiology 1991;181(3): 655–60.
[40] Debatin JF, Ting RH, Wegmuller H, et al. Renal artery blood flow: quantitation with phase-contrast MR imaging with and without breath holding. Radiology 1994;190(2):371–8.
[41] Pelc LR, Pelc NJ, Rayhill SC, et al. Arterial and venous blood flow: noninvasive quantitation with MR imaging. Radiology 1992;185(3):809–12.
[42] Saloner D. Flow and motion. Magn Reson Imaging Clin N Am 1999;7(4):699–715.
[43] Cerqueira MD, Weissman NJ, Dilsizian V, et al. Standardized myocardial segmentation and nomenclature for tomographic imaging of the heart: a statement for healthcare professionals from the Cardiac Imaging Committee of the Council on Clinical Cardiology of the American Heart Association. Circulation 2002;105(4): 539–42.

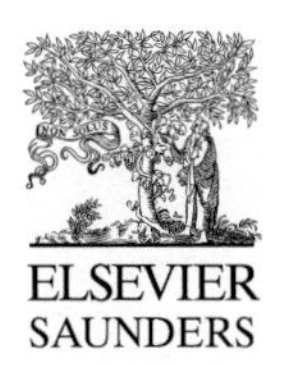

ELSEVIER
SAUNDERS

Cardiol Clin 25 (2007) 15–33

CARDIOLOGY
CLINICS

Assessment of Ventricular Function with Cardiovascular Magnetic Resonance

Thomas F. Walsh, MD[a], W. Gregory Hundley, MD, FACC, FAHA[a,b,*]

[a]*Department of Internal Medicine, Wake Forest University School of Medicine, Bowman Gray Campus, Medical Center Boulevard, Winston-Salem, NC 27157-1045, USA*

[b]*Department of Radiology, Wake Forest University School of Medicine, Bowman Gray Campus, Medical Center Boulevard, Winston-Salem, NC 27157-1045, USA*

Management of patients who have cardiovascular disorders depends on assessments of global and regional left ventricular (LV) and right ventricular (RV) function. The high spatial and temporal resolution of cardiovascular magnetic resonance (CMR) images makes it well-suited for use in the assessment of RV and LV function. This article reviews CMR methods used to assess regional and global ventricular function.

Image acquisition techniques

Gradient echo

Gradient echo, also known as fast low-angle shot or FLASH [1] imaging, is the most extensively studied technique for assessing ventricular wall motion, volumes, and ejection fraction [2]. With gradient-echo imaging, the movement of the blood pool provides bright contrast against the gray appearance of the myocardium [3]. Previous studies have demonstrated the utility of gradient-echo imaging in the assessment of RV and LV volumes, mass, and ejection fraction [4–10].

True fast imaging with steady-state free precession

Fast imaging with steady-state precession refocuses the signal between excitations resulting in heightened blood pool—myocardial tissue contrast [11]. This technique can be used to acquire cine images with short repetition (<3 milliseconds) and echo (<1.5 milliseconds) times [12–16]. As can be seen in Fig. 1, the contrast between the LV endocardial surface and blood pool appears high even when LV systolic function is reduced [17].

Echo planar imaging

Gradient echo planar imaging (EPI) sequences acquire single snapshots of LV wall motion during 40- to 60-millisecond intervals. By placing these acquisitions in series, LV wall motion can be visualized in near real time. Importantly, chemical shift artifacts, and the relatively long temporal resolution of current techniques (60 milliseconds) inhibit identification of end systole for determination of ejection fraction and LV end systolic volume when heart rates are high [18].

Sensitivity-encoding scheme

With the sensitivity-encoding scheme (SENSE), the resonance signal is encoded by spatially varying the receiver sensitivity of the phased array elements [19]. Using simultaneous signal acquisition with multiple parallel receiver coils, the speed of data collection is not limited by sequential data from gradient encoding acquisitions. For this reason, scan times can be reduced by a factor related to the number of coils in the array [20,21]. In one study

Dr. Hundley is supported in part by National Institutes of Health R21CA109224, and R21/R33CA121296, and an industrial grant from Bracco Diagnostics.

* Corresponding author. Department of Internal Medicine (Cardiology Section), Wake Forest University School of Medicine, Bowman Gray Campus, Medical Center Boulevard, Winston-Salem, NC 27157-1045.

E-mail address: ghundley@wfubmc.edu (W.G. Hundley).

0733-8651/07/$ - see front matter
doi:10.1016/j.ccl.2007.01.002

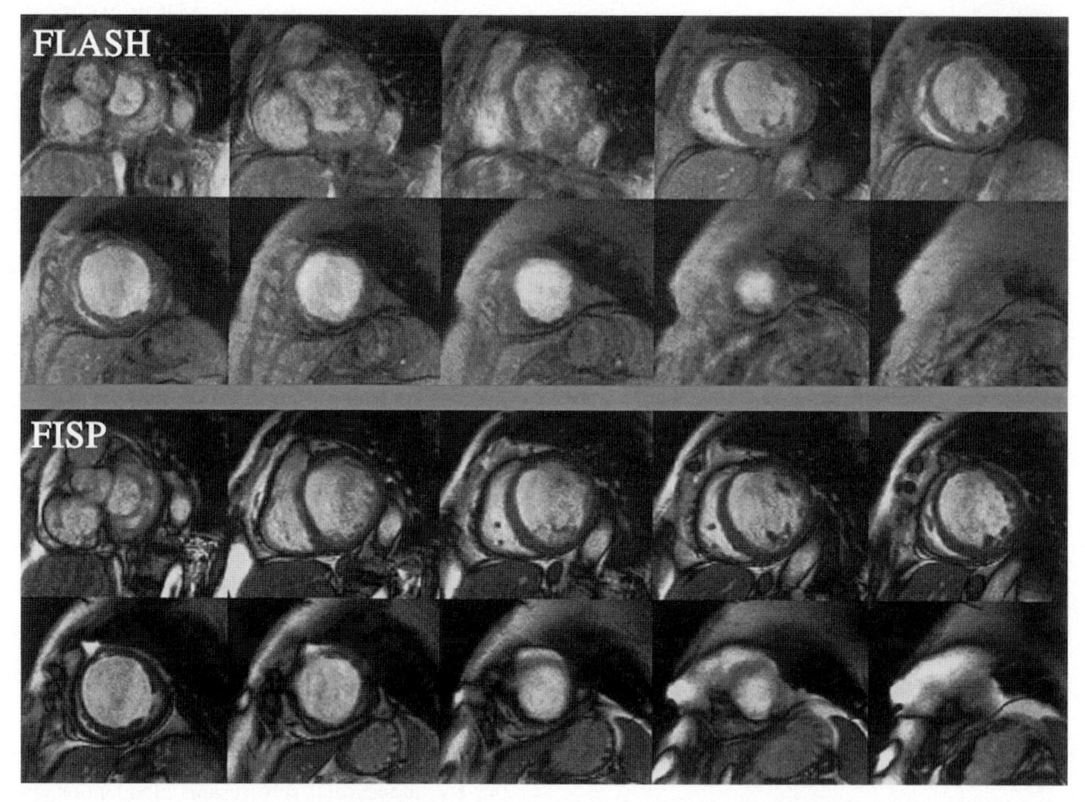

Fig. 1. Gradient echo and steady-state free precession. Images from a patient who presented to an emergency room with chest pain. The top panel is a gradient echo also known as a fast low-angle shot (FLASH) image. The bottom panel illustrates the superior image quality of SSFP. (*From* Moon JC, Lorenz CH, Francis JM, et al. Breath-hold FLASH and fast imaging with steady-state precession cardiovascular imaging: left ventricular volume differences and reproducibility. Radiology 2002;223:789–97; with permission.)

by Pruessmann and colleagues [22], a temporal resolution of 13 milliseconds was acquired with three parallel slices. This technique may lead to further improvements in providing real-time images of cardiovascular function.

Tissue tagging

With myocardial tissue tagging, radiofrequency pulses are used to create regular dark banks of selective saturation before initiation of the remainder of the imaging sequence. Consequently, motion of material can be tracked as the saturation bands deform [4]. Using this technique, termed spatial modulation magnetization (SPAMM), myocardial contraction or relaxation can be quantified. Tagging bands usually disappear after 400 to 500 milliseconds. Therefore a tagging grid can be obtained, followed by a saturation pulse (termed: complimentary spatial modulation magnetization [CSPAMM]) to create a negative grid in the second or diastolic portion of the imaging acquisition (Fig. 2) [23–25].

Displacement encoding with simulated echos

Recently, a new technique termed displacement encoding with simulated echoes (DENSE) has been described that allows one to track myocardial motion data using phase-reconstructed images. Similar to tagging, DENSE uses spatial modulation of magnetization to position encode magnetization at a point in time and follow tissue displacement during a subsequent portion of the cardiac cycle [26,27]. Compared with CSPAMM, DENSE allows one to differentiate LV regional function within the endocardium, midmyocardium, and epicardium (Fig. 3).

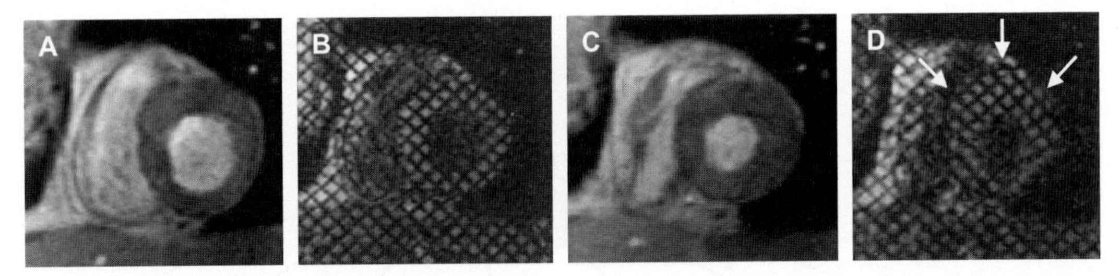

Fig. 2. Tagging of the left ventricle. Images of a patient without (*A*) and with (*B*) tagging during the diastolic phase of a normal left ventricle at rest. (*C, D*) are comparative images at peak stress. There is akinesea of the anterior, anterior–septal, and septal walls indicating ischemia. (*From* Wahl A, Paetsch I, Roethemeyer S, et al. High-dose dobutamine–atropine stress cardiovascular MR imaging after coronary revascularization in patients with wall motion abnormalities at rest. Radiology 2004;233:210–6; with permission.)

Phase contrast MRI

Measurement of motion with MRI also can be done through velocity phase mapping [28–32]. With this method, the change in phase of the net magnetization inside each pixel is related to the velocity of the tissue in the direction parallel to the magnetic field. With this technique, the entire cardiac cycle can be evaluated without an elaborate pulse sequence, as it is insensitive to T1 relaxation [33–38]. To date, this technique has received limited use because of lengthy scan times and time-consuming analyses of the acquired image data.

Rest measures of right and left ventricular volume and ejection fraction

Left ventricular volume and ejection fraction

There are several different methods available for measuring left ventricular volume and ejection fraction with CMR. The two most common include the Simpson's rule technique and area-length technique. With the Simpson's rule technique, LV volumes are determined by summing the endocardial area within multiple short axial slices spanning the base to the apex of the heart and multiplying each area determination by slice thickness (Fig. 4) [5,39,40]. This technique is

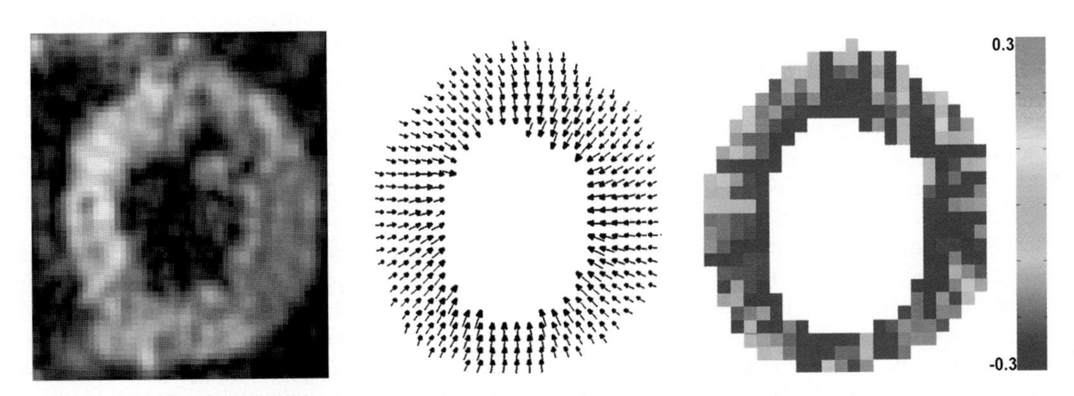

Fig. 3. Short axis displacement encoding with simulated echoes images of the left ventricle. These figures were obtained in single breath hold in a healthy volunteer. The far left figure is of a magnitude reconstruction of the short axis view of the left ventricle. The middle figure is a two-dimensional displacement map computed from a phase-reconstructed image with each vector in the map representing the end–diastolic to end–systolic motion of the myocardium as depicted in a single pixel. The far right figure demonstrates circumferential shortening as computed from the displacement field as a color-coded myocardial strain map. (*From* Kim D, Gilson WD, Kramer CM, et al. Myocardial tissue tracking with two-dimensional cine displacement-encoded MR imaging: development and initial evaluation. Radiology 2004:230:862–71; with permission.)

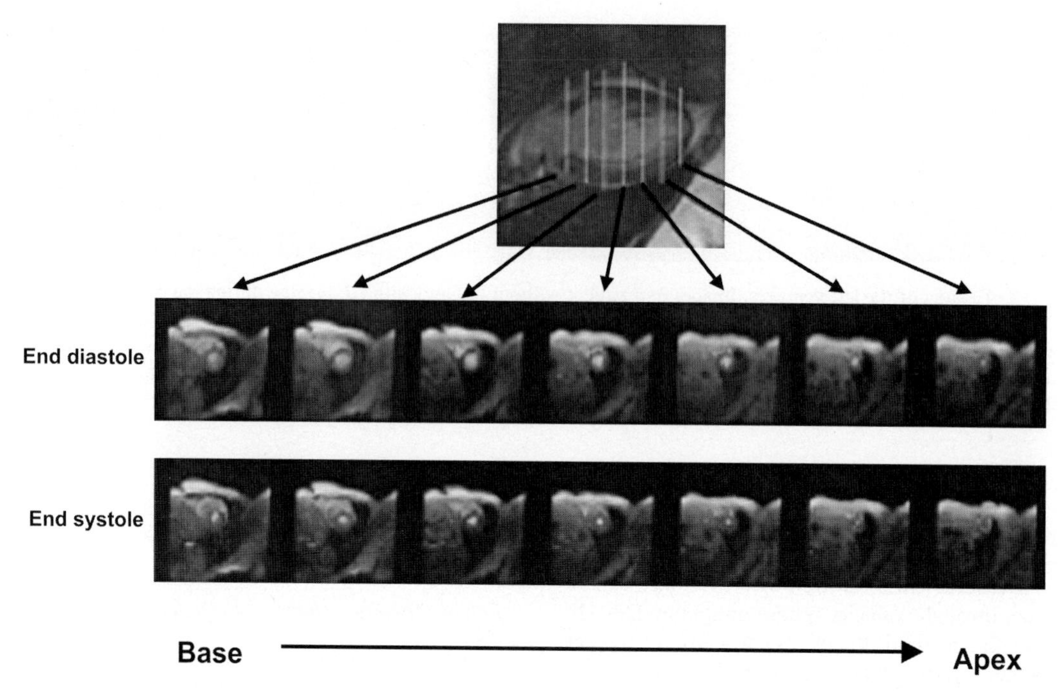

Fig. 4. Gradient echo images of sequential multiple slices of the left ventricle in short-axis planes (from base to apex) are displayed for determining left ventricle volume by Simpson's rule. Endocardial area in each segment is measured at end diastole (top row) and end–systole (bottom row). Left ventricular volume is calculated by the summing the endocardial area within each slice and multiplying by the slice thickness. Left ventricular ejection fraction equals (end–diastolic volume−end–systolic volume)/end–diastolic volume.

advantageous, because one can calculate LV volumes without using formulae that require assumptions about LV shape. For this reason, the Simpson's rule technique is useful in patients who have cardiomyopathy or regional wall motion abnormalities.

The area length techniques are based on formulae that assume the left ventricle exhibits the shape of a prolate ellipse. With the single-plane or biplane area-length methods, only one or two slice acquisitions are required, and image analysis time is short [41,42]. Because patients who have distorted LV geometry caused by dilated cardiac chambers or resting regional wall motion abnormalities do not exhibit left ventricles in the shape of a prolate ellipse, LV volume determinations may be less precise than those generated with the Simpson's rule method [43]. With both methods, LV ejection fraction is calculated by subtracting end–diastolic volume from end–systolic volume and dividing by end–diastolic volume.

Assessments of LF volumes measured with the Simpson's rule technique have been validated with cadaver studies. In 1985, Rehr and colleagues [39] used cadaver hearts and created latex casts of excised human left ventricles to compare CMR measurements derived from scanning the casts with actual volume measurements from the casts themselves. They found excellent correlation between CMR-determined measurements and cast measurements ($r = 0.997$, standard error of the estimate equal to 4.3 to 4.9 mL over a range of 26 to 190 mL [Fig. 5]). Other studies have performed similar analyses from autopsy series and found excellent correlations also [5].

Data from animal models have confirmed the findings in phantom and cadaver studies. Keller and colleagues [44] examined canine hearts and found a close correlation ($r = 0.98$) between LV mass and volumes measured with CMR and those calculated by the volume of displacement method. In another study by Koch and colleagues [45], eight porcine hearts were explanted and prepared by removal of the atria. The correlation between measures obtained from both ventricles and the CMR-derived measures was greater than 0.99. Multiple studies have been performed in canine,

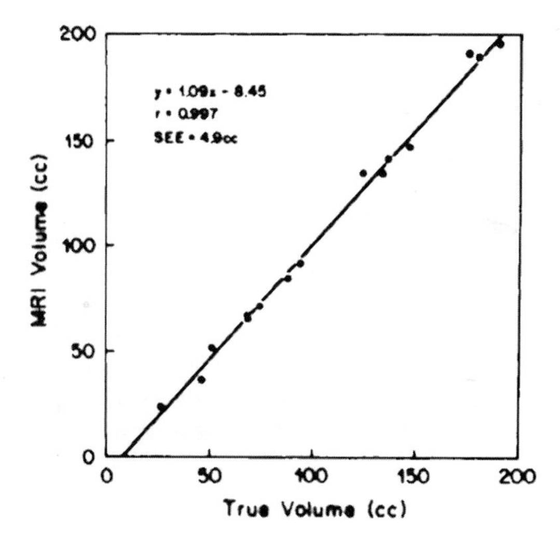

Fig. 5. Cardiovascular magnetic resonance of human casts. Relation between volume calculated using MRI and true volume (superimposed on regression line relating the two) for the images obtained using normal resolution. Regression line is calculated using all 15 casts. (*From* Rehr RB, Malloy CR, Filipchuk NG, et al. Left ventricular volumes measured by MR imaging. Radiology 1985;156:717–9; with permission.)

porcine, rat, and mice models to confirm excellent correlation between CMR-calculated ventricular volumes and actual volumes measured by timed volume collections [46–49].

Assessment of LV volumes and EF with CMR using cine gradient echo techniques in people in vivo with both normal and abnormal LF morphology is highly reproducible and exhibits low intraobserver and interobserver variability [50–53]. Ventricular volumes, mass, and ejection fraction also can be assessed with a high degree of accuracy in patients who have congestive heart failure. As small as a 5% difference in LV ejection fraction with 90% power and $\alpha = 0.05$ can be detected in subjects who have impaired LV function.

Because of the heightened reproducibility and low variance of this method, small sample sizes can be used when a change in LV volumes or EF by CMR serve as a study endpoint. In comparison with sample sizes required through the use of area-length methods acquired through other invasive and noninvasive imaging modalities, CMR measures have been demonstrated to be more precise and reproducible [54]. For this reason, studies using CMR measures of LV volumes and ejection fraction require sample sizes that are 80% to 90% smaller then the sample sizes needed with other modalities [54].

The white blood imaging technique used to assess LV volumes may influence the calculated measures derived from CMR. One study comparing short axis cine magnetic resonance (MR) images with steady-state free precession and gradient-echo techniques indicated that LV ejection fraction was lower and LV mass, end-systolic, and stroke volumes were higher in the steady-state free precession technique when compared with the measures from the gradient-echo sequences. The heightened contrast between the blood and myocardial border are thought to be the source of these discrepancies [55].

Right ventricular volume and ejection fraction

Because of the shape and location of the right ventricle beneath the sternum, quantification of RV volumes and ejection fraction is difficult with echocardiography or radionuclide ventriculography. With CMR, there are no limitations imposed by body habitus, and thus, as with LV functional measures, RV volumes and ejection fraction can be determined accurately [56–60]. In studies with normal volunteers, there has been low intraobserver, interobserver, and interstudy variability (5% to 6%) [61].

Two studies have reported normative CMR values for the right ventricle. Rominger and colleagues [60] reported an average RV end–diastolic volume index of 78 plus or minus 15 mL/m^2, an average end–systolic volume index of 30 plus or minus 9 mL/m^2, and an average ejection fraction of 62% plus or minus 6% in 52 healthy volunteers aged 18 to 58 years. Lorenz and colleagues [61] found similar results in 75 healthy participants ranging in age from 8 to 55 years. In this study, the RV end–diastolic volume index averaged 75 plus or minus 13 mL/m^2, and the RV ejection fraction averaged 61% plus or minus 7%.

Assessment of left ventricular regional function

Wall motion

CMR is an excellent technique for visualizing wall motion. Using various white blood imaging techniques, cine loops can be constructed during 3- to 4-second periods of breath holding. Because CMR can acquire images in virtually any tomographic plane, standard apical (long axis, four-chamber, and two-chamber) and short-axis (basal, middle, and apical) views of LV wall motion can be obtained without limitation imposed by body habitus (Fig. 6).

Wall thickening

Two primary methods have been described for the assessment of LV wall thickening: the center line method and myocardial tissue tagging [62–64]. With the center line technique, a line is created in the center of the myocardium equidistant from the epicardial and endocardial borders. Perpendicular to the center line, multiple chords are evenly distributed circumferentially around the LV myocardium at specified intervals, with the length of each chord identifying local wall thickness (defined as the ratio of the length of the chord at end systole to end diastole) [37]. After myocardial infarction (MI), this technique has been used to identify abnormal thickening associated with the site and extent of the infarct [48,65]. This technique also has been used during dobutamine MR stress testing to identify abnormal thickening in association with myocardial ischemia. The sensitivity of detecting luminal narrowings of greater than 50% in one, two, and three epicardial arteries was 88%, 91%, and 100%, respectively [66]. A limitation of this technique is the fact that when the imaging slice is not positioned perpendicular to the long axis of the left ventricle, local wall thickness (and consequently,

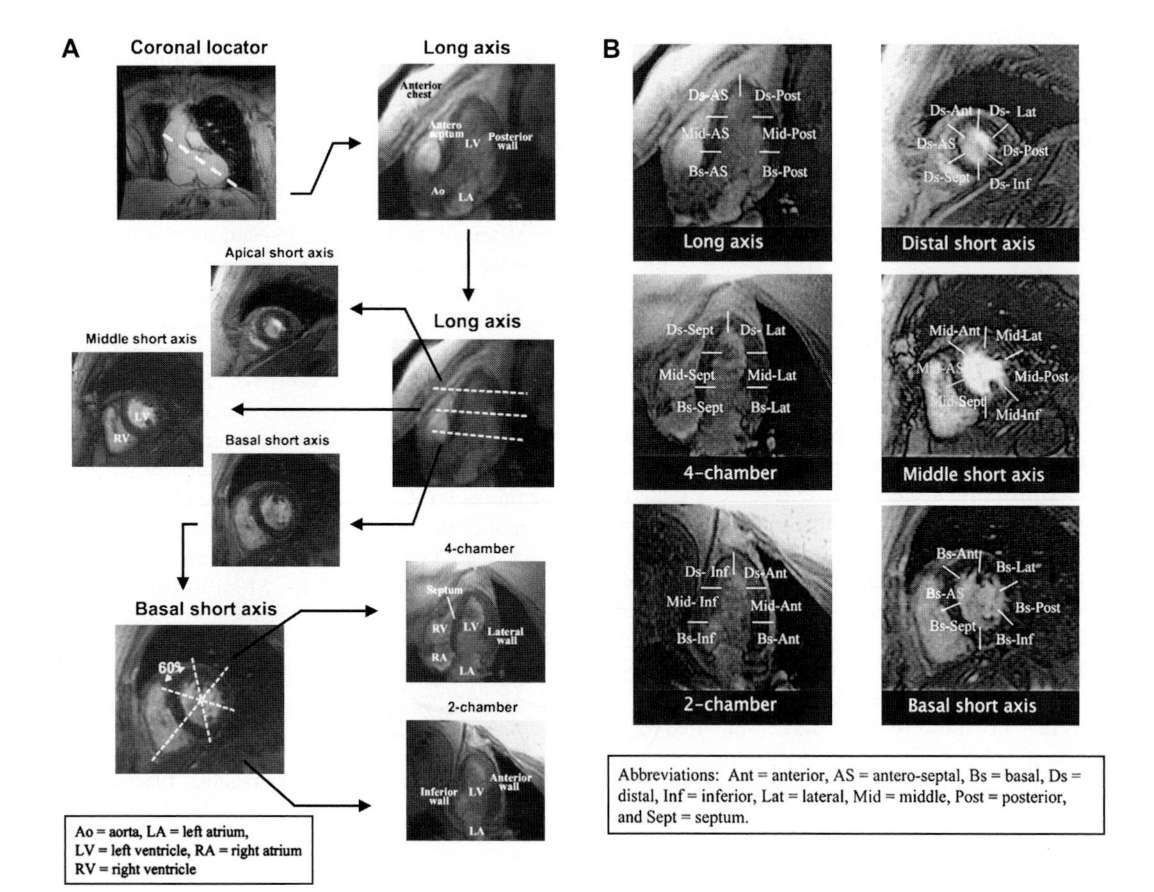

Fig. 6. Method for obtained standard views. (*A*) Illustration of a method for obtaining three short-axis (basal, middle, and apical) and three apical (long-axis, four-chamber, and two-chamber) cardiovascular magnetic resonance views of the left ventricle. In all images, the myocardium is gray, and the blood pool white. The white dotted lines on the coronal locator, long-axis view, and basal short-axis view indicate the slice positions for obtaining the subsequent views demarcated by the black arrows. (*B*) The 18 myocardial segments are demarcated by white lines. (*From* Hundley WG, Morgan TM, Neagle CM, et al. Magnetic resonance imaging determination of cardiac prognosis. Circulation 2002;106(18): 2328–33; with permission.)

wall thickening) may be overestimated. Additionally, through-plane myocardial motion is not accounted for as the heart translates from diastole to systole [66].

Tagging can be used to monitor wall thickening throughout the cardiac cycle. By tracking the side-to-side separation of tag lines or tag line intersections or the change in distance between line pairs, myocardial shortening or elongation can be observed [67]. With this approach, it is possible to measure wall thickness across the LV myocardium [67,68].

Left ventricular strain

Measurements of LV strain are useful in that they are not dependent on volume loading or preload in the determination of ventricular relaxation [69]. Strain analysis can be used to characterize regional deformation of the myocardium. Strain can be defined as the percent change in length per unit of initial length. Normal strains can be analyzed in radial (E_{rr}), longitudinal (E_{ll}), and circumferential (E_{cc}) axes. Shear strains are defined in the plane between two coordinate axes in which the strain between the circumferential and longitudinal axis is E_{cl}; the strain between the circumferential and radial axis is E_{cr}; and the strain between the longitudinal and radial axis is E_{lr} [67,70]. To date, strain has been assessed with both CSPAMM and DENSE techniques. Using sonomicrometric measurement techniques, measurements of myocardial thickening and strain by tagged MR imaging have been validated [71]. In a recent study examining LV diastolic dysfunction in patients who had type 2 diabetes mellitus and normal LV ejection fractions, it was found that peak LV systolic circumferential and longitudinal shortening values were lower in the patients who had diabetes compared with normal controls [72]. In hypertensive patients who have LV hypertrophy, it has been found that intramural myocardial strain is abnormal [73]. Investigators in other studies have used myocardial strain assessments and tissue tagging to evaluate patients who have myocardial ischemia, infarction, hibernating or stunned myocardium, or postinfarction remodeling (Fig. 7) [74,75].

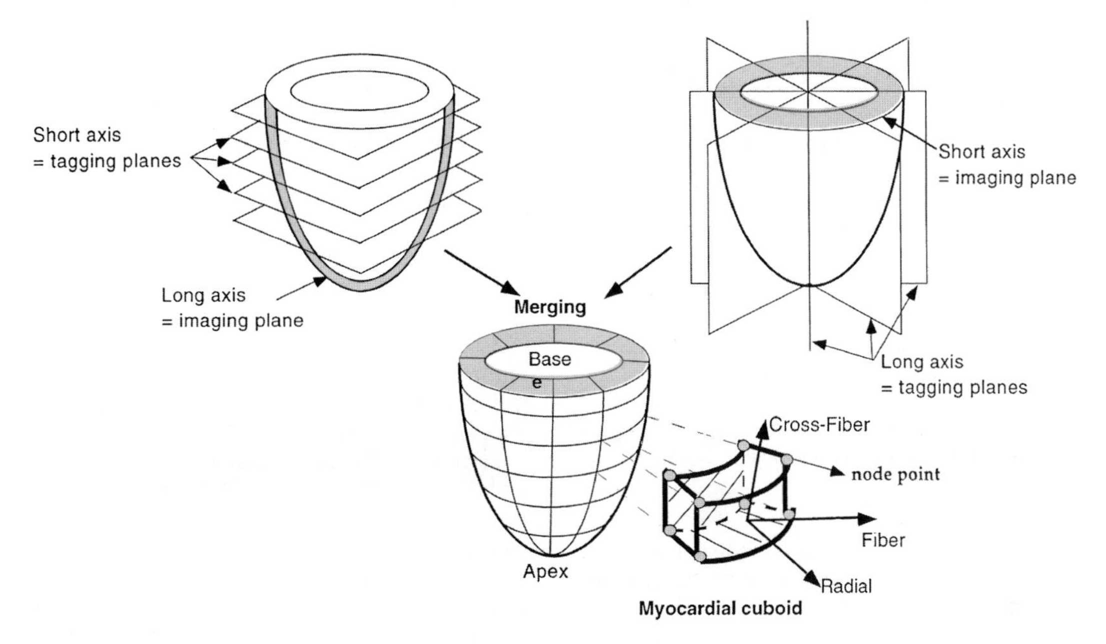

Fig. 7. Magnetic resonance (MR) tagging used for regional strain analysis. The left ventricle is divided into 32 small cuboids by means of a combination of MR tagging along five cardiac short- and four long-axis planes. Each cuboid is constructed from four subendocardial and four subepicardial node points. Strains are expressed in local cardiac coordinate system for each subepicardial and subendocardial node point. Axes are radial (R) using the direction perpendicular to wall; fiber (F), tangent to surface and parallel to local fiber direction at either epicardium or endocardium; and cross-fiber (X), tangent to surface and perpendicular to F. (*From* Bogaert J, Maes A, Van de Werf F, et al. Functional recovery of subepicardial myocardial tissue in transmural myocardial infarction after successful reperfusion: an important contribution to the improvement of regional and global left ventricular function. Circulation 1999;99(1):37; with permission.)

Regional relaxation

Relaxation is a highly ATP-dependent process, and thus if abnormalities of relaxation can be measured, they may be more sensitive markers of abnormal LV performance than measures reliant upon assessments of LV systole. Paetsch and colleagues [76] evaluated the diastolic parameters from myocardial tagging of 25 patients who had low- and high-dose dobutamine stress to identify patients with flow-limiting epicardial coronary arterial luminal narrowings. They showed that myocardial tagging helps in a quantitative analysis of systolic and diastolic function during low- and high-dose dobutamine stress. They concluded that the diastolic parameter of time to peak untwist assessed during low-dose dobutamine stress was the most promising global parameter for identification of patients who had flow-limiting epicardial coronary arterial luminal narrowings.

Assessment of right ventricular regional function

CMR has been used to assess RV function in patients who have congenital heart disease [77–79], pulmonary hypertension [80–82], and other disorders such as arrhythmogenic RV cardiomyopathy (ARVC) [83–85]. Keller and colleagues [86] studied 36 patients who had suspected ARVC. The diagnosis was confirmed by CMR in 16 of 18 patients who had a clinical diagnosis of ARVC (sensitivity 89%), and correctly excluded in 14 of 17 patients who had clinically excluded ARVC (specificity 82%). Importantly, in ARVC, CMR is suited well for assessing fatty infiltration of the RV free wall and the consequent regional wall motion abnormality associated with the fatty infiltration (Fig. 8).

Dynamic measures of left ventricular function

Detection of ischemia

Over the last decade, software and hardware advances have enabled investigators to demonstrate the clinical utility of CMR wall motion stress testing in patients referred for cardiovascular care. This has been accomplished using phased-array surface coils, fast scans with short repetition and echo times, advanced gating systems, specialized software for image display during stress testing, and intravenous administration and hemodynamic measurement (heart rate, oxygen saturation, blood pressure) equipment that allow for the safe monitoring of patients during the course of stress testing [87]. To date, in general, LV wall motion during CMR stress testing has been assessed across LV myocardial segments (as recommended by the American Heart Association) using a four-point scoring system (1 is normal; 2 is hypokinetic;3 is akinetic, and 4 is dyskinetic) similar to that used with dobutamine stress echo (DSE). A deterioration score of 1 or higher is used to identify ischemia.

The first clinical use of CMR for the detection of inducible ischemia was reported by Pennell and colleagues [88]. In this study, CMR was compared with thallium-201 single photon emission CT (PET) and coronary angiography. Twenty-five study subjects received dobutamine infusions of up to 20 μg/kg/min and underwent conventional gradient-echo cine CMR. Twenty-two participants had significant coronary artery disease (CAD) with angiography, and of these 20 had wall motion abnormalities as per CMR compared with 21 identified as having reversible ischemia by dobutamine thallium tomography. Consequently, the sensitivity of CMR for detection of significant CAD in this study was 91%. Between PET and CMR, there was a 96% agreement at rest, 90% agreement during stress, and 91% agreement for the assessment of reversible ischemia. This study was the first to demonstrate in patients who had CAD that CMR could be used effectively to assess LV regional function.

In another early study, Baer and colleagues [89]. This source is incorrect. Please see below compared stress dobutamine CMR results with those obtained using dipyridamole CMR testing in 61 patients who had a normal ejection fraction and known 70% stenoses of one of three epicardial coronary arteries. Thirty-three patients had wall motion assessed after high-dose dipyridamole infusion (0.75 mg/kg over 10 min), and 28 patients underwent wall motion assessments with dobutamine infusion (5, 10, 15, and 20 μg/kg/min). In basal and midventricular short-axis planes, segmental wall motion analysis was performed. The sensitivity of dipyridamole CMR and dobutamine CMR for detecting coronary artery luminal narrowing greater than 70% was 84% and 85%, respectively.

van Rugge and colleagues [90] used patients who had known wall motion abnormalities to assess the efficacy of quantitative measurements during dobutamine stress CMR for detection and localization of myocardial ischemia. Thirty-nine patients with prior wall motion abnormalities

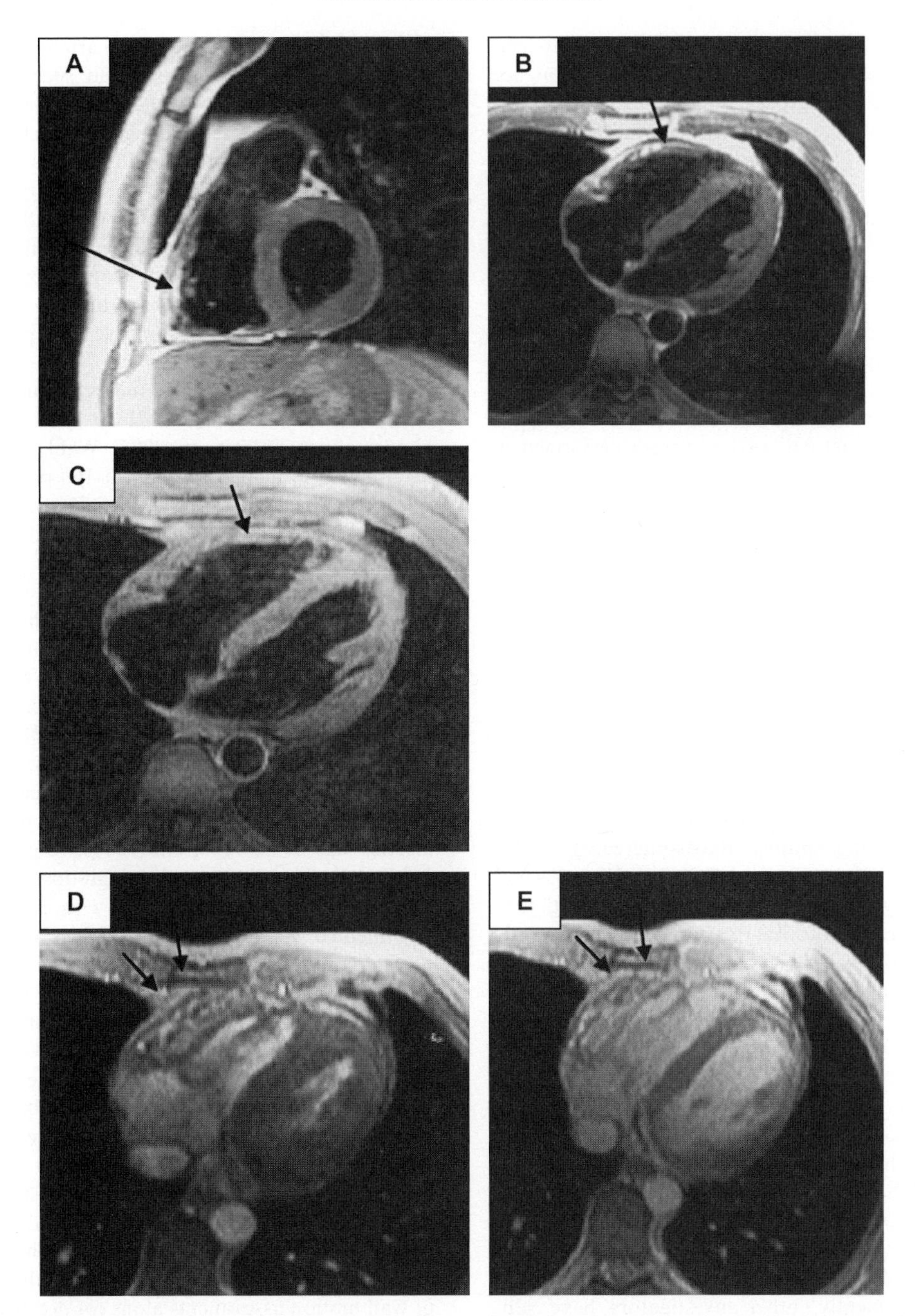

Fig. 8. Cardiovascular magnetic resonance imaging for the diagnosis of arrhythmogenic right ventricular dysplasia. T1-weighted turbo spin–echo sequences show the high signal intensity (bright) region within the right ventricular (RV) anterior wall in a left ventricular (LV) short-axis (*A*) and axial (*B*) view (arrows). Signal intensity of this region is comparable to that of subcutaneous fat. With application of a fat suppression pulse, the bright signal of the fatty infiltrates disappear, again comparable with subcutaneous fat (*C*) (arrow). End–systolic (*D*) and end–diastolic (*E*) frames from a cine gradient echo sequence demonstrate the RV dilation and the impaired inward motion and systolic thickening of the RV anterior wall (arrows). (*From* Keller D, Osswald S, Bremerich J, et al. Arrhythmogenic right ventricular dysplasia: diagnostic and prognostic value of cardiac MRI in relation to arrhythmia free survival. Int J Card Imaging 2003;19:537; with permission.)

and 10 without were assessed with gradient-echo dobutamine cardiovascular magnetic resonance at rest and during peak dobutamine stress (infusion rate of 20 μg/kg/min). They found excellent sensitivity (91%) and specificity (80%) for the detection of significant CAD (diameter stenosis ≥50%) with dobutamine stress CMR [91].

Each of these early studies demonstrated the diagnostic utility of stress CMR for detection of wall motion abnormalities in patients who had known disease. They were limited by wall motion analysis at baseline compared only with peak stress and not continuously throughout testing. As noted previously, these studies were relatively small (20 to 60 patients) and were performed in a single institution. In addition, infusions were terminated prematurely when patients developed chest pain. Nevertheless, this series of small studies highlighted the feasibility of dobutamine administration in the CMR environment and showed that diagnostic utility of these techniques may be high.

Two major studies were performed that demonstrated the feasibility of DCMR in patients with known or suspected CAD without awareness of the extent of coronary arteriosclerosis before testing. Nagel and colleagues [92] compared DSE with DCMR in 208 patients referred for contrast coronary angiography (cross-reference). CMR provided better sensitivity (89% versus 74%) and specificity (86% versus 70%) for detecting 50% or more cases of coronary arterial luminal narrowing with coronary angiography compared with DSE. In a second study, Hundley and colleagues [87] used DCMR to study patients who had poor acoustic windows that prevented the use of second harmonic DSE imaging. When compared with contrast coronary angiography, the sensitivity and specificity were 83% for detecting coronary arterial luminal narrowing of greater than 50% [93]. Assessment of myocardial perfusion and wall motion during DMR imaging appears to improve the diagnostic accuracy of MRI stress tests compared with wall motion analysis alone [94].

Subsequently, other investigators have substantiated the utility of CMR wall motion stress testing. Sensky and colleagues [95] examined the accuracy of CMR results when compared with angiography in identifying regions of ischemia in patients who had multivessel coronary arteriosclerosis before coronary artery revascularization. Using steady-state free precession sequences combined with parallel imaging acquisitions, Paetsch and colleagues [96] acquired images to identify at least 50% of coronary arterial luminal narrowings with a sensitivity and specificity of 89% and 80%, respectively. Zoghbi and colleagues [97] emphasized the high diagnostic accuracy, feasibility, versatility, and relatively low cost and high sensitivity (91%) and specificity (85%) for diagnosing CAD compared with DSE (with a sensitivity of 85%). In these studies, implementation of newer white blood imaging techniques reduced scan times by factors of three to four, allowing the acquisition of multiple slice positions during a single breath hold.

Although many earlier studies excluded patients who had a prior MI or wall motion abnormalities at rest, in 2004, Wahl and colleagues [98] evaluated a group of 160 patients to document the utility of DCMR in patients who had previously documented resting wall motion abnormalities. The subjects were difficult to assess with DSE because of the variability in interpreting wall motion with poor visualization. Additionally, they had prior revascularization with underlying resting LV wall motion abnormalities. The sensitivity and specificity of DCMR for detecting coronary luminal narrowing of at least 50% in this patient population was 89% and 84%, respectively. In addition, the sensitivity of detecting luminal narrowing of one, two, or three epicardial arteries was 87%, 91%, and 100%, respectively. This study demonstrated that high-dose DCMR can be useful even in patients with previously documented wall motion abnormalities and a history of coronary revascularization.

In 2003, Kuijpers and colleagues [99] reported on the qualitative assessment of tagged images in comparison with nontagged cine CMR. One hundred ninety-four patients referred for the evaluation of chest pain underwent tagged dobutamine stress wall motion analyses and contrast coronary angiography. Tagged DCMR images detected new wall motion abnormalities in 68 patients, compared with 58 patients without tagged images. This was the first study to demonstrate that high-dose DCMR with tagging may improve the utility of wall motion assessments alone for detecting inducible LV wall motion abnormalities indicative of ischemia during dobutamine CMR stress testing. As shown in Table 1, multiple studies have been performed that demonstrate the clinical utility of CMR wall motion stress testing in diagnosing more than 50% of epicardial coronary arterial luminal narrowings. Combing the results from all studies, the sensitivity and specificity of dobutamine stress CMR was 86% and 84%,

Table 1
Sensitivity and specificity analysis for stress dobutamine cardiovascular magnetic resonance in detection of ≥50% coronary arterial luminal narrowings

Author/ year	Dose (μg/kg/ min)	Number of patients	Sensitivity	Specificity
Pennell, et al 1992 [88]	20	25	91	—
van Rugge, et al 1993 [66,90]	20	45	81	100
van Rugge, et al 1994 [91]	20	39	91	80
Nagel, et al 1999 [92]	20	208	86	86
Baer, 1994 [89]	20	35	84	-
Nagel, 1999 [92]	40 + atropine	172	86	86
Hundley, et al 1999 [87]	40 + atropine	163	83	83
Wahl, 2004 [98]	40 + atropine	160	89	84
Summary		847	86	84

respectively, for identifying at least 50% of epicardial coronary arterial luminal narrowings with contrast coronary arteriography.

Detection of viability

CMR also has been used for identifying left ventricular myocardial segments that, because of myocardial stunning or hibernation, display abnormal wall motion at rest and will improve in contractility after coronary arterial revascularization procedures. Early studies examining viability compared CMR with other modalities including DSE and radioisotope studies. Development of tagging has enabled better quantitative assessment of LV wall thickening indicative of viability. Recently, there have been several studies looking at specific characteristics of the myocardium, including movement of individual layers, circumferential shortening, and wall thickening, all of which represent important determinants of potential recovery after revascularization.

After an MI, the transmural extent of necrosis and decrease in LV ejection fraction can vary considerably. Using CMR tagging to regionally quantify fiber strains, wall thickening, and ejection fraction, Bogaert and colleagues [100] assessed 12 patients who had single-vessel disease 1 week and 3 months after successful reperfusion of a first transmural anterior MI. Improved subepicardial fiber shortening at the 3-month mark was associated with an improved regional LV wall motion and global LV ejection fraction.

Geskin and colleagues [101] demonstrated that myocardial function recovery at 8 weeks after MI was predicted by an increase in circumferential shortening in resting dysfunctional segments during dobutamine infusion. In a group of 20 patients with first reperfused MI, they noted that midmyocardial response and subepicardial response to dobutamine were predictive of subsequent functional recovery, but improvement in subendocardial layers was not.

Using tissue tagging, Sayad and colleagues [102] demonstrated how low-dose dobutamine CMR analysis of LV thickening predicts future recovery of systolic thickening after revascularization of epicardial coronary arteries, supplying regions of hibernating and stunned myocardium (Fig. 9). In a group of 10 patients with segmental wall motion abnormalities at rest, they found that CMR had a sensitivity of 89%, a specificity of 93%, a negative predictive value of 82%, and a positive predictive value of 96% for recovery of segmental function after revascularization. Although not the focus of their study, the authors alluded to the excellent correlation between end–systolic wall thickness at peak dobutamine infusion and after revascularization.

Dendale and colleagues [103] evaluated the feasibility of stress CMR use for the detection of viability after acute MI. CMR images were analyzed for wall motion abnormalities during low-dosage dobutamine stimulation in 37 patients who had recent MI. The authors concluded that low-dosage dobutamine CMR is a safe and accurate predictor recovery of wall motion abnormalities after MI, but this study was limited by the lack of quantitative analysis of the CMR images.

In a quantitative analysis, Saito and colleagues [104] showed that CMR was as effective as DSE

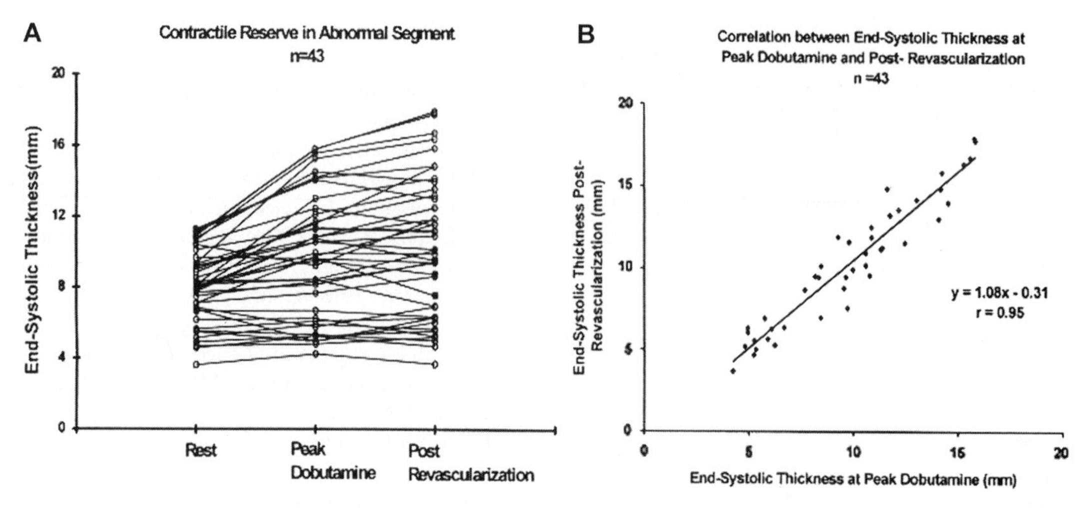

Fig. 9. Contractile reserve. (*A*) Plot of end–systolic wall thickening at rest, peak dobutamine, and after revascularization in all 43 abnormal segments. Squares represent the three segments that had contractile reserve with dobutamine, but no recovery of function after revascularization. Triangles represent the segment without contractile reserve, but this improved after revascularization. No segment with end–systolic wall thickness less than 7 mm had contractile reserve or improved after revascularization. (*B*) Regression line for end–systolic wall thickening at peak dobutamine and after revascularization. (*From* Sayad DE, Willett DL, Hundley WG, et al. Dobutamine magnetic resonance imaging with myocardial tagging quantitatively predicts improvement in regional function after revascularization. Am J Cardiol 1998;82(9):1149–51, A10; with permission.)

for identifying myocardial viability in subjects who had LV dysfunction at rest. Dobutamine CMR and stress echo had similar results in 86% of the patients for detecting myocardial viability. Sensitivity (76%) and specificity (86%) with CMR compared well with the sensitivity (66%) and specificity for DSE (100%). The sensitivity of DCMR with tagging was noted to be 76%, whereas that of DSE was 66%. The specificity of DCMR was 86%, and that of DSE was 100%. The accuracy of DCMR was 78%; that of DSE was 72%.

Dobutamine CMR has been compared with metabolic assessment of viability obtained during radionuclide studies. Baer and colleagues [89] reported that implementation of dobutamine stress provided further information regarding viability than resting LV end–diastolic wall thickness. End–diastolic wall thickness at rest and dobutamine-induced systolic wall thickening assessed by DCMR were compared with positron emission tomography (PET). They concluded that DCMR was a better predictor of residual metabolic activity, with sensitivity of 81%, specificity of 95%, and positive predictive accuracy of 96%, than PET, with a sensitivity of 72%. specificity of 89%, and positive predictive accuracy of 91%.

Delayed hyperenhancement techniques also have been used to identify myocardial necrosis and an absence of myocellular viability. In several small studies of 10 to 30 subjects, delayed enhancement imaging has been compared with dobutamine wall motion analyses for predicting the return of LV systolic function after coronary arterial revascularization [105–108]. In the most widely referenced of these studies, Wellnhofer and colleagues [108] compared recovery of systolic thickening as measured by CMR with delayed-enhancement imaging in 29 patients. Increased thickening during dobutamine CMR was more likely than delayed enhancement to identify improvement in contractility after revascularization in myocardial segments with the transmural extent of infarction less than 50%. For those with no or extensive infarcts, the techniques had similar efficacy.

Prognosis

Assessments of LV wall motion and ejection fraction can be used to predict long-term prognosis. In 2002, Hundley and colleagues [110] reported on the utility of dobutamine CMR for

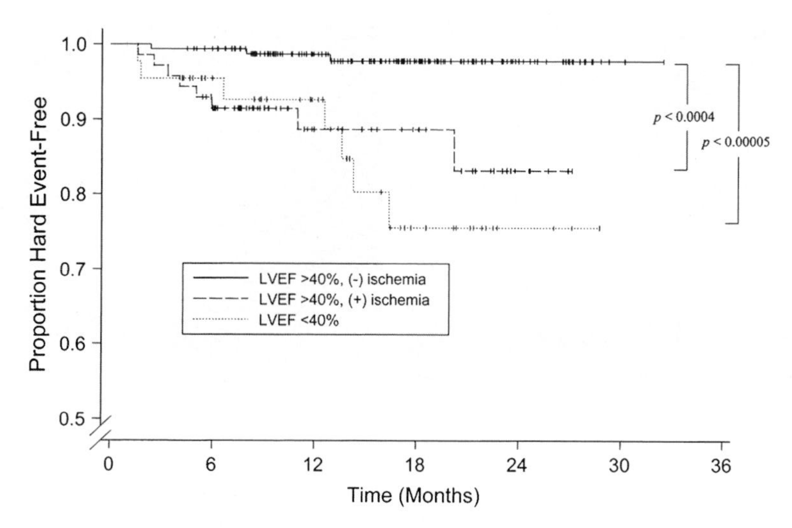

Fig. 10. Cardiovascular magnetic resonance prognosis. Kaplan-Meier event-free survival curves in patients who had an left ventricular ejection fraction (LVEF) less than 40% and greater than 40% with and without inducible ischemia. In patients who had an LVEF greater than 40%, the event-free survival was significantly lower in patients who had inducible ischemia compared with those who did not ($P < .0004$). An even greater difference was found between patients with patients who had an LVEF with 40% evidence of inducible ischemia compared with those with an LVEF less than 40% ($P < .00005$). (*From* Hundley WG, Morgan TM, Neagle CM, et al. Magnetic resonance imaging determination of cardiac prognosis. Circulation 2002;106(18):2328–33; with permission.)

identifying future myocardial infarction and cardiac death in 279 patients who were followed over an average of 20 months. In a multivariate analysis, inducible ischemia, contractile reserve, or low LV ejection fraction were associated with cardiac death and future MI, independent of the presence of risk factors for coronary arteriosclerosis or MI (Fig. 10).

CMR also has been used to determine preoperative cardiovascular risk in patients referred for noncardiac surgery. Rerkpattanapipat and colleagues [111] followed a group of 102 consecutive patients for the occurrence of cardiac death, MI, or congestive heart failure during or after noncardiac surgery. Six patients experienced a cardiac event (death in four, nonfatal myocardial

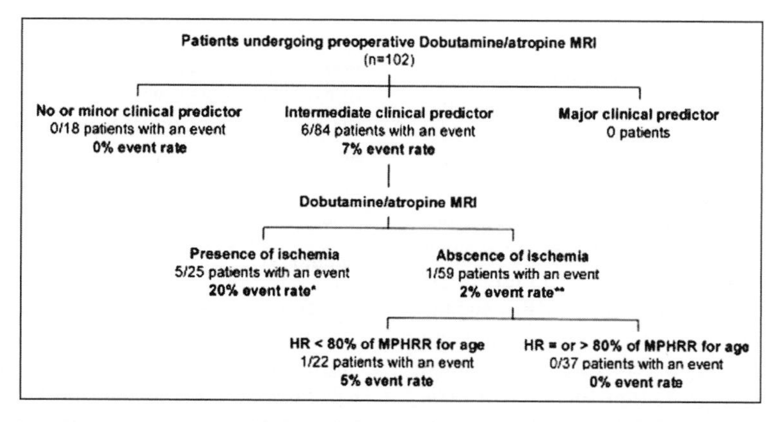

Fig. 11. Preoperative evaluation with cardiovascular magnetic resonance. The number of events and event rates for participants in the authors' study. As shown, those with inducible ischemia during dobutamine magnetic resonance imaging had a significant increase in the incidence of cardiac events. *Abbreviations:* HR, heart rate; MPHRR, maximal predicted heart rate response. (*From* Rerkpattanapipat P, Morgan TM, Neagle CM, et al. Assessment of preoperative cardiac risk with magnetic resonance imaging. Am J Cardiol 2002;90(4):416–9; with permission.)

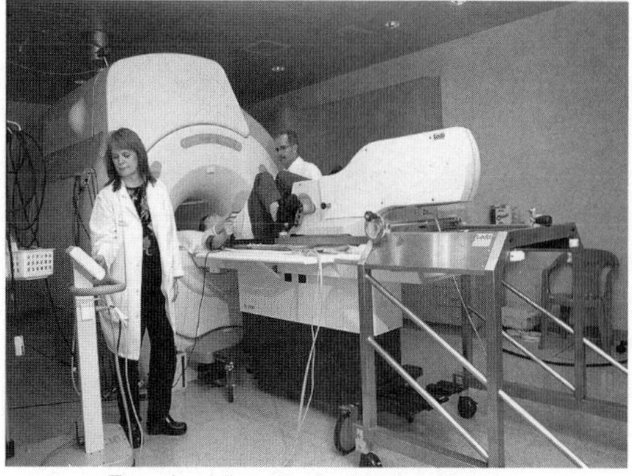

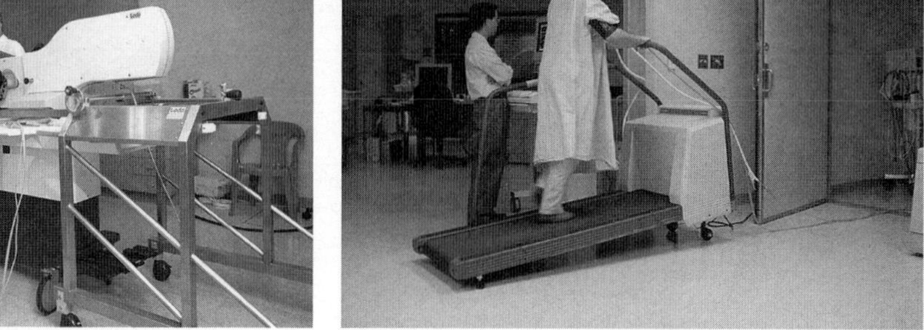

Fig. 12. Exercise cardiovascular magnetic resonance (CMR). Diagrammatic representation of an exercise bike used for CMR stress studies made from nonferromagnetic materials (left panel). In the right panel, a treadmill positioned outside of the magnetic resonance scanner. With this treadmill approach, heightened diagnostic accuracy is achieved when images are collected within a minute of exercise cessation.

infarction in one, and congestive heart failure in one) during surgery or in their postoperative course. Five of 26 patients who had evidence of inducible ischemia during DCMR underwent revascularization before surgery (one sustained an event, and four did not). In patients who had intermediate clinical predictors of events as defined by the American College of Cardiology and the American Heart Association, evidence of inducible ischemia during CMR imaging was associated with a significant increase in perioperative cardiac events (Fig. 11).

Exercise stress testing

As with echocardiography, it may be possible to implement exercise instead of pharmacologic stress to obtain imaging. Studies have been conducted looking at both the bicycle and treadmill exercise as stress agents. Bicycle exercise has the advantage of reduction in stress protocol duration and acquisition of data regarding functional capacity. In one study, Roest and colleagues [112] studied 16 healthy volunteers (eight women and eight men, mean age 18 ± 2 years) with bicycle exercise in the supine position on a MR-compatible bicycle ergometer at 1.5 T. By breath holding at end expiration, image blurring was avoided because of respiratory motion for all short-axis images. Stroke volume and ejection fraction increased in both ventricles in response to exercise; as would be expected, the end–systolic volume of the two ventricles decreased, while the end–diastolic volumes remained the same This study demonstrates that exercise CMR, in normal patients, can be used to assess physiologic changes in both the left and right ventricles simultaneously (Fig. 12).

Although the previous study used supine bicycle exercise, Rerkpattanapipat and colleagues [109] used upright treadmill in 27 patients who had images obtained less than 1 minute after exercise (see Fig. 12). Ischemia was appreciated in 14 patients, with good overall sensitivity and specificity of detecting epicardial artery luminal narrowings greater than 50% of 79% and 85%, respectively. This study was limited, however, in that comprehensive coverage of the myocardium was not achieved, and results were acquired on a small number of subjects. Further studies are needed in this area to determine the clinical utility of exercise-induced wall motion abnormalities for the assessment of patients who have cardiovascular disease.

Summary

Several imaging techniques are available for assessing global and regional LV and RV function during cardiovascular MRI examinations. These techniques can be used to provide accurate and reproducible measures of ventricular volumes and ejection fraction. In those who can undergo CMR, it may be the most accurate noninvasive imaging test for determining LV or RV volumes or ejection fraction.

CMR also can be used to provide information about regional LV function including: wall motion, thickening, and strain. To date, these regional function measures have been acquired at rest and with stress, and they have been shown to be useful for identifying myocardial ischemia, injury, and viability. In addition, changes in regional function observed during dobutamine stress CMR are useful for assessing cardiac prognosis and preoperative cardiac risk assessment for noncardiac surgery.

References

[1] Haase A, Frahm J, Mathaei D. Rapid three-dimensional MR imaging using the FLASH technique J Comput Assist Tomogr 1986;67:256–66.
[2] Balaban R. The physics of image generation by magnetic resonance. In: Manning WJ, Pennell DJ, editors. Cardiovascular magnetic resonance. 1st edition. Philadelphia: Churchill Livingstone; 2002. p. 3–17.
[3] Mirowitz S, Eilenberg S, White R. Cardiac MR imaging techniques and strategies. In: Gutierrez F, Brown J, Mirowitz S, editors. Cardiovascular magnetic resonance imaging. Chicago: Mosby; 1992. p. 17–22.
[4] Masood S, Yang GZ, Pennell DJ, et al. Investigating intrinsic myocardial mechanics: the role of MR tagging, velocity phase mapping, and diffusion imaging. J Magn Reson Imaging 2000;12:873–83.
[5] Longmore DB, Klipstein RH, Underwood SR, et al. Dimensional accuracy of magnetic resonance in studies of the heart. Lancet 1985;1(8442):1360–2.
[6] Semelka RC, Tomei E, Wagner S, et al. Normal left ventricular dimensions and function: interstudy reproducibility of measurements with cine MR imaging. Radiology 1990;174(3 Pt 1):763–8.
[7] Debatin JF, Nadel SN, Paolini JF, et al. Cardiac ejection fraction: phantom study comparing cine MR imaging, radionuclide blood pool imaging, and ventriculography. J Magn Reson Imaging 1992;2(2):135–42.
[8] Germain P, Roul G, Kastler B, et al. Interstudy variability in left ventricular mass measurement. Comparison between M-mode echography and MRI. Eur Heart J 1992;13(8):1011–9.
[9] Sandstede J, Lipke C, Beer M, et al. Age- and gender-specific differences in left and right ventricular cardiac function and mass determined by cine magnetic resonance imaging. Eur Radiol 2000;10(3): 438–42.
[10] Salehian O, Schwerzmann M, Merchant N, et al. Assessment of systemic right ventricular function in patients with transposition of the great arteries using the myocardial performance index: comparison with cardiac magnetic resonance imaging. Circulation 2004;110(20):3229–33.
[11] Nitz W. Fast and ultrafast nonecho–planar MR imaging techniques. Eur Radiol 2002;12(12): 2866–82.
[12] Oppelt A, Graumann R, Barfuss A, et al. FISP: a new fast MRI sequence. Electromedica 1986;3: 15–8.
[13] Zur Y, Wood ML, Neuringer LJ. Motion-insensitive, steady-state free precession imaging. Magn Reson Med 1990;16:444–59.
[14] Duerk JL, Lewin JS, Wendt M, et al. Remember true FISP? A high SNR, near 1-second imaging method for T2-like contrast in interventional MRI at .2 T. J Magn Reson Imaging 1998;8:203–8.
[15] Chung YC, Merkle EM, Lewin JS, et al. Fast T(2)-weighted imaging by PSIF at 0.2 T for interventional MRI. Magn Reson Med 1999;42:335–44.
[16] Wendt M, Wacker F, Wolf KJ, et al. [Keyhole-true FISP: fast T2-weighted imaging for interventional MRT at 0.2 T]. Rofo 1999;170:391–3 [in German].
[17] Barkhausen J, Ruehm SG, Goyen M, et al. MR evaluation of ventricular function: true fast imaging with steady-state precession versus fast low-angle shot cine MR imaging: feasibility studyRadiology 2001;219:264–9.
[18] Fischer H, Ladebeck R. Echo-planar imaging image artifacts. In: Schmitt F, Stehling MK, Turner R, editors. Echo-planar imaging: theory, technique, and application. New York: Springer; 1998. p. 179–210.
[19] Weiger M, Pruessmann KP, Boesiger P. Cardiac real-time imaging using SENSE: sensitivity-encoding scheme. Magn Reson Med 2000;43:177–84.
[20] Pruessmann KP, Weiger M, Bornert P, et al. Advances in sensitivity encoding with arbitrary k-space trajectories. Magn Reson Med 2001;46: 638–51.
[21] Weiger M, Pruessmann KP, Leussler C, et al. Specific coil design for SENSE: a six-element cardiac array. Magn Reson Med 2001;45:495–504.
[22] Pruessmann KP, Weiger M, Boesiger P. Sensitivity-encoded cardiac MRI. J Cardiovasc Magn Reson 2001;3:1–9.
[23] Huang J, Abendschein D, Davila-Roman VG, et al. Spatio–temporal tracking of myocardial deformations with a 4-D B-spline model from tagged MRI. IEEE Trans Med Imaging 1999;18:957–72.
[24] Fischer SE, McKinnon GC, Maier SE, et al. Improved myocardial tagging contrast. Magn Reson Med 1993;30:191–200.
[25] Fischer SE, Stuber M, Dam J, et al. Late diastolic tag persistence with slice followed echo planar imaging. In: Proceedings of the 4th Scientific Meeting, New York: International Society of Magnetic Resonance 1; 1996:297.
[26] Aletras AH, Wen H. Mixed echo train acquisition displacement encoding with stimulated echoes: an optimized DENSE method for in vivo functional imaging of the human heart. Magn Reson Med 2001;46:523–34.

[27] Kim D, Gilson WD, Kramer CM, et al. Myocardial tissue tracking with two-dimensional cine displacement-encoded MR imaging: development and initial evaluation. Radiology 2004;230(3):862–71.

[28] Rumancik W, Naidich D, Chandra R, et al. Cardiovascular disease: evaluation with MR phase imaging. Radiology 1988;166:63–8.

[29] Pelc LR, Sayre J, Yun K, et al. Evaluation of myocardial motion tracking with cine-phase contrast magnetic resonance imaging. Invest Radiol 1994;29:1038–42.

[30] Jung B, Zaitsev M, Hennig J, et al. Navigator gated high temporal resolution tissue phase mapping of myocardial motion. Magn Reson Med 2006;55:937–42.

[31] Markl M, Schneider B, Hennig J. Fast phase contrast cardiac magnetic resonance imaging: improved assessment and analysis of left ventricular wall motion. J Magn Reson Imaging 2002;15:642–53.

[32] Jung B, Foll D, Bottler P, et al. Detailed analysis of myocardial motion in volunteers and patients using high temporal resolution MR tissue phase mapping. J Magn Reson Imaging 2006;24:1033–9.

[33] van Dijk P. Direct cardiac NMR imaging of heart wall and blood flow velocity. J Comput Assist Tomogr 1984;8:429–36.

[34] Wedeen VJ. Magnetic resonance imaging of myocardial kinematics. Technique to detect, localize, and quantify the strain rates of the active human myocardium. Magn Reson Med 1992;27:52–67.

[35] Nayler GL, Firmin DN, Longmore DB. Blood flow imaging by cine magnetic resonance. J Comput Assist Tomogr 1986;10:715–22.

[36] Petersen SE, Jung BA, Wiesmann F, et al. Myocardial tissue phase mapping with cine phase-contrast MR imaging: regional wall motion analysis in healthy volunteers. Radiology 2006;238:816–26.

[37] Van der Geest RJ, Reiber JH. Quantification in cardiac, MRI. J Magn Reson Imaging 1999;10:602–8.

[38] Wedeen VJ, Weisskoff RM, Reese TG, et al. Motionless movies of myocardial strain—rates using stimulated echoes. Magn Reson Med 1995;33:401–8.

[39] Rehr RB, Malloy CR, Filipchuk NG, et al. Left ventricular volumes measured by MR imaging-Radiology 1985;156:717–9.

[40] Chuang ML, Hibberd MG, Salton CJ, et al. Importance of imaging method over imaging modality in noninvasive determination of left ventricular volumes and ejection fraction: assessment by two- and three-dimensional echocardiography and magnetic resonance imaging. J Am Coll Cardiol 2000;35:477–84.

[41] Cranney GB, Lotan CS, Dean L, et al. Left ventricular volume measurement using cardiac axis nuclear magnetic resonance imaging. Validation by calibrated ventricular angiography. Circulation 1990;82:154–63.

[42] Lawson MA, Blackwell GG, Davis ND, et al. Accuracy of biplane long-axis left ventricular volume determined by cine magnetic resonance imaging in patients with regional and global dysfunction. Am J Cardiol 1996;77:1098–104.

[43] Martin ET, Fuisz AR, Pohost GM. Imaging cardiac structure and pump function. Cardiol Clin 1998;16:135–60.

[44] Keller AM, Peshock RM, Malloy CR, et al. In vivo measurement of myocardial mass using nuclear magnetic resonance imaging. J Am Coll Cardiol 1986;8(1):113–7.

[45] Koch JA, Poll LW, Godehardt E, et al. Right and left ventricular volume measurements in an animal heart model in vitro: first experiences with cardiac MRI at 1.0 T. Eur Radiol 2000;10(3):455–8.

[46] Nahrendorf M, Hiller KH, Hu K, et al. Cardiac magnetic resonance imaging in small animal models of human heart failure. Med Image Anal 2003;7(3):369–75.

[47] Caputo G, Tscholakoff D, Sechtem U, et al. Measurement of canine left ventricular mass by using MR imaging. AJR Am J Roentgenol 1987;148:33–8.

[48] Holman ER, Vliegen HW, van der Geest RJ, et al. Quantitative analysis of regional left ventricular function after myocardial infarction in the pig assessed with cine magnetic resonance imaging. Magn Reson Med 1995;34:161–9.

[49] Rudin M, Pedersen B, Umemura K, et al. Determination of rat heart morphology and function in vivo in two models of cardiac hypertrophy by means of magnetic resonance imaging. Basic Res Cardiol 1991;86(2):165–74.

[50] Pattynama PM, Lamb HJ, van der Velde EA, et al. Left ventricular measurements with cine and spin echo MR imaging: a study of reproducibility with variance component analysis. Radiology 1993;187:261–8.

[51] Semelka RC, Tomei E, Wagner S, et al. Interstudy reproducibility of dimensional and functional measurements between cine magnetic resonance studies in the morphologically abnormal left ventricle. Am Heart J 1990;119:1367–73.

[52] Stratemeier EJ, Thompson R, Brady TJ, et al. Ejection fraction determination by MR imaging: comparison with left ventricular angiography. Radiology 1986;158:775–7.

[53] Shapiro EP, Rogers WJ, Beyar R, et al. Determination of left ventricular mass by MRI in hearts deformed by acute infarction. Circulation 1989;79:706–11.

[54] Meyer S, Curry G, Donsky M, et al. Influence of dobutamine on hemodynamics and coronary blood flow in patients with and without coronary artery disease. Am J Cardiol 1976;38:103–8.

[55] Lee VS, Resnick D, Bundy JM, et al. Cardiac function: MR evaluation in one breath hold with real-time true fast imaging with steady-state precession. Radiology 2002;222:835–42.
[56] Boxt LM, Katz J. Magnetic resonance imaging for quantitation of right ventricular volume in patients with pulmonary hypertension. J Thorac Imaging 1993;8:92–7.
[57] Doherty NE III, Fujita N, Caputo GR, et al. Measurement of right ventricular mass in normal and dilated cardiomyopathic ventricles using cine magnetic resonance imaging. Am J Cardiol 1992;69: 1223–8.
[58] Katz J, Whang J, Boxt LM, et al. Estimation of right ventricular mass in normal subjects and in patients with primary pulmonary hypertension by nuclear magnetic resonance imaging. J Am Coll Cardiol 1993;21:1475–81.
[59] Pattynama PM, Lamb HJ, van der Velde EA, et al. Reproducibility of MRI-derived measurements of right ventricular volumes and myocardial mass. Magn Reson Imaging 1995;13:53–63.
[60] Rominger MB, Bachmann GF, Pabst W, et al. Right ventricular volumes and ejection fraction with fast cine MR imaging in breath-hold technique: applicability, normal values from 52 volunteers, and evaluation of 325 adult cardiac patients. J Magn Reson Imaging 1999;10:908–18.
[61] Lorenz CH, Walker ES, Morgan VL, et al. Normal human right and left ventricular mass, systolic function, and gender differences by cine magnetic resonance imaging. J Cardiovasc Magn Reson 1999;1:7–21.
[62] Azhari H, Sideman S, Weiss JL, et al. Three-dimensional mapping of acute ischemic regions using MRI: wall thickening versus motion analysis. Am J Physiol 1990;259:1492–503.
[63] Henschke CI, Risser TA, Sandor T, et al. Quantitative computer-assisted analysis of left ventricular wall thickening and motion by two-dimensional echocardiography in acute myocardial infarction. Am J Cardiol 1983;52:960–4.
[64] Lieberman AN, Weiss JL, Jugdutt BI, et al. Two-dimensional echocardiography and infarct size: relationship of regional wall motion and thickening to the extent of myocardial infarction in the dog. Circulation 1981;63:739–46.
[65] Holman ER, van Jonbergen HP, van Dijkman PR, et al. Comparison of magnetic resonance imaging studies with enzymatic indexes of myocardial necrosis for quantification of myocardial infarct size. Am J Cardiol 1993;71:1036–40.
[66] van Rugge FP, Holman ER, van der Wall EE, et al. Quantitation of global and regional left ventricular function by cine magnetic resonance imaging during dobutamine stress in normal human subjects. Eur Heart J 1993;14:456–63.
[67] Reichek N. MRI myocardial tagging. J Magn Reson Imaging 1999;10:609–16.
[68] Wang J, Urheim S, Korinek J, et al. Analysis of postsystolic myocardial thickening work in selective myocardial layers during progressive myocardial ischemia. J Am Soc Echocardiogr 2006;19(9): 1102–11.
[69] Edvardsen T, Rosen BD, Pan L, et al. Regional diastolic dysfunction in individuals with left ventricular hypertrophy measured by tagged magnetic resonance imaging—the Multi-Ethnic Study of Atherosclerosis (MESA). Am Heart J 2006; 151(1):109–14.
[70] Lima JA, Jeremy R, Guier W, et al. Accurate systolic wall thickening by nuclear magnetic resonance imaging with tissue tagging: correlation with sonomicrometers in normal and ischemic myocardium. J Am Coll Cardiol 1993;21:1741–51.
[71] Yeon SB, Reichek N, Tallant BA, et al. Validation of in vivo myocardial strain measurement by magnetic resonance tagging with sonomicrometry J Am Coll Cardiol 2001;38:555–61.
[72] Fonseca CG, Dissanayake AM, Doughty RN, et al. Three-dimensional assessment of left ventricular systolic strain in patients with type 2 diabetes mellitus, diastolic dysfunction, and normal ejection fraction. Am J Cardiol 2004;94(11):1391–5.
[73] Palmon LC, Reichek N, Yeon SB, et al. Intramural myocardial shortening in hypertensive left ventricular hypertrophy with normal pump function. Circulation 1994;89:122–31.
[74] Bogaert J, Bosmans H, Maes A, et al. Remote myocardial dysfunction after acute anterior myocardial infarction: impact of left ventricular shape on regional function: a magnetic resonance myocardial tagging study. J Am Coll Cardiol 2000;35:1525–34.
[75] Marcus JT, Gotte MJ, Van Rossum AC, et al. Myocardial function in infarcted and remote regions early after infarction in man: assessment by magnetic resonance tagging and strain analysis. Magn Reson Med 1997;38:803–10.
[76] Paetsch I, Foll D, Kaluza A, et al. Magnetic resonance stress tagging inischemic heart disease. Am J Physiol Heart Circ Physiol 2005;288:H2708–14.
[77] Rebergen SA, Ottenkamp J, Doornbos J, et al. Postoperative pulmonary flow dynamics after Fontan surgery: assessment with nuclear magnetic resonance velocity mapping. J Am Coll Cardiol 1993;21:123–31.
[78] Holmqvist C, Oskarsson G, Stahlberg F, et al. Functional evaluation of extracardiac ventriculopulmonary conduits and of the right ventricle with magnetic resonance imaging and velocity mapping. Am J Cardiol 1999;83:926–32.
[79] Fogel MA. Assessment of cardiac function by magnetic resonance imaging. Pediatr Cardiol 2000;21: 59–69.
[80] Saito H, Dambara T, Aiba M, et al. Evaluation of cor pulmonale on a modified short-axis section of the heart by magnetic resonance imaging. Am Rev Respir Dis 1992;146:1576–81.

[81] Pattynama PM, Willems LN, Smit AH, et al. Early diagnosis of cor pulmonale with MR imaging of the right ventricle. Radiology 1992;182:375–9.
[82] Boxt LM. MR imaging of pulmonary hypertension and right ventricular dysfunction. Magn Reson Imaging Clin N Am 1996;4:307–25.
[83] Casolo GC, Poggesi L, Boddi M, et al. ECG-gated magnetic resonance imaging in right ventricular dysplasia. Am Heart J 1987;113:1245–8.
[84] Blake LM, Scheinman MM, Higgins CB. MR features of arrhythmogenic right ventricular dysplasia. Am J Roentgenol 1994;162:809–12.
[85] McKenna WJ, Thiene G, Nava A, et al. Diagnosis of arrhythmogenic right ventricular dysplasia/cardiomyopathy. Task Force of the Working Group Myocardial and Pericardial Disease of the European Society of Cardiology and of the Scientific Council on Cardiomyopathies of the International Society and Federation of Cardiology. Br Heart J 1994;71:215–8.
[86] Keller D, Osswald S, Bremerich J, et al. Arrhythmogenic right ventricular dysplasia: diagnostic and prognostic value of cardiac MRI in relation to arrhythmia-free survival. Int J Card Imaging 2003;19:537–43.
[87] Hundley WG, Hamilton CA, Thomas MS, et al. Utility of fast cine magnetic resonance imaging and display for the detection of myocardial ischemia in patients not well-suited for second harmonic stress echocardiography. Circulation 1999;100:1697–702.
[88] Pennell DJ, Underwood SR, Manzara CC, et al. Magnetic resonance imaging during dobutamine stress in coronary artery disease. Am J Cardiol 1992;70(1):34–40.
[89] Baer FM, Theissen P, Smolarz K, et al. Dobutamine versus dipyridamole magnetic resonance tomography: safety and sensitivity in the detection of coronary stenosis. Z Kardiol 1993;82:494–503.
[90] van Rugge FP, van der Wall EE, de Roos A, et al. Dobutamine stress magnetic resonance imaging for detection of coronary artery disease. J Am Coll Cardiol 1993;22:431–9.
[91] van Rugge FP, van der Wall EE, Spanjersberg SJ, et al. Magnetic resonance imaging during dobutamine stress for detection and localization of coronary artery disease. Quantitative wall motion analysis using a modification of the centerline method. Circulation 1994;90:127–38.
[92] Nagel E, Lehmkuhl HB, Bocksch W, et al. Noninvasive diagnosis of ischemia-induced wall motion abnormalities with the use of high-dose dobutamine stress magnetic resonance imaging: comparison with dobutamine stress echocardiography. Circulation 1999;99:763–70.
[93] Wahl A, Roethemeyer S, Paetsch I, et al. High-dose dobutamine stress MRI for follow-up after coronary revascularization procedures in patients with wall motion abnormalities at rest. J Cardiovasc Magn Reson 2002;4:22–3.
[94] Wahl A, Roethemeyer S, Paetsch I, et al. Simultaneous assessment of wall motion and myocardial perfusion during high-dose dobutamine stress MRI improves diagnosis of ischemia in patients with known coronary artery disease. J Cardiovasc Magn Reson 2002;4:136–7.
[95] Sensky PR, Jivan A, Hudson N, et al. Coronary artery disease: combined stress MR imaging protocol—one-stop evaluation of myocardial perfusion and function. Radiology 2000;215:608–14.
[96] Paetsch I, Jahnke C, Wahl A, et al. Comparison of dobutamine stress magnetic resonance, adenosine stress magnetic resonance, and adenosine stress magnetic resonance perfusion. Circulation 2004; 110:835–42.
[97] Zoghbi WA, Barasch E, Dobutamine MRI. A serious contender in pharmacological stress imaging? Circulation 1999;99(6):730–2.
[98] Wahl A, Paetsch I, Roethemeyer S, et al. High-dose dobutamine–atropine stress cardiovascular MR imaging after coronary revascularization in patients with wall motion abnormalities at rest. Radiology 2004;233:210–6.
[99] Kuijpers D, Ho KY, van Dijkman PR, et al. Dobutamine cardiovascular magnetic resonance for the detection of myocardial ischemia with the use of myocardial tagging. Circulation 2003; 107(12):1592–7.
[100] Bogaert J, Maes A, Rademakers FE. Functional recovery of subepicardial myocardial tissue in transmural myocardial infarction after successful reperfusion: an important contribution to the improvement of regional and global left ventricular function. Circulation 1999;99(1):36–43.
[101] Geskin G, Kramer CM, Rogers WJ, et al. Quantitative assessment of myocardial viability after infarction by dobutamine magnetic resonance tagging. Circulation 1998;98(3):217–23.
[102] Sayad DE, Willett DL, Hundley WG, et al. Dobutamine magnetic resonance imaging with myocardial tagging quantitatively predicts improvement in regional function after revascularization. Am J Cardiol 1998;82(9):1149–51, A10.
[103] Dendale PA, Franken PR, Waldman GJ, et al. Low-dosage dobutamine magnetic resonance imaging as an alternative to echocardiography in the detection of viable myocardium after acute infarction. Am Heart J 1995;130(1):134–40.
[104] Saito I, Watanabe S, Masuda Y. Detection of viable myocardium by dobutamine stress tagging magnetic resonance imaging with three-dimensional analysis by automatic trace method. Jpn Circ J 2000;64(7):487–94.
[105] Motoyasu M, Sakuma H, Ichikawa Y, et al. Prediction of regional functional recovery after acute myocardial infarction with low-dose dobutamine stress cine MR imaging and contrast-enhanced MR imaging. J Cardiovasc Magn Reson 2003; 5(4):563–74.

[106] Kaandorp TA, Bax JJ, Schuijf JD, et al. Head-to-head comparison between contrast-enhanced magnetic resonance imaging and dobutamine magnetic resonance imaging in men with ischemic cardiomyopathy. Am J Cardiol 2004;93(12): 1461–4.

[107] Rerkpattanapipat P, Little WC, Clark HP, et al. Effect of the transmural extent of myocardial scar on left ventricular systolic wall thickening during intravenous dobutamine administration. Am J Cardiol 2005;95(4):495–8.

[108] Wellnhofer E, Olariu A, Nagel E, et al. Magnetic resonance low-dose dobutamine test is superior to SCAR quantification for the prediction of functional recovery. Circulation 2004;109(18):2172–4.

[109] Rerkpattanapipat P, Darty SN, Hundley WG, et al. Feasibility to detect severe coronary artery stenoses with upright treadmill exercise magnetic resonance imaging. Am J Cardiol 2003;92(5):603–6.

[110] Hundley WG, Morgan TM, Neagle CM, et al. Magnetic resonance imaging determination of cardiac prognosis. Circulation 2002;106(18):2328–33.

[111] Rerkpattanapipat P, Morgan TM, Neagle CM, et al. Assessment of preoperative cardiac risk with magnetic resonance imaging. Am J Cardiol 2002; 90(4):416–9.

[112] Roest AA, Kunz P, Lamb HJ, et al. Biventricular response to supine physical exercise in young adults assessed with ultrafast magnetic resonance imaging. Am J Cardiol 2001;87:601–5.

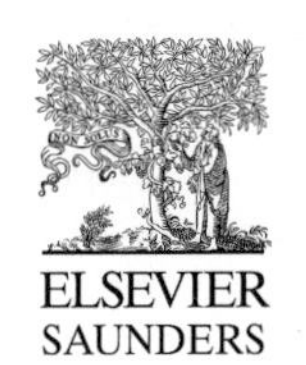

ELSEVIER
SAUNDERS

Cardiol Clin 25 (2007) 35–56

CARDIOLOGY
CLINICS

MRI for the Assessment of Myocardial Viability

Jonathan W. Weinsaft, MD[a,*], Igor Klem, MD[b], Robert M. Judd, PhD[b]

[a]*Greenberg Division of Cardiology, Weill Medical College of Cornell University, 525 East 68th Street, Starr-4, New York, NY 10021, USA*

[b]*Duke Cardiovascular Magnetic Resonance Center, Duke University Medical Center, Box 3934, Durham, NC 27710, USA*

Clinical significance of viable and infarcted myocardium

Accurate distinction between viable and infarcted myocardium holds important clinical implications for patients who have cardiac dysfunction. In patients who have ischemic heart disease and substantial viable myocardium, left ventricular (LV) dysfunction can improve following coronary revascularization [1–6] and myocardial functional improvements may be accompanied by survival benefits [7–11]. Identification of infarcted myocardium is also important because infarcted myocardium provides a substrate for ventricular tachyarrhythmias [12–14], which are a leading cause of sudden cardiac death. Thus, identification of viable myocardium capable of response to revascularization and of infarcted myocardium capable of arrhythmogenesis holds important clinical implications for patients who have cardiac dysfunction.

This article reviews the role of MRI for assessment of myocardial viability, providing a detailed overview of experimental and clinical data concerning the utility of delayed-enhancement MRI (DE-MRI) for detection of viable and infarcted myocardium.

Definition of myocardial viability

Viable myocardium is intrinsically defined by the presence of living myocytes, irrespective of contractile function or response to extrinsic stimuli. The disconnect between myocardial viability and myocardial contractility is well established. Studies have demonstrated that viable myocardium may be hypocontractile in the setting of chronic myocardial hypoperfusion or acute myocardial ischemia [5,6,15–17]. Terms such as "hibernating" or "stunned" myocardium have been used to describe the phenomenon of viable but dysfunctional myocardium.

The absence of myocardial viability is most often a consequence of myocardial infarction resulting from coronary artery occlusion. A number of parameters can be used to determine whether infarction has occurred and, if so, how much of the affected myocardial territory has not been infarcted and may be salvaged. In a review, Kaul [18] summarized clinical markers of infarction and ranked them from least to most precise (Fig. 1). For example, presence of a wall motion abnormality alone does not provide information regarding infarction because hibernating or stunned myocardium may be viable but hypocontractile. ECG may insensitive to small infarctions that may not produce Q-waves or other diagnostically specific changes [19,20]. Serum markers such as creatine kinase or troponin cannot be used to localize the location or to determine the chronicity of a myocardial infarction. Changes in myocyte cellular integrity and tissue composition are highly sensitive indices of viability that have traditionally been assessed based on pathology examination. The presence or absence of living myocytes can be established by light microscopy, electron microscopy, or by the use of histologic stains such as triphenyl tetrazolium chloride (TTC) [21]. As testing for viability based on microscopy or

* Corresponding author.
E-mail address: jww2001@med.cornell.edu (J.W. Weinsaft).

0733-8651/07/$ - see front matter
doi:10.1016/j.ccl.2007.02.001

Markers of Infarct Size
Less Precise
• Wall motion abnormality
• Q waves
• Total enzyme leak
• No-reflow or low-reflow
• Change in tissue composition
More Precise
• Myocyte integrity

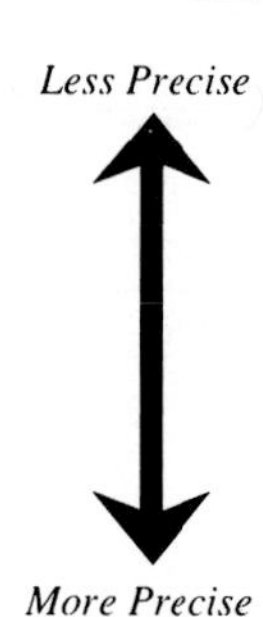

Fig. 1. Clinical and physiologic markers to determine the size of infarction. (*Adapted from* Kaul SN. Assessing the myocardium after attempted reperfusion: should we bother? Circulation 1998;98:625; with permission.)

histologic staining is not practical in a clinical setting, several less precise definitions of viability have been developed that are based on parameters that are more easily measured in patients.

Improvement in contractile function following coronary revascularization has traditionally been used as a surrogate measure of myocardial viability. Although convenient for clinical purposes, this definition can be inaccurate. If contractility improves following revascularization, then it is reasonable to assume that there is a significant amount of viable myocardium in a given territory. The converse, however, is not necessarily true. Analysis of transmural needle biopsy specimens taken during coronary artery bypass graft surgery have demonstrated that substantial viable myocardium may be present in some regions that do not demonstrate contractile improvement following revascularization. In a study in which myocardial tissue samples of dysfunctional segments were obtained, Dakik and colleagues [22] found that mean extent of viability was nearly 70% of segmental myocardium in territories that did not improve following coronary artery bypass graft surgery. The paradox of viable myocardium that does not functionally improve following revascularization may be due to several factors. First, the use of a single time point on which to assess recovery of function may not account to the true rate of functional recovery, which may require up to 14 months following revascularization [23]. Second, coronary revascularization may be incomplete, particularly in patients who have diffuse coronary atherosclerosis. Third, tethering of regions that have extensive scar to those that have predominant viability may alter ventricular geometry and thereby inhibit the postrevascularization contractile response of viable regions.

MRI techniques for assessment of myocardial viability

MRI has the ability to assess viable and infarcted myocardium by a variety of different techniques. For instance, spectroscopy techniques can detect viability by measuring the presence of subcellular components required to maintain cellular integrity. Studies have shown that phosphorus 31 spectroscopy [24–28], water-suppressed proton spectroscopy [29], or direct sodium 23 [30–33] or potassium 39 [34] imaging can be used to distinguish between viable and infarcted myocardium. The primary limitations of these metabolic approaches are poor signal-to-noise ratio, poor spatial resolution, and long imaging times [35].

Studies examining intrinsic proton relaxation times have shown that acutely infarcted myocardium has long T1 and T2 [36–38]. These changes are typically visualized on T2-weighted images, with the clinical interpretation being that regions of elevated image intensity (long T2) correspond to regions of acute infarction. This approach provides higher signal-to-noise ratio and spatial resolution compared with spectroscopy and does not require administration of a contrast agent. A major limitation of this approach is that changes in T1 and T2 are not specific for irreversible injury because some studies have demonstrated increased image intensity in areas of reversible injury [35]. Additional limitations include the fact that chronic infarcts cannot be detected and that even in acute infarcts, regional differences in image intensity are usually modest, resulting in increased interobserver variability regarding image interpretation [35].

Assessment of resting wall thickness and thickening by cine-MRI can be used to assess viability. The underlying hypothesis is that regions of myocardial thinning reflect chronic myocardial infarction [39,40]. Information regarding wall thickness is often combined with information regarding systolic wall thickening to improve the sensitivity and specificity of the technique [39]. This approach suffers from several limitations. First, it does not account for the phenomenon of myocardial stunning or hibernation in which wall thickening may be absent despite preserved viability [5,6,15–17]. Second, it is not intended to examine viability following recent infarction, whereby wall thickness may remain unchanged or increase by as much as 50% [41]. Third, in the setting of chronic myocardial hypoperfusion, wall thinning may be present in regions that have a substantial amount of viable myocardium [42]. Although the mechanism for differential thinning of viable territories remains poorly understood, emerging data suggest that thinned regions of viable myocardium can respond to coronary revascularization, with improvement in wall thickness and contractile function [43].

Cine-MRI performed during dobutamine infusion can be used to assess potential for contractile response to coronary revascularization [39,44–47]. This approach is predicated on the hypothesis that viable myocardium, unlike infarcted tissue, will respond to inotropic stimulation by increasing systolic wall thickening, which can be detected on cine-MRI. One limitation of this approach concerns the fact that contractile reserve may have reduced sensitivity for viable myocardium in the setting of severe resting dysfunction. Experimental studies have shown that some viability regions may have severe reductions in perfusion with exhausted coronary flow reserve such that any inotropic stimulation merely results in ischemia and precludes the ability for enhanced contractility [48]. There are also several practical constraints associated with use of dobutamine for viability assessment: inotropic stimulation in patients who have coronary disease is associated with risk of exacerbating myocardial ischemia, and the positioning of patients within an MRI magnet limits patient–physician interactions. In addition, the diagnostic waveform of the ECG may be altered by magnetic fields, thereby limiting monitoring for ischemia. Clinical data concerning the diagnostic utility of dobutamine-based viability assessment are discussed at length in a subsequent section (see "Comparison of delayed-enhancement MRI to other imaging techniques/Dobutamine stress imaging").

Reports of imaging of myocardial injury using T1-weighted pulse sequences after the administration of gadolinium contrast media have been in the literature since the mid-1980s [49–51]. This approach is predicated on the concept that infarcted tissue accumulates gadolinium and appear as hyperenhanced or "bright" regions on T1-weighted images acquired at least 10 minutes after gadolinium injection. A major limitation of the initial technique was insufficient differential image intensity between normal and infarcted myocardium. Suboptimal image quality was likely a factor leading to early suggestions that hyperenhancement not only occurs in regions of acute infarction but also in regions of injured but viable myocardium [52,53], a concept that has not been supported by histopathology data. More recently, a segmented inversion-recovery gradient echo sequence has been developed that significantly improves in-vivo detection of hyperenhanced regions [54,55]. This technique (DE-MRI) provides high spatial resolution imaging of acute and chronic myocardial infarctions with a near exact correlation with histopathology-evidenced size of infarcted and viable myocardium [54–56]. With standard imaging parameters, DE-MRI is capable of detecting infarcts involving as little as one thousandth of total LV myocardial mass [57] that are undetectable by techniques that assess myocardial perfusion or contractile function [56,58].

Delayed-enhancement MRI

Technical considerations

The procedure for viability assessment using DE-MRI is relatively simple (Fig. 2). It can be performed in a single brief examination, requires only a peripheral intravenous catheter, and does not require pharmacologic or physiologic stress. After obtaining scout images to delineate the short- and long-axis views of the heart, cine images are acquired to provide a matched assessment of LV morphology and contractile function with the viability characterization from DE-MRI. Short-axis views (eg, 6-mm slice thickness with 4-mm gap to match delayed contrast-enhanced images) are taken every 10 mm from mitral valve insertion to the LV apex, along with two to three long-axis views to encompass the entire LV. The patient is then given a bolus of 0.10 to 0.20 mmol/kg intravenous gadolinium.

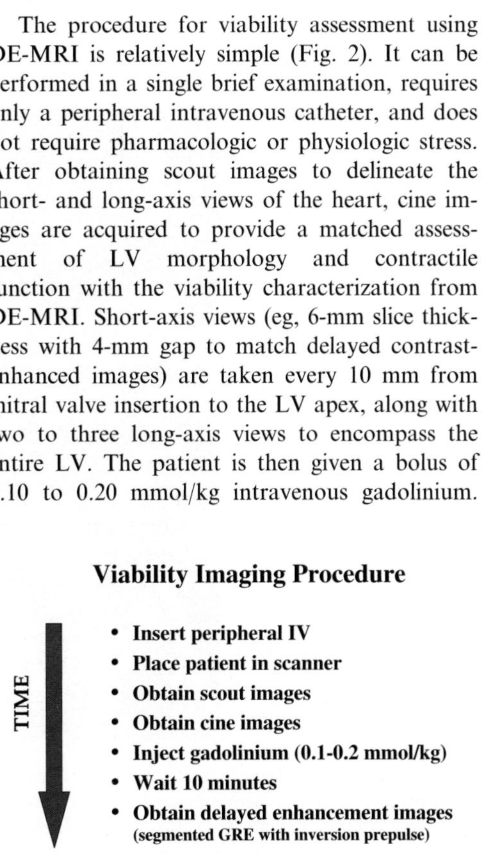

Viability Imaging Procedure

TIME

- **Insert peripheral IV**
- **Place patient in scanner**
- **Obtain scout images**
- **Obtain cine images**
- **Inject gadolinium (0.1-0.2 mmol/kg)**
- **Wait 10 minutes**
- **Obtain delayed enhancement images** **(segmented GRE with inversion prepulse)**

Fig. 2. Overall sequence of events for performing infarction/viability imaging. IV, intravenous.

After a 10- to 15-minute delay to allow the contrast media to distribute, delayed enhancement images of the heart are obtained at the same slice locations as the cine images using a segmented inversion-recovery gradient echo sequence [55]. Each delayed enhancement image is acquired during an 8- to 10-second breath hold, and the imaging time for the entire examination is generally 30 to 40 minutes. Fig. 3 demonstrates cine and DE-MRI images from a typical patient scan.

Physiologic basis

Although the cellular mechanisms for myocardial hyperenhancement have not been fully elucidated, the physiologic processes responsible for this phenomenon are believed to relate to myocyte cellular alterations that produce an increase in local gadolinium concentration within areas of infarcted myocardium. Fig. 4 illustrates this hypothesized mechanism, showing that in the acute and chronic settings, hyperenhancement is believed to directly result from an absence of viable myocytes. Resultant increases in gadolinium extracellular volume of distribution produce T1 shortening, which manifests as hyperenhancement on DE-MRI.

Experimental data support the concept that hyperenhancement results from myocardial tissue changes as a consequence of cellular necrosis. Animal studies have demonstrated that local concentrations of gadolinium-based contrast agents are increased in areas of acute myocardial infarction (AMI) [59,60]. Whole-body data suggest that in normal myocardial regions, gadolinium is excluded from the myocyte intracellular space by intact sarcolemmal membranes [61,62]. In the setting of acute cell death, sarcolemmal membrane integrity is disrupted, thereby providing a mechanism for extravasation of gadolinium and resultant hyperenhancement. Loss of sarcolemmal membrane integrity is thought to be closely related to cell death [63–65], and the thought that an event specific to cell death is related to hyperenhancement explains the near exact relationship of hyperenhancement to myocyte necrosis (Fig. 5).

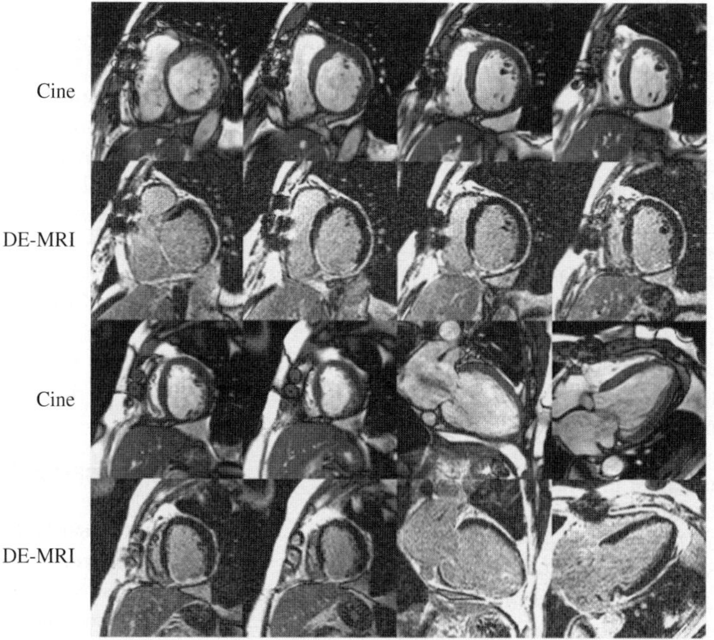

Fig. 3. Images from a typical patient scan. Cine and delayed-enhancement images are acquired at six to eight short-axis locations and at two to three long-axis locations during repeated breath holds. Images are interpreted with the cine images (cine-MRI) immediately adjacent to the delayed-enhancement images (DE-MRI). In this patient example, DE-MRI demonstrates a myocardial infarction involving the inferior wall and inferoseptum of the left ventricle. (*From* Kim RJ, Shah DJ, Judd RM. How we perform delayed enhancement imaging. J Cardiovasc Magn Reson 2003;5:506; with permission.)

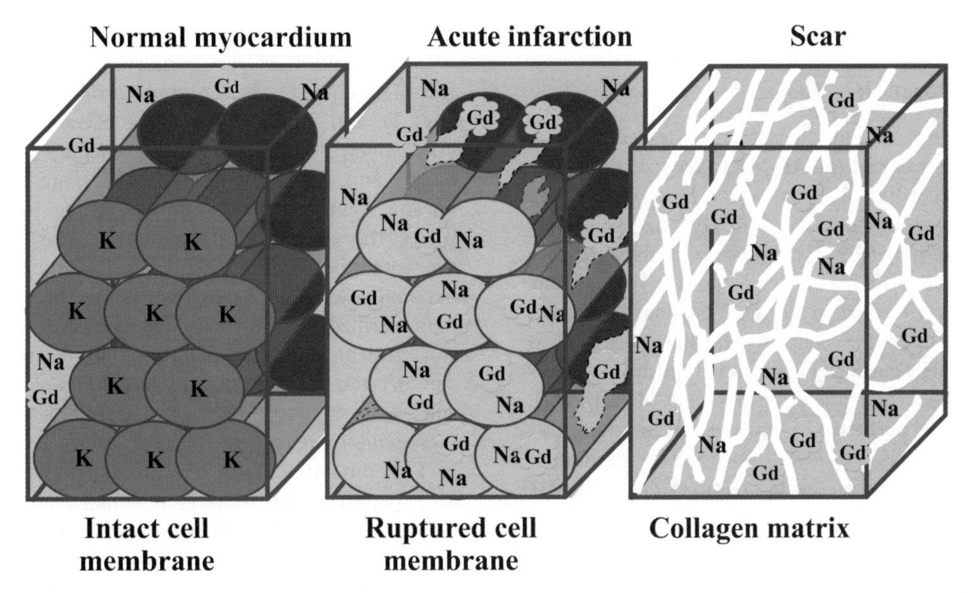

Fig. 4. Potential mechanisms of hyperenhancement. In the acute and chronic infarct settings, hyperenhancement is hypothesized to directly result from consequences of myocyte cell death, with associated increase in extracellular volume of distribution for gadolinium-based contrast agents.

In the chronic setting, myocardial scar is characterized by relative increases in extracellular collagen content [66,67]. On a cellular level, the interstitial space between collagen fibers may be greater than the space between densely packed living myocytes that is characteristic of viable myocardium. This space would be expected to produce an increase in concentration of gadolinium in scar versus normal myocardium due to the expanded volume of distribution. Histopathology data support this proposed mechanism. In analysis of a heart explanted shortly after MRI, Moon and colleagues [68] demonstrated that myocardial areas that hyperenhanced on DE-MRI exhibited increased collagen content on histopathology, with a linear relationship between the degree of collagen content and the percentage of hyperenhanced pixels.

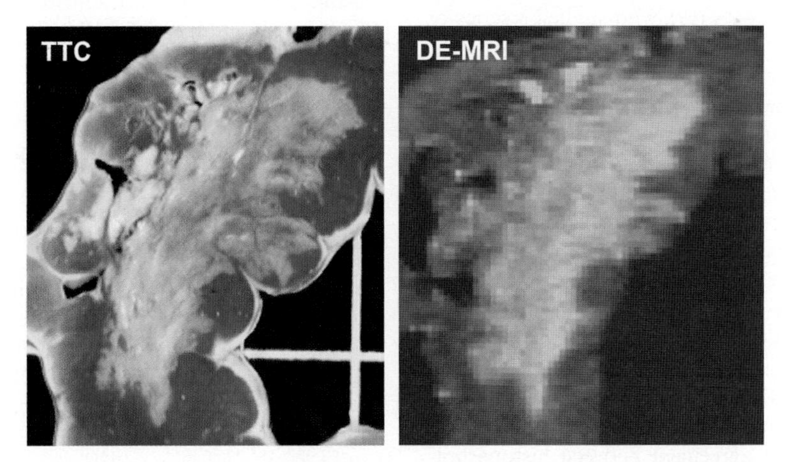

Fig. 5. Comparison of high-resolution ex vivo DE-MRI (*right*) with acute myocyte necrosis defined by histopathology (*left*). Note that the size and shape of the infarcted region (*yellowish-white region*) defined histologically by TTC stain is nearly exactly matched by the size and shape of the hyperenhanced (*bright*) region of DE-MRI. (*Adapted from* Kim RJ, Fieno DS, Parrish TB, et al. Relationship of MRI delayed contrast enhancement to irreversible injury, infarct age, and contractile function. Circulation 1999;100:1996; with permission.)

Delayed-enhancement MRI validation: correlation between delayed-enhancement MRI and histopathology findings

Multiple studies have demonstrated that hyperenhancement on DE-MRI is a specific marker of myocardial necrosis, which closely correlates histopathology-evidenced infarct size and morphology [54,56,69–71]. These concepts were demonstrated by Kim and colleagues [54] in a study of dogs subjected to transient coronary occlusion (to produce transient myocardial ischemia) or permanent coronary ligation (to produce irreversible myocardial injury). In vivo cine-MRI and DE-MRI were performed at various time points (1 day, 3 days, 8 weeks) following coronary manipulation. Animals were then sacrificed and ex vivo DE-MRI was performed before histopathology analysis using TTC staining for determination of infarct size. In animals subjected to coronary ligation, there was a near exact correlation between DE-MRI and histopathology-evidenced infarct size in the acute ($r = 0.99$, $P < .001$) and chronic ($r = 0.97$, $P < .001$) infarct settings. DE-MRI also provided accurate assessment of infarct morphology, closely replicating histopathology-evidenced infarct shape and contours. Conversely, in animals subjected to transient coronary occlusion, affected coronary territories did not demonstrate hyperenhancement or histopathology-evidenced infarct despite transient impairment in myocardial contractility.

Further demonstration of the accuracy of DE-MRI for distinguishing between infarcted and reversibly injured myocardium was provided by Fieno and colleagues [69], who studied a series of dogs subjected to coronary occlusion with or without reperfusion. In animals that had reperfused infarcts, coronary reocclusion was performed before sacrifice, and fluorescent microparticles were then injected into the heart to identify areas of jeopardized but viable myocardium at risk of infarction. In vivo DE-MRI was performed at serial time points (1 day to 8 weeks) before animal sacrifice with ex vivo DE-MRI and subsequent histopathology analysis (TTC stain) performed for quantification of infarcted and viable myocardium. Consistent with prior studies, in vivo and ex vivo DE-MRI provided near identical findings for quantification of infarct size ($r = 0.99$), with near exact agreement between histopathology-evidenced and DE-MRI–evidenced infarct size (lowest $r = 0.95$, largest bias 1.7% of total LV area). Findings from this study also demonstrated that areas of "at-risk" myocardium do not demonstrate hyperenhancement. Fig. 6 provides illustration of this concept: corresponding DE-MRI (row 1), TTC stained gross pathology (row 2), and fluorescent imaging of radiolabeled microspheres (row 3) are shown on the left panels and light microscopy images are shown on the right panels. As shown in the top left panel, the region of myocardium "at risk but not infarcted" (zone 2) does not demonstrate hyperenhancement. Light microscopy of this region verified that normal myocyte architecture was present. Findings from this study strongly support the concept that hyperenhancement results from myocyte necrosis and is not present in regions of reversible ischemic injury.

Experimental clinical and animal studies have also demonstrated that hyperenhancement on DE-MRI is highly reproducible if postcontrast inversion time is appropriately adjusted following gadolinium administration. Using a canine infarct model in which DE-MRI was performed before ex vivo histopathology determination of infarct size, Amado and colleagues [71] demonstrated a close correlation between histopathology and DE-MRI findings ($r^2 = 0.94$, $P < .001$). Adjustment of inversion time on DE-MRI provided accurate assessment of infarct size throughout 30 minutes of postcontrast imaging, without significant difference in mean infarct size between DE-MR images obtained at 6 minutes (15.2 $\pm$ 2.9%) and at 30 minutes (14.5 $\pm$ 4.2%). These findings have also been replicated in the clinical setting, with studies of patients in the acute and chronic infarct settings demonstrating that with adjustment of postcontrast inversion time, DE-MRI provides highly reproducible measurements of infarct size [72,73].

Delayed-enhancement MRI validation: prediction of functional response to therapy

Transmural extent of infarction (TEI), as evident on DE-MRI, has been shown to be a powerful predictor of contractile response to revascularization and medical therapy. The following sections review the data that have established the predictive utility of DE-MRI in the context of acute and chronic myocardial contractile dysfunction.

Acute ischemic heart disease

In the context of AMI, prompt restoration of coronary blood flow has been shown to result in

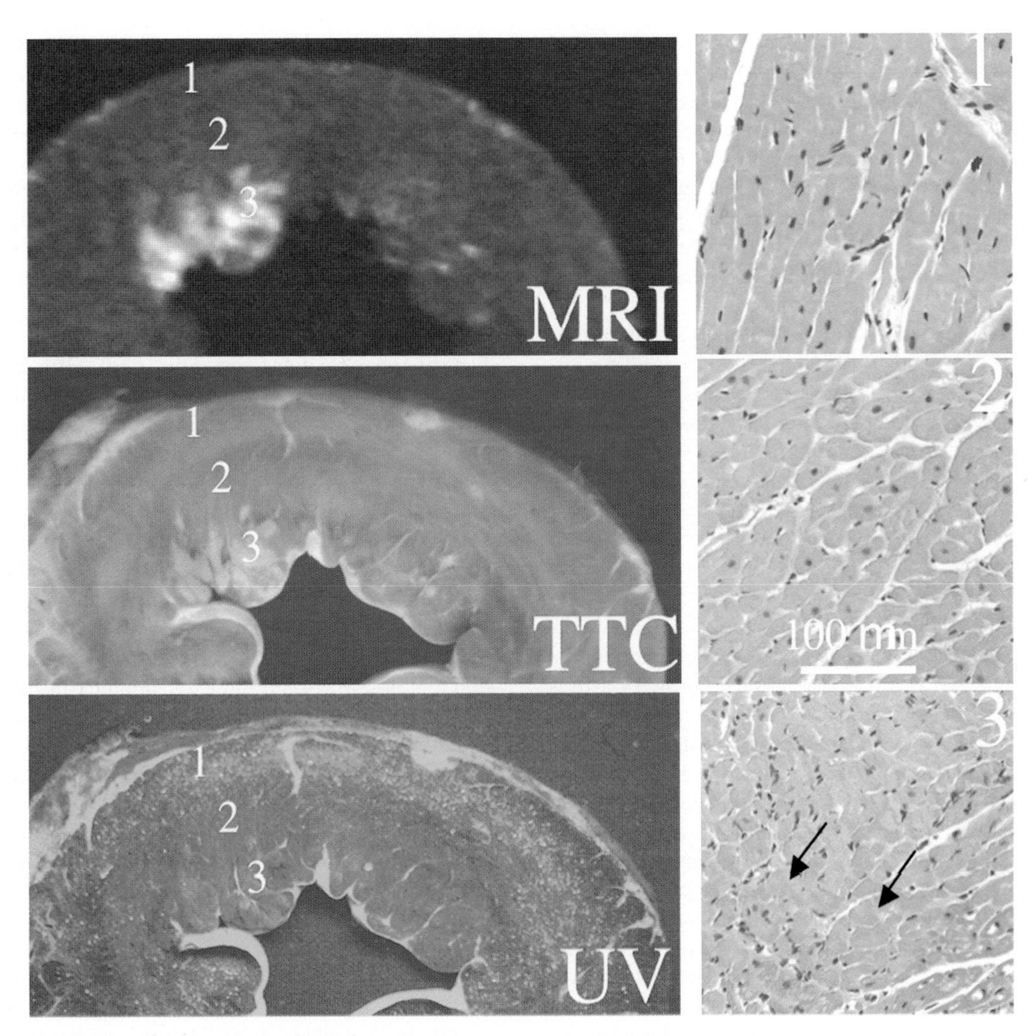

Fig. 6. Comparison of MRI hyperenhancement (*upper left*), TTC staining (*middle left*), and the myocardium at risk (region without fluorescent microparticles; *lower left*) in an animal with a 1-day-old reperfused infarction. Light microscopy views of region 1 (not at risk, not infarcted; *upper right*), region 2 (at risk but not infarcted; *middle right*), and region 3 (infarcted; *lower right*) are shown. Arrows point to contraction bands. See text for details. (*Adapted from* Fieno DS, Kim RJ, Chen EL, et al. Contrast-enhanced magnetic resonance imaging of myocardium at risk: distinction between reversible and irreversible injury throughout infarct healing. J Am Coll Cardiol 2000;36:1989; with permission from the American College of Cardiology Foundation.)

salvage of viable myocardium, improvement in LV ejection fraction (LVEF), and long-term improvement in survival [74–78]. Even after successful coronary reperfusion has been restored, myocardial dysfunction may persist and it is important to distinguish whether it is due to myocardial necrosis or stunning. Differentiation between these conditions is important because patients who have substantial viable but stunned myocardium would be expected to have marked functional and clinical improvement with restoration of coronary blood flow to affected myocardial territories.

DE-MRI has been shown to predict functional improvement after reperfused AMI. This concept was demonstrated by Choi and colleagues [79] in a study of consecutive patients who presented with their first myocardial infarction and were successfully revascularized. All patients underwent cine-MRI and DE-MRI within 7 days of their infarction, with cine-MRI repeated 8 to 12 weeks following myocardial infarction. TEI, as measured by DE-MRI, was highly predictive of improvement in wall motion following infarction ($P < .001$). When quantified on a segmental basis, 77% (213/275) of segments without infarction showed improvement, whereas 5% (3/64) of segments with 75% to 100% TEI showed improvement. In addition to predicting segmental functional recovery, DE-MRI predicted improvement in global function: the presence of dysfunctional but viable myocardium (<25% TEI) was directly related to change in mean wall-thickening score ($r = 0.87$, $P < .0001$) and ejection fraction ($r = 0.65$, $P = .002$). Other studies of DE-MRI in the acute infarct setting have provided similar findings, providing confirmatory evidence that TEI DE-MRI predicts functional improvement following AMI [80,81].

Chronic ischemic heart disease

DE-MRI–evidenced TEI has been shown to predict response to myocardial revascularization in patients who have established coronary artery disease. This concept was demonstrated by Kim and colleagues [82], who performed cine and DE-MRI in consecutive patients who had LV dysfunction prior to surgical or percutaneous revascularization. Similar to findings in the acute setting, likelihood of functional improvement was inversely related in a progressive stepwise fashion to TEI. Among all dysfunctional segments, the proportion of segments with improved contractility decreased as TEI increased ($P < .001$). When volume of dysfunctional but viable myocardium was calculated on a per-patient basis, this parameter predicted the magnitude of improvement in LV function following revascularization, as measured by mean wall motion score and ejection fraction ($P < .001$ for both). Similarly, in a patient cohort that had more severe LV dysfunction (mean LVEF, 28 ± 10%), Schvartzman and colleagues [83] demonstrated an inverse relationship ($P < .002$) between TEI and postrevascularization functional recovery.

These data demonstrate that there is a progressive relationship between the likelihood of contractile response to revascularization and the TEI, as evidenced by DE-MRI. Thus, use of a single cutoff value on which to base predictions of functional improvement would not have a physiologic basis and would be suboptimal. The ability to grade myocardial viability as a continuum rather than in a binary fashion is one of the greatest strengths of DE-MRI. For example, according to the data of Kim and colleagues [82], if a cutoff value of 25% hyperenhancement is chosen, then the positive and negative predictive accuracy rates for functional improvement would be 71% and 79%, respectively. Although these predictive accuracy rates compare favorably with those reported using other imaging modalities [84], the full diagnostic information portrayed by DE-MRI is not used through the use of a single arbitrary cutoff value. Consider the situation in which a region has greater than 75% hyperenhancement. The data from Kim and colleagues [82] demonstrate that 57 of 58 such segments did not improve—a negative predictive value of 98%. Thus, in this example, rather than assuming that the negative predictive value of DE-MRI remains at 79% (using a dichotomous cutoff of 25% hyperenhancement), approaching viability as a continuum allows the negative predictive value to be raised to 98%. This example highlights an important advantage of DE-MRI over other imaging modalities used to assess viability. Myocardial regions are not interpreted in a binary fashion as viable or nonviable; rather, the transmural extent of viable and infarcted myocardium is directly visualized. Knowledge of infarct transmurality can then be used to predict functional improvement more accurately, as in the preceding example, and can also be used to understand the underlying physiology of functional response to coronary revascularization.

Chronic heart failure

DE-MRI–evidenced TEI has been shown to predict response to medical therapy in patients who have contractile dysfunction. This concept was demonstrated by Bello and colleagues [85] in a study in which MRI was performed in patients who had chronic systolic heart failure (mean LVEF, 26 ± 11%) before and 6 months after initiation of β-blocker maintenance therapy. Similar to findings in patients undergoing coronary revascularization, an inverse relationship was found between baseline TEI and likelihood of functional improvement after β-blocker therapy. Contractility improved in 56% (674/1207) of segments with no hyperenhancement but in only 3% (8/232) of segments with more than 75% hyperenhancement. On a per-patient basis, the percentage of LV myocardium that was dysfunctional but viable was directly related to improvement in ejection fraction ($r = 0.57$, $P = .0003$) and mean wall motion score ($r = 0.70$, $P < .001$). This DE-MRI parameter was also directly related to improvement in LV reverse remodeling, as measured by a decrease in end diastolic volume index (r = 0.45, P = .007) and end systolic volume index (r = 0.64, P = .007).

Overview of validative data

The data presented in the preceding sections strongly support the following statements:

- In the setting of acute and chronic infarction, hyperenhancement is exclusively associated with myocyte necrosis.
- Regions within myocardial "areas at risk" but outside of "areas of infarction" do not exhibit hyperenhancement.
- Regions subjected to severe but reversible ischemic injury do not hyperenhance, even in the presence of myocardial stunning.
- In patients who have ischemic heart disease undergoing revascularization procedures and in those who have chronic heart failure being treated with β-blocker therapy, transmural extent of hyperenhancement can predict those regions that are most likely (minimal hyperenhancement) or least likely (predominant hyperenhancement) to improve in function.
- The extent of dysfunctional but nonhyperenhanced myocardium can predict on a case-by-case basis those patients who are most likely to experience an improvement in LVEF.

Comparison of delayed-enhancement MRI to other viability techniques

DE-MRI offers an alternative means of viability assessment to several noninvasive imaging techniques have been used for this purpose. These include dobutamine stress with cine-MRI, dobutamine stress echocardiography (DSE), radionuclide imaging by way of positron emission tomography (PET) or single-photon emission CT (SPECT), and CT. Unlike modalities such as dobutamine or radionuclide imaging that can assess for presence or absence of viable myocardium, DE-MRI concomitantly detects infarcted and normal myocardium within a given myocardial segment and thereby allows extent of viability to be assessed as a continuum based on TEI. When only viable myocardium can be visualized, the percentage of viability in a given segment is assessed indirectly and generally refers to the amount of viable myocardium in the segment normalized to the segment with the maximum amount of viable myocardium. Conversely, when viable and infarcted myocardium are visualized, the "percentage of viability" can be assessed directly and expressed as the amount of viability in the segment normalized to the amount of viability plus infarction in the same segment. This difference can alter clinical interpretations [86], as is illustrated in Fig. 7. In this example, MRI images were obtained in a patient who had chronic coronary artery disease and an akinetic anterior wall. Although the anterior wall was thinned, only a small subendocardial portion of the anterior wall was infarcted. In this case, indirect visualization would show that the anterior wall is only 39% viable (compared with the remote region), whereas direct visualization would show that the anterior wall infarction is 70% viable. Based on this assessment, the indirect method would predict no recovery of wall motion, whereas the direct method would predict recovery. The postrevascularization images (see Fig. 7, bottom right panel) illustrate the predictive accuracy of the direct method.

DE-MRI provides other advantages for infarct characterization beyond direct assessment size of infarcted and viable myocardium. For example, the presence of regions of microvascular obstruction ("no reflow zones") within hyperenhanced areas is an important parameter that has been shown to predict impaired LV remodeling and adverse clinical prognosis following acute infarct setting. In a study of patients who had AMI, Gerber and colleagues [87] found that DE-MRI–evidenced microvascular obstruction predicted impairment in functional recovery, as assessed at 7 months following AMI. Similarly, in a study of patients who underwent MRI following AMI (mean 6.1 ± 2.2 days), Hombach and colleagues [88] demonstrated that DE-MRI–evidenced microvascular obstruction, infarct size, and TEI each predicted subsequent adverse LV remodeling, as defined by a greater than 20% increase in LV end-diastolic volume on follow-up MRI (mean 225 ± 92 days post AMI). During clinical follow-up, presence of microvascular obstruction (P = .04), increased LV end-diastolic volume (P = .04), and impaired LVEF ($P < .01$) were each found to be independent predictors of adverse clinical events, as defined by death, myocardial infarction, heart failure–related hospitalization, or follow-up coronary revascularization (total model $P < .01$).

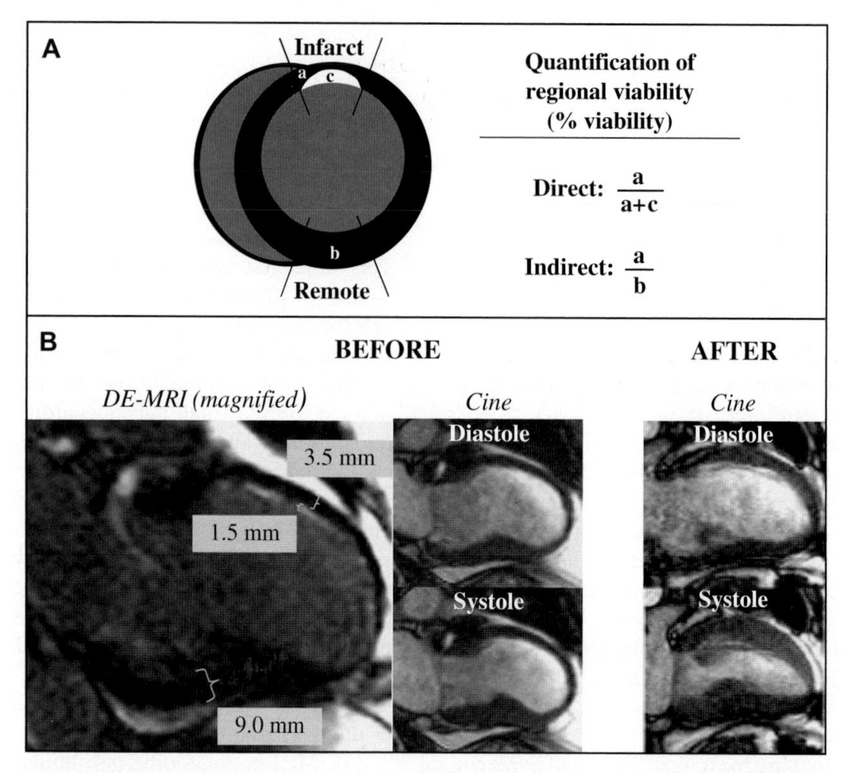

Fig. 7. (*A*) Cartoon illustrating the differences between a direct and an indirect method of quantifying regional viability. Viable myocardium is displayed in black; infarcted myocardium is displayed in white. (*B*) Long-axis MRI views of a patient before and 2 months after revascularization. Although the akinetic anterior wall is "thinned" (diastolic wall thickness = 5 mm; remote zone = 9 mm), DE-MRI demonstrates that there is only a subendocardial infarction (1.5 mm thick). A direct assessment of viability would show that the anterior wall is predominantly viable (3.5 mm/5 mm = 70% viable), whereas an indirect assessment would show that the anterior wall is predominantly nonviable (3.5 mm/9 mm = 39% viable). CineMR images obtained following coronary revascularization demonstrate full recovery of wall motion and diastolic wall thickness. Full-motion movies can be viewed at http://dcmrc.duhs.duke.edu/NF10. (*Modified from* Kim RJ, Shah DJ. Fundamental concepts in myocardial viability assessment revisited: when knowing how much is "alive" is not enough. Heart 2004;90:139; with permission).

The following sections provide an overview of studies that have compared DE-MRI to other noninvasive imaging modalities for assessment of myocardial viability.

Dobutamine stress imaging

Dobutamine infusion has been used to determine myocardial viability based on inotropic response of hypocontractile segments. Echocardiography has traditionally been used for assessment of contractile response to dobutamine. In a meta-analysis including over 400 patients, low-dose DSE had a positive predictive accuracy of 83% and a negative predictive accuracy of 81% for predicting recovery of contractile function following coronary revascularization [84]. DSE has been found to provide improved specificity but decreased sensitivity for functional response to revascularization in comparison to thallium SPECT [89–91].

DE-MRI has been directly compared with DSE. In a series of patients who had postinfarction LV dysfunction in whom both tests were performed within a 2-week interval, Nelson and colleagues [92] found that there was an inverse relationship between TEI by DE-MRI and contractile reserve by DSE ($P < .001$). In this study, however, presence of complete viability by DE-MRI did not preclude absence of contractile reserve by DSE. Although few regions with transmural or nearly transmural infarction by DE-MRI had contractile reserve by

DSE (8/68, 12%), half (76/152, 50%) of all segments that were fully (100%) viable by DE-MRI had absence of contractile reserve. Although the underlying mechanism for absence of contractile reserve in regions of viable myocardium remains undetermined, possible explanations for this phenomenon include tethering of viable regions to areas of scar, myocyte cellular adaptations that impair dobutamine response, and absence of coronary flow reserve in chronically hypoperfused regions of viable but dysfunctional myocardium.

Myocardial contractile reserve can also be assessed if dobutamine is administered during acquisition of cine-MRI images. Steady-state free precession imaging sequences are conventionally used for this purpose. This approach provides potential advantages over DSE because steady-state free precession provides excellent endocardial border definition [93] and superior reproducibility in comparison to echocardiography [94]. The utility of dobutamine stress MRI for viability assessment was recently studied by Wellnhoffer and colleagues [44], who compared the technique to DE-MRI in 29 patients who had ischemic cardiomyopathy and were undergoing coronary revascularization. Based on receiver operating curve (ROC) characteristics, the investigators concluded that dobutamine cine-MRI was superior to DE-MRI for prediction of postrevascularization functional recovery. In their report, however, the investigators employed a flawed method for ROC curve analysis [95]. In addition, DE-MRI viability was graded as a dichotomous variable, thereby discounting one of the greatest strengths of DE-MRI: the ability to assess viability as a continuum in relation to transmural extent of infarction.

Positron emission tomography

Cardiac PET uses radiotracer uptake patterns to identify viable myocardium based on evidence of preserved metabolic function. DE-MRI has been compared with PET in several studies. Klein and colleagues [96] studied patients who had ischemic cardiomyopathy (LVEF 28 $\pm$ 9%) and underwent DE-MRI and PET within a 1-week interval. Nonviable tissue (infarct) was defined by PET as a region with matched reduction in blood flow (N-13 ammonia) and metabolism (F-18 fludeoxyglucose). There was correlation between the two tests for visual ($r = 0.91$, $P < .0001$) and quantitative ($r = 0.81$, $P < .0001$) assessment of infarct size. In another study of patients who had advanced ischemic cardiomyopathy (LVEF 31 $\pm$ 11%), Kuhl and colleagues [97] found an inverse correlation between TEI by DE-MRI and segmental glucose uptake by PET ($r = -0.86$, $P < .001$). In both of these studies, however, DE-MRI detected more infarcts than PET. Klein and colleagues [96] reported that more than half (55%) of subendocardial infarcts detected by DE-MRI were classified as normal by PET, whereas Kuhl and colleagues [97] reported that DE-MRI detected subendocardial infarcts in 36% of segments classified as normal by PET.

Single-photon emission CT

SPECT imaging identifies viable and infarcted myocardium based on regional differences in radiotracer uptake, with segments classified as viable as a consequence of preserved mitochondrial function (sestamibi SPECT) or preserved membrane integrity (thallium SPECT). Prior studies comparing DE-MRI to SPECT have reported that DE-MRI provides improved sensitivity and specificity for infarct detection. This may relate to differences in spatial resolution, which is approximately 60-fold greater for DE-MRI compared with SPECT. The expected improvement in infarct detection for DE-MRI versus SPECT was demonstrated by Wagner and colleagues [56], who performed both imaging tests in a canine infarct model. Animals were sacrificed following DE-MRI and SPECT, with histopathology used as a "gold standard" measure for extent of viable and infarcted myocardium. Level of agreement between DE-MRI and SPECT varied according to TEI. Among segments in which the histologically demonstrated infarct size was greater than 75% of wall thickness, all showed evidence of infarction by both DE-MRI and by SPECT. Conversely, among segments identified by histopathology as having a subendocardial infarction (<50% wall thickness), DE-MRI detected infarction in 92%, whereas SPECT demonstrated infarction in only 28%. Fig. 8 provides representative examples of three animals that had subendocardial infarcts detected by DE-MRI and histology but not by SPECT.

Wagner and colleagues [56] also compared DE-MRI with SPECT in patients who had coronary artery disease (n = 109). Both techniques were performed within a narrow interval (10 $\pm$ 17 days), and interpretation was performed blinded to the results of the other modality. Similar to animal data in this study, patient data

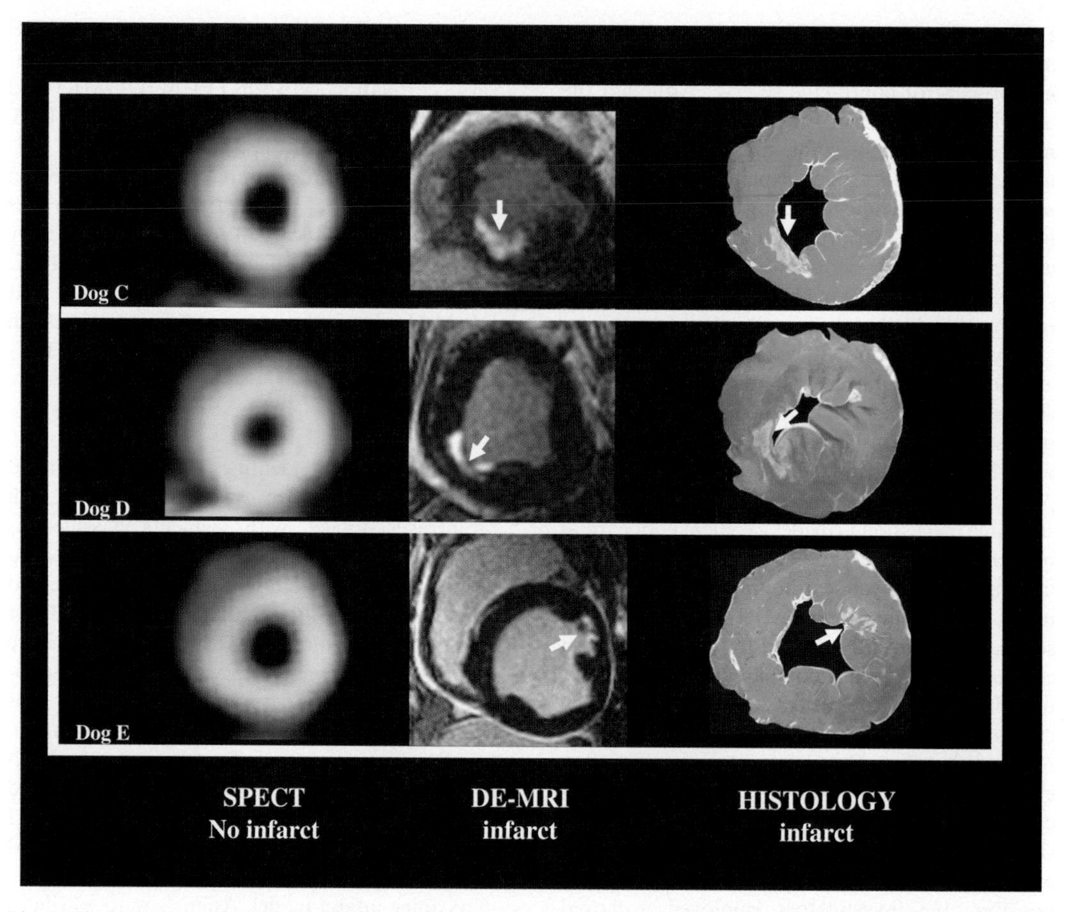

Fig. 8. Short-axis views from three dogs that had subendocardial infarctions. Note that unlike SPECT images, DE-MRI readily demonstrates the infarcted regions (*arrowheads*). (*Adapted from* Wagner A, Mahrholdt H, Holly TA, et al. Contrast-enhanced MRI and routine single photon emission computed tomography (SPECT) perfusion imaging for detection of subendocardial myocardial infarcts: an imaging study. Lancet 2003;361:376; with permission.)

demonstrated that SPECT detection of DE-MRI–evidenced infarcts varied according to transmural extent. Among segments with near transmural hyperenhancement (involving >75% wall thickness), all showed evidence of infarct by SPECT. Among segments with subendocardial hyperenhancement (involving ≤50% wall thickness), SPECT detected infarct in only 53%. Based on these results, the investigators concluded that DE-MRI and SPECT detect transmural infarcts at similar rates, whereas DE-MRI systematically detects subendocardial infarcts that are missed by SPECT.

Other studies have provided confirmatory evidence that DE-MRI identifies myocardial infarctions that are undetected by SPECT. In a study of patients who had equivocal SPECT findings, Lee and colleagues [98] performed DE-MRI in 20 patients who had fixed defects but preserved wall motion on stress–rest sestamibi SPECT. DE-MRI confirmed infarction in 10 of 41 (24%) equivocal segments in 8 patients (40%). An additional 29 segments in 8 patients (40%) had DE-MRI–evidenced infarctions that were not detected by SPECT. All infarctions undetected by SPECT except 1 were nontransmural on DE-MRI.

DE-MRI has also been shown to provide improved prediction of response to revascularization compared with SPECT. This concept was demonstrated by Kitagawa and colleagues [99], who performed DE-MRI and thallium 201 SPECT imaging in patients following myocardial infarction. Cine-MRI was performed following the initial DE-MRI scan (mean 67 ± 17 days) for assessment of functional recovery. Although viability assessment by MRI and by SPECT was significantly correlated with improvement in regional wall thickening, the sensitivity, specificity, and accuracy of DE-MRI was superior to SPECT (98% versus 90%, $P < .01$; 75% versus 54%, $P < .05$; 92% versus 81%, $P < .001$, respectively).

Computed tomography

CT can assess myocardial viability based on relative tissue contrast concentrations on delayed postcontrast imaging. Similar to DE-MRI, CT provides high spatial resolution imaging and concomitantly identifies infarcted and viable myocardium based on localized differences in contrast pharmacokinetics. Unlike DE-MRI, however, postcontrast CT images are not acquired though the use of an inversion pulse that serves to increase differential signal intensity between viable and infarcted myocardium. Consistent with this, prior studies directly comparing DE-MRI to postcontrast CT have reported that DE-MRI provides approximately a threefold to fivefold greater difference in image intensity between infarcted and viable myocardium [100,101]. In addition, unlike CT, MRI does not involve exposure to ionizing radiation or potentially nephrotoxic iodinated contrast dye. Such exposures may present prohibitive risks for patients who have advanced vascular disease for whom coronary revascularization procedures are being considered.

In studies using animal infarct models, several investigators have reported close correlations between postcontrast CT and DE-MRI, as well as, histopathology-evidenced (TTC) evidenced infarct size. In a study using canine and porcine models imaged 90 minutes or 8 weeks following myocardial infarction, Lardo and colleagues [102] found that postcontrast CT–evidenced infarct volume was closely matched by pathology findings in acute (mean difference 0.7% LV volume) and chronic (mean difference 0.8% LV volume) infarct settings. Similarly, in a study in which postcontrast CT and DE-MRI were performed in the acute infarct setting, Baks and colleagues [100] demonstrated that postcontrast CT ($r^2 = 0.96$, $P < .001$) and DE-MRI ($r^2 = 0.93$, $P < .001$) closely correlated with histopathology-evidenced infarct size. Mean image intensity of infarcted to viable myocardium, however, was 2.9-fold greater for DE-MRI compared with DE-CT.

Although few clinical studies have directly compared DE-MRI to postcontrast CT, available data suggest that the techniques closely agree with regard to measurement of overall infarct size but may occasionally differ with regard to infarct transmurality. In a study of 28 patients who had reperfused myocardial infarctions, Mahnken and colleagues [101] performed DE-MRI and postcontrast CT within a 5-day interval. Mean infarct size (measured per short-axis LV slice) closely agreed between postcontrast CT (33.3 ± 23.8%) and DE-MRI (31.2 ± 22.5%); however, there was disagreement with regard to TEI. Eighty-two percent of all segments with subendocardial infarctions based on DE-MRI were classified as having subendocardial infarctions based on postcontrast CT, with CT not demonstrating any infarct in 13% of these segments. Conversely, only 71% of all segments with transmural infarcts based on DE-MRI were classified as having transmural infarcts based on postcontrast CT. The utility of postcontrast CT–evidenced TEI as a predictor of response to coronary revascularization has not been reported.

Emerging applications of delayed-enhancement MRI

With its high spatial resolution and ability to directly image infarcted and viable myocardium, DE-MRI provides novel information that can be applied to a broad variety of clinical scenarios beyond that of viability assessment as related to potential coronary revascularization. The following sections provide an overview of emerging data concerning the utility of DE-MRI for two important clinical applications: diagnostic assessment of cardiomyopathies and arrhythmic risk stratification.

Delayed-enhancement MRI for cardiomyopathy assessment

The ability of DE-MRI to noninvasively assess myocardial substrate in patients who have cardiomyopathies provides potential advantages over traditional diagnostic techniques. For example, although coronary angiography has traditionally been used to distinguish between ischemic and nonischemic cardiomyopathies [103], presence or absence of coronary obstruction may not necessarily correspond to tissue changes within the myocardium. Autopsy studies of patients who had idiopathic dilated cardiomyopathy have demonstrated gross pathology–evidenced myocardial infarctions in 12% to 14% of patients despite absence of epicardial coronary artery disease [104,105]. Even endomyocardial biopsy, which has been considered a diagnostic gold standard, can be limited for cardiomyopthy assessment because the technique may be compromised by sampling error [106].

The utility of DE-MRI for diagnostic assessment of cardiomyopathies is predicated on the concept that the presence and the pattern of scar can be used to discriminate between myopathic processes. The typical pattern of hyperenhancement that occurs in patients who have myocardial infarction and, thus, ischemic cardiomyopathy can be explained by the pathophysiology of myocardial ischemia. Following approximately 15 minutes of coronary occlusion, a wave front of myocardial necrosis begins in the subendocardium and progresses transmurally with increasing duration of occlusion. Therefore, hyperenhancement can be classified as "ischemic" or "nonischemic" type, and the former should always involve the subendocardium (ie, subendocardial or transmural) and be located in a region that is consistent with the perfusion territory of an epicardial coronary artery. Using this approach, McCrohon and colleagues [107] reported that 13% of patients who had idiopathic dilated cardiomyopathy had ischemic-type hyperenhancement, whereas 28% had nonischemic type. Similarly, Bello and colleagues [85] reported that 12% of patients who had dilated cardiomyopathy had ischemic-type hyperenhancement.

Hyperenhancement pattern has been shown to provide diagnostic utility for distinguishing between ischemic and nonischemic cardiomyopathies. An evaluation of this approach was recently provided by Patel and colleagues [108] in patients who had advanced systolic dysfunction and who underwent coronary angiography within 6 months of MRI. A nonischemic DE-MRI scar pattern was diagnosed as midmyocardial or epicardial hyperenhancement, whereas an ischemic DE-MRI scar pattern was diagnosed as subendocardial or transmural hyperenhancement in a typical coronary anatomic distribution. Although the simple presence of scar was sensitive (94%) for the diagnosis of ischemic cardiomyopathy, specificity was relatively poor (60%). When ischemic- or nonischemic-type scar pattern was considered in as an adjunctive diagnostic criteria, sensitivity remained high (92%), whereas specificity was improved (93%) ($P < .0001$).

Although classification of cardiomyopathies as ischemic or nonischemic is an important means of dichotomizing patients who have systolic dysfunction, prior studies have found that disease-specific differences in etiology of myocardial dysfunction alter prognosis and therapy [109,110]. Among patients who have nonischemic cardiomyopathies, therapeutic options include corticosteroids for treatment of cardiac sarcoid or myocarditis, alkyloids in the setting of cardiac amyloid, α-galactosidase enzyme replacement therapy in the setting of Anderson-Fabry's disease, and septal ablation or myomectomy in the setting of hypertrophic cardiomyopathy (HCM). DE-MRI–evidenced hyperenhancement can occur in all of these conditions, having been reported in inflammatory conditions such as myocarditis [111,112], infiltrative cardiomyopathies such as sarcoid [113–115], systemic processes such as amyloid [116] or Chagas' disease [117], and genetic abnormalities such as HCM [118,119] or Anderson-Fabry's disease [120–122]. Each of these conditions results in myocardial dysfunction as a result of diverse pathologic processes and has associated differences in hyperenhancement patterns. For example, in the setting of LV hypertrophy, the presence of midwall hyperenhancement at the junctions of the interventricular septum and the right ventricular free wall is a compelling argument for the diagnosis of HCM [7], whereas midwall or epicardial hyperenhancement in the inferolateral wall suggests Anderson-Fabry's disease [122]. Fig. 9 provides representative examples of hyperenhancement patterns, along with a differential diagnosis of associated disease processes.

In addition to diagnostic applications, presence of myocardial scar on DE-MRI holds the potential to be used as a marker of disease severity. This concept has been studied in patients who have HCM, a condition associated with myocardial scarring and an increased risk of arrhythmic events [123,124]. Necropsy studies performed in patients who have HCM have reported associations between scar or fibrosis size and indices of disease severity [123,125] and sudden death risk [126]. Studies using DE-MRI for assessment of scar have also reported a relationship between hyperenhancement burden and disease severity. Among a cohort of patients who had HCM, Moon and colleagues reported a greater extent of hyperenhancement (15.7% versus 8.6% of LV mass, $P = .02$) among patients who had more than two sudden death risk factors (defined by unexplained syncope, ventricular tachycardia,

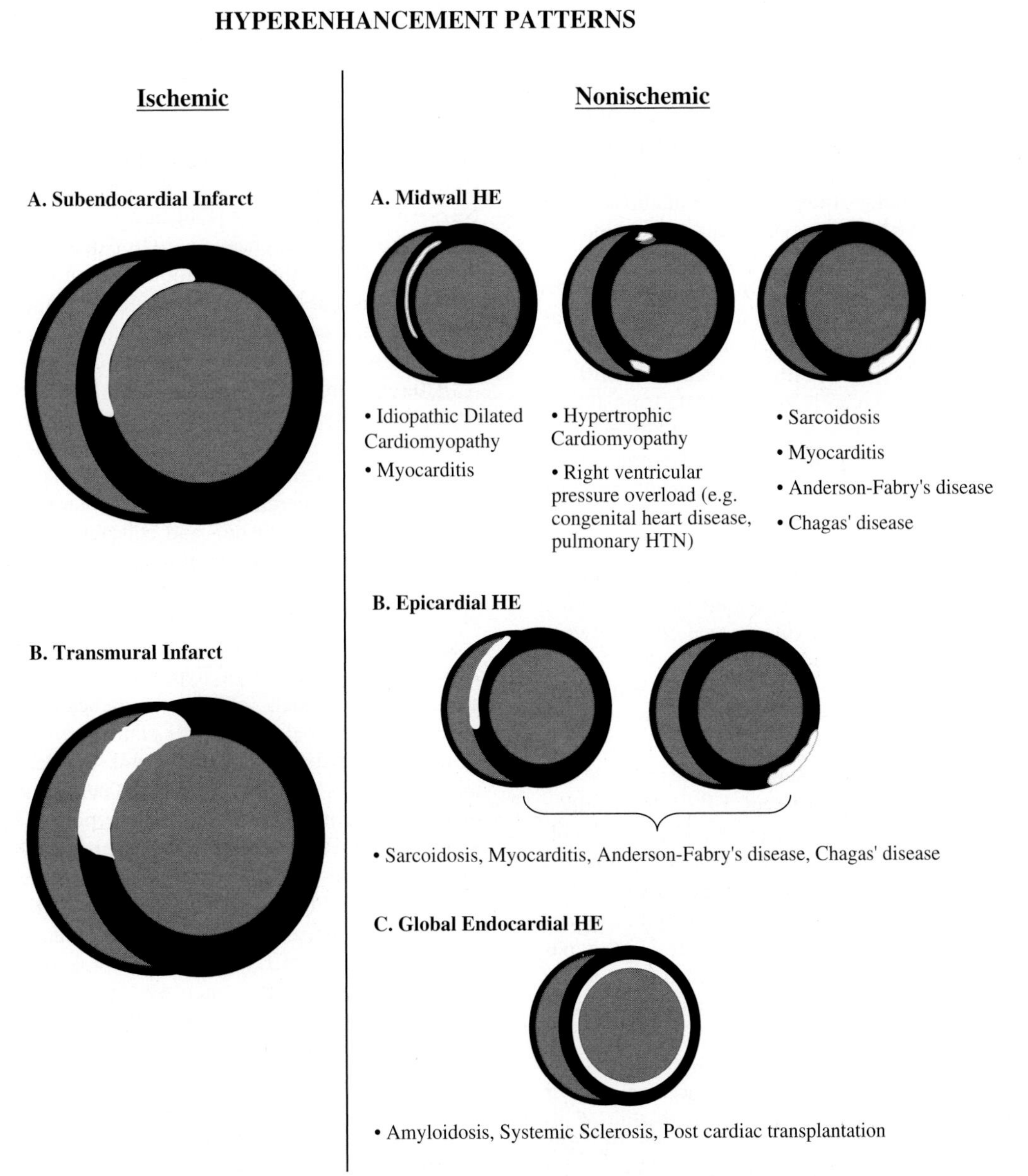

HYPERENHANCEMENT PATTERNS

Ischemic

A. Subendocardial Infarct

B. Transmural Infarct

Nonischemic

A. Midwall HE

- Idiopathic Dilated Cardiomyopathy
- Myocarditis

- Hypertrophic Cardiomyopathy
- Right ventricular pressure overload (e.g. congenital heart disease, pulmonary HTN)

- Sarcoidosis
- Myocarditis
- Anderson-Fabry's disease
- Chagas' disease

B. Epicardial HE

- Sarcoidosis, Myocarditis, Anderson-Fabry's disease, Chagas' disease

C. Global Endocardial HE

- Amyloidosis, Systemic Sclerosis, Post cardiac transplantation

Fig. 9. Representations of hyperenhancement patterns that are characteristic for ischemic and nonischemic disorders. Because myocardial necrosis due to coronary artery disease progresses as a "wave front" from the endocardium to the epicardium, when hyperenhancement is present (*white regions*), the endocardium should be involved in patients who have ischemic heart disease. Isolated midwall or epicardial hyperenhancement strongly suggests a nonischemic etiology. HE, hyperenhancement; HTN, hypertension. (*From* Shah DJ, Judd RM, Kim RJ, et al. Magnetic resonance of myocardial viability. In: Edelman RR, Hesselink JR, Zlatkin MI, editors. Clinical Magnetic Resonance Imaging (3rd ed.). New York, NY: Elsevier; 2005.)

abnormal hemodynamic response to exercise, family history of sudden death, or LV wall thickness ≥ 30 mm). These findings are in agreement with those reported by Mahrholdt and colleagues [127], who found a progressive stepwise relationship between hyperenhancement size and clinical risk factors for sudden death ($P < .001$ for trend) among patients who had HCM.

Delayed-enhancement MRI for arrhythmic risk stratification

Myocardial scar forms a substrate for ventricular tachyarrhythmias [12–14], with a relationship between scar morphology and arrhythmic risk demonstrated in experimental and epidemiologic studies. Imaging studies using modalities other than DE-MRI have reported an association between scar size and arrhythmic risk. For example, SPECT-evidenced infarct size has been shown to be associated with risk of inducible ventricular tachycardia during electrophysiology study (EPS) [128,129] and death and recurrent ventricular tachyarrhythmias [130–132]. Data from animal studies indicate that scar size [13,133] and scar morphology [133] influence arrhythmic risk. DE-MRI–evidenced hyperenhancement provides highly accurate assessment of scar size and morphology [54,69–71], with improved scar detection in comparison to other modalities such as SPECT [56]. Thus, DE-MRI provides an important noninvasive tool for studying associations between scar characteristics and arrhythmic risk.

The relationship between hyperenhancement and arrhythmogenic potential is supported by findings from several investigations. In a study of patients who had established coronary artery disease and who underwent EPS-based sudden cardiac death risk stratification, Bello and colleagues [134] found that size (mass 49 ± 5 g versus 28 ± 5 g, $P < .005$) and surface area (172 ± 15 cm^2 versus 93 ± 14 cm^2, $P < .0005$) of hyperenhanced myocardium was greater among patients who had inducible sustained ventricular tachycardia compared with patients who were noninducible. In this study, logistic regression and ROC analysis demonstrated that risk stratification on the basis of hyperenhancement size or surface area provided improved prediction of inducible ventricular tachycardia versus ejection fraction alone. The relationship between hyperenhancement and arrhythmogenic substrate has also been reported in patients who have nonischemic cardiomyopathy. Klem and colleagues [135] performed DE-MRI before EPS in a heterogeneous population of patients, 52% of whom had no evidence of coronary artery disease. Patients who had inducible ventricular tachycardia had larger mean size of hyperenhanced myocardium ($P < .05$) than noninducible patients, with ROC analysis demonstrating hyperenhancement size to be a better predictor of inducibility than ejection fraction ($P<.01$). Absence of hyperenhancement identified a low-risk group as characterized by the fact that none of the patients who did not have hyperenhancement (31% of study population) manifested inducible ventricular tachycardia during EPS. Studies have also reported that infarct morphology influences arrhythmogenic substrate. This concept was demonstrated by Nazarian and colleagues [136] in a study of patients who had nonischemic cardiomyopathy undergoing EPS. In this population, predominance of nontransmural hyperenhancement predicted inducible ventricular tachycardia ($P = .02$), even after adjustment for LVEF.

Although investigations have yet to directly study the utility of DE-MRI for arrhythmic risk stratification in unselected patient populations, existing data in at-risk cohorts support a relationship between hyperenhancement and mortality risk. In a study by Kwong and colleagues [137], DE-MRI was performed in 195 patients without clinical history of myocardial infarction. Presence of hyperenhancement was associated with increased cardiac mortality risk (hazard ratio 10.9, $P < .0001$). Inclusion of hyperenhancement in multivariable models provided significant improvement to models comprising clinical variables alone for prediction of mortality risk (model χ^2 improved from 5.97 to 23.78, $P < .0001$). These findings are consistent with results reported by Kim and colleagues [19], who performed DE-MRI in a series of consecutive patients who did not have clinical history of myocardial infarction. In this study, presence of hyperenhancement involving over 15% of LV myocardium was associated with subsequent increase in all-cause mortality (hazard ratio 6.55, $P = .02$).

Data also suggest that hyperenhancement pattern influences clinical event risk. In a study of patients who had established coronary artery disease and DE-MRI–evidenced myocardial infarction, Yan and colleagues [138] found that the presence of extensive peri-infarct regions of intermediate hyperenhancement (defined by hyperenhancement with signal intensity 2 to 3 SD above normal) conferred increased mortality risk. Patients who had above-median volumes of peri-infarct regions were at highest risk for subsequent death (28% versus 13%, $P < .01$). Even after adjustment for LVEF and patient age, relative volume of peri-infarct regions was independently associated with all-cause mortality (adjusted hazard ratio 1.42 per 10% increase, $P = .005$) and cardiovascular mortality (adjusted hazard ratio 1.49, $P = .01$). Although Yan and colleagues

[138] studied a particularly high-risk cohort (20% mortality during 2.4-year median follow-up), findings from this study provide further evidence of a relationship between hyperenhancement and event risk and support the need for additional study of the utility of DE-MRI for arrhythmic risk stratification in a broad at-risk population. This hypothesis is currently under investigation by several groups and is likely to become an important focus of research.

Summary

MRI is capable of assessing myocardial viability through several different methods. These methods include assessment of myocardial function, morphology, and tissue characteristics. Through the technique of DE-MRI, presence or absence of hyperenhancement distinguishes infarcted from viable myocardium in a manner that highly correlates with histopathology findings. DE-MRI provides high-resolution imaging capable of identifying myocardial infarcts that are undetected by viability imaging techniques such as SPECT, PET, and echocardiography. By concomitantly imaging infarcted and viable myocardium, DE-MRI assesses viability as a continuum based on transmural thickness of hyperenhancement, a parameter that has been shown to predict contractile response to revascularization and medical therapy in patients who have LV systolic dysfunction. Presence and pattern of hyperenhancement has been shown to have diagnostic utility in identifying etiology of LV systolic dysfunction and assessing disease severity in nonischemic myopathic processes such as HCM. Emerging data suggest that presence of hyperenhancement can be used to assess arrhythmogenic potential and mortality risk among patients who have ischemic and nonischemic cardiomyopathies.

References

[1] Arnese M, Cornel JH, Salustri A, et al. Prediction of improvement of regional left ventricular function after surgical revascularization. A comparison of low-dose dobutamine echocardiography with 201Tl single-photon emission computed tomography. Circulation 1995;91:2748–52.

[2] Ragosta M, Beller GA, Watson DD, et al. Quantitative planar rest-redistribution 201Tl imaging in detection of myocardial viability and prediction of improvement in left ventricular function after coronary bypass surgery in patients with severely depressed left ventricular function. Circulation 1993;87:1630–41.

[3] Dilsizian V, Rocco TP, Freedman NM, et al. Enhanced detection of ischemic but viable myocardium by the reinjection of thallium after stress-redistribution imaging. N Engl J Med 1990;323:141–6.

[4] Tillisch J, Brunken R, Marshall R, et al. Reversibility of cardiac wall-motion abnormalities predicted by positron tomography. N Engl J Med 1986;314:884–8.

[5] Braunwald E, Rutherford JD. Reversible ischemic left ventricular dysfunction: evidence for the "hibernating myocardium." J Am Coll Cardiol 1986;8:1467–70.

[6] Rahimtoola SH. A perspective on the three large multicenter randomized clinical trials of coronary bypass surgery for chronic stable angina. Circulation 1985;72:V123–35.

[7] Chaudhry FA, Tauke JT, Alessandrini RS, et al. Prognostic implications of myocardial contractile reserve in patients with coronary artery disease and left ventricular dysfunction. J Am Coll Cardiol 1999;34:730–8.

[8] Di Carli MF, Maddahi J, Rokhsar S, et al. Long-term survival of patients with coronary artery disease and left ventricular dysfunction: implications for the role of myocardial viability assessment in management decisions. J Thorac Cardiovasc Surg 1998;116:997–1004.

[9] Haas F, Haehnel CJ, Picker W, et al. Preoperative positron emission tomographic viability assessment and perioperative and postoperative risk in patients with advanced ischemic heart disease. J Am Coll Cardiol 1997;30:1693–700.

[10] Pagley PR, Beller GA, Watson DD, et al. Improved outcome after coronary bypass surgery in patients with ischemic cardiomyopathy and residual myocardial viability. Circulation 1997;96:793–800.

[11] Allman KC, Shaw LJ, Hachamovitch R, et al. Myocardial viability testing and impact of revascularization on prognosis in patients with coronary artery disease and left ventricular dysfunction: a meta-analysis. J Am Coll Cardiol 2002;39:1151–8.

[12] Wetstein L, Mark R, Kaplinsky E, et al. Histopathologic factors conducive to experimental ventricular tachycardia. Surgery 1985;98:532–9.

[13] Wilber DJ, Lynch JJ, Montgomery D, et al. Postinfarction sudden death: significance of inducible ventricular tachycardia and infarct size in a conscious canine model. Am Heart J 1985;109:8–18.

[14] Josephson ME, Zimetbaum P, Huang D, et al. Pathophysiologic substrate for sustained ventricular tachycardia in coronary artery disease. Jpn Circ J 1997;61:459–66.

[15] Bolli R. Myocardial 'stunning' in man. Circulation 1992;86:1671–91.

[16] Vanoverschelde JL, Wijns W, Depre C, et al. Mechanisms of chronic regional postischemic dysfunction in humans. New insights from the study of noninfarcted collateral-dependent myocardium. Circulation 1993;87:1513–23.
[17] Buxton DB. Dysfunction in collateral-dependent myocardium. Hibernation or repetitive stunning? Circulation 1993;87:1756–8.
[18] Kaul S. Assessing the myocardium after attempted reperfusion: should we bother? Circulation 1998; 98:625–7.
[19] Kim HW, Wu E, Meyers SN, et al. Prognostic-significance of unrecognized myocardial infarction detected by contrast MRI. Circulation 2002; 106(supplement 2):389.
[20] Moon JC, De Arenaza DP, Elkington AG, et al. The pathologic basis of Q-wave and non-Q-wave myocardial infarction: a cardiovascular magnetic resonance study. J Am Coll Cardiol 2004;44:554–60.
[21] Fishbein MC, Meerbaum S, Rit J, et al. Early phase acute myocardial infarct size quantification: validation of the triphenyl tetrazolium chloride tissue enzyme staining technique. Am Heart J 1981;101: 593–600.
[22] Dakik HA, Howell JF, Lawrie GM, et al. Assessment of myocardial viability with 99mTc-sestamibi tomography before coronary bypass graft surgery: correlation with histopathology and postoperative improvement in cardiac function. Circulation 1997;96:2892–8.
[23] Haas F, Augustin N, Holper K, et al. Time course and extent of improvement of dysfunctioning myocardium in patients with coronary artery disease and severely depressed left ventricular function after revascularization: correlation with positron emission tomographic findings. J Am Coll Cardiol 2000;36:1927–34.
[24] Pohost GM. Is 31P-NMR spectroscopic imaging a viable approach to assess myocardial viability? Circulation 1995;92:9–10.
[25] Rehr RB, Tatum JL, Hirsch JI, et al. Reperfused-viable and reperfused-infarcted myocardium: differentiation with in vivo P-31 MR spectroscopy. Radiology 1989;172:53–8.
[26] Rehr RB, Fuhs BE, Lee F, et al. Differentiation of reperfused-viable (stunned) from reperfused-infarcted myocardium at 1 to 3 days postreperfusion by in vivo phosphorus-31 nuclear magnetic resonance spectroscopy. Am Heart J 1991;122:1571–82.
[27] Wroblewski LC, Aisen AM, Swanson SD, et al. Evaluation of myocardial viability following ischemic and reperfusion injury using phosphorus 31 nuclear magnetic resonance spectroscopy in vivo. Am Heart J 1990;120:31–9.
[28] Yabe T, Mitsunami K, Inubushi T, et al. Quantitative measurements of cardiac phosphorus metabolites in coronary artery disease by 31P magnetic resonance spectroscopy. Circulation 1995;92: 15–23.
[29] Bottomley PA, Weiss RG. Non-invasive magnetic-resonance detection of creatine depletion in non-viable infarcted myocardium. Lancet 1998;351: 714–8.
[30] Cannon PJ, Maudsley AA, Hilal SK, et al. Sodium nuclear magnetic resonance imaging of myocardial tissue of dogs after coronary artery occlusion and reperfusion. J Am Coll Cardiol 1986;7:573–9.
[31] Kim RJ, Lima JA, Chen EL, et al. Fast 23Na magnetic resonance imaging of acute reperfused myocardial infarction. Potential to assess myocardial viability. Circulation 1997;95:1877–85.
[32] Kim RJ, Judd RM, Chen EL, et al. Relationship of elevated 23Na magnetic resonance image intensity to infarct size after acute reperfused myocardial infarction. Circulation 1999;100:185–92.
[33] Hillenbrand HB, Becker LC, Kharrazian R, et al. 23Na MRI combined with contrast-enhanced 1H MRI provides in vivo characterization of infarct healing. Magn Reson Med 2005;53:843–50.
[34] Fieno DS, Kim RJ, Rehwald WG, et al. Physiological basis for potassium (39K) magnetic resonance imaging of the heart. Circ Res 1999;84:913–20.
[35] Kim RJ, Hillenbrand HB, Judd RM. Evaluation of myocardial viability by MRI. Herz 2000;25: 417–30.
[36] Been M, Smith MA, Ridgway JP, et al. Serial changes in the T1 magnetic relaxation parameter after myocardial infarction in man. Br Heart J 1988;59:1–8.
[37] Johnston DL, Homma S, Liu P, et al. Serial changes in nuclear magnetic resonance relaxation times after myocardial infarction in the rabbit: relationship to water content, severity of ischemia, and histopathology over a six-month period. Magn Reson Med 1988;8:363–79.
[38] Higgins CB, Herfkens R, Lipton MJ, et al. Nuclear magnetic resonance imaging of acute myocardial infarction in dogs: alterations in magnetic relaxation times. Am J Cardiol 1983;52:184–8.
[39] Baer FM, Theissen P, Schneider CA, et al. Dobutamine magnetic resonance imaging predicts contractile recovery of chronically dysfunctional myocardium after successful revascularization. J Am Coll Cardiol 1998;31:1040–8.
[40] Cwajg JM, Cwajg E, Nagueh SF, et al. End-diastolic wall thickness as a predictor of recovery of function in myocardial hibernation: relation to rest-redistribution Tl-201 tomography and dobutamine stress echocardiography. J Am Coll Cardiol 2000;35:1152–61.
[41] Haendchen RV, Corday E, Torres M, et al. Increased regional end-diastolic wall thickness early after reperfusion: a sign of irreversibly damaged myocardium. J Am Coll Cardiol 1984;3:1444–53.
[42] Perrone-Filardi P, Bacharach SL, Dilsizian V, et al. Metabolic evidence of viable myocardium in regions with reduced wall thickness and absent wall thickening in patients with chronic ischemic left

ventricular dysfunction. J Am Coll Cardiol 1992; 20:161–8.

[43] James O, Kim HW, Weinsaft J, et al. Demonstration and prediction of the potential reversible nature of thinned myocardium by CMR. J Cardiovasc Magn Reson 2005;7(1):69.

[44] Wellnhoffer E, Olariu A, Klein C, et al. Magnetic resonance low-dose dobutamine test is superior to SCAR quantification for the prediction of functional recovery. Circulation 2004;109:2172–4.

[45] Dendale PA, Franken PR, Waldman GJ, et al. Low-dosage dobutamine magnetic resonance imaging as an alternative to echocardiography in the detection of viable myocardium after acute infarction. Am Heart J 1995;130:134–40.

[46] Gunning MG, Anagnostopoulos C, Knight CJ, et al. Comparison of 201Tl, 99mTc-tetrofosmin, and dobutamine magnetic resonance imaging for identifying hibernating myocardium. Circulation 1998;98:1869–74.

[47] Sandstede JJ, Bertsch G, Beer M, et al. Detection of myocardial viability by low-dose dobutamine Cine MR imaging. Magn Reson Imaging 1999;17: 1437–43.

[48] Sansoy V, Glover DK, Watson DD, et al. Comparison of thallium-201 resting redistribution with technetium-99m-sestamibi uptake and functional response to dobutamine for assessment of myocardial viability. Circulation 1995;92:994–1004.

[49] Rehr RB, Peshock RM, Malloy CR, et al. Improved in vivo magnetic resonance imaging of acute myocardial infarction after intravenous paramagnetic contrast agent administration. Am J Cardiol 1986;57:864–8.

[50] McNamara MT, Tscholakoff D, Revel D, et al. Differentiation of reversible and irreversible myocardial injury by MR imaging with and without gadolinium-DTPA. Radiology 1986;158:765–9.

[51] Eichstaedt HW, Felix R, Dougherty FC, et al. Magnetic resonance imaging (MRI) in different stages of myocardial infarction using the contrast agent gadolinium-DTPA. Clin Cardiol 1986;9: 527–35.

[52] Baer FM, Theissen P, Schneider CA, et al. Magnetic resonance tomography imaging techniques for diagnosing myocardial vitality [German]. Herz 1994;19:51–64.

[53] Saeed M, Wendland MF, Takehara Y, et al. Reperfusion and irreversible myocardial injury: identification with a nonionic MR imaging contrast medium. Radiology 1992;182:675–83.

[54] Kim RJ, Fieno DS, Parrish TB, et al. Relationship of MRI delayed contrast enhancement to irreversible injury, infarct age, and contractile function. Circulation 1999;100:1992–2002.

[55] Simonetti OP, Kim RJ, Fieno DS, et al. An improved MR imaging technique for the visualization of myocardial infarction. Radiology 2001;218: 215–23.

[56] Wagner A, Mahrholdt H, Holly TA, et al. Contrast-enhanced MRI and routine single photon emission computed tomography (SPECT) perfusion imaging for detection of subendocardial myocardial infarcts: an imaging study. Lancet 2003;361: 374–9.

[57] Wu E, Judd RM, Vargas JD, et al. Visualisation of presence, location, and transmural extent of healed Q-wave and non-Q-wave myocardial infarction. Lancet 2001;357:21–8.

[58] Ricciardi MJ, Wu E, Davidson CJ, et al. Visualization of discrete microinfarction after percutaneous coronary intervention associated with mild creatine kinase-MB elevation. Circulation 2001;103:2780–3.

[59] Schaefer S, Malloy CR, Katz J, et al. Gadolinium-DTPA-enhanced nuclear magnetic resonance imaging of reperfused myocardium: identification of the myocardial bed at risk. J Am Coll Cardiol 1988;12:1064–72.

[60] Rehwald WG, Fieno DS, Chen EL, et al. Myocardial magnetic resonance imaging contrast agent concentrations after reversible and irreversible ischemic injury. Circulation 2002;105:224–9.

[61] Weinmann HJ, Brasch RC, Press WR, et al. Characteristics of gadolinium-DTPA complex: a potential NMR contrast agent. AJR Am J Roentgenol 1984;142:619–24.

[62] Koenig SH, Spiller M, Brown RD 3rd, et al. Relaxation of water protons in the intra- and extracellular regions of blood containing Gd(DTPA). Magn Reson Med 1986;3:791–5.

[63] Reimer KA, Jennings RB. Myocardial ischemia, hypoxia and infarction. In: Fozzard HA, Haber E, Jennings RB, et al, editors. The heart and cardiovascular system. New York: Raven Press; 1992. p. 1875–973.

[64] Jennings RB, Schaper J, Hill ML, et al. Effect of reperfusion late in the phase of reversible ischemic injury. Changes in cell volume, electrolytes, metabolites, and ultrastructure. Circ Res 1985;56:262–78.

[65] Whalen DA Jr, Hamilton DG, Ganote CE, et al. Effect of a transient period of ischemia on myocardial cells. I. Effects on cell volume regulation. Am J Pathol 1974;74:381–97.

[66] McCormick RJ, Musch TI, Bergman BC, et al. Regional differences in LV collagen accumulation and mature cross-linking after myocardial infarction in rats. Am J Physiol 1994;266:H354–9.

[67] Jugdutt BI, Joljart MJ, Khan MI. Rate of collagen deposition during healing and ventricular remodeling after myocardial infarction in rat and dog models. Circulation 1996;94:94–101.

[68] Moon JC, Reed E, Sheppard MN, et al. The histologic basis of late gadolinium enhancement cardiovascular magnetic resonance in hypertrophic cardiomyopathy. J Am Coll Cardiol 2004;43: 2260–4.

[69] Fieno DS, Kim RJ, Chen EL, et al. Contrast-enhanced magnetic resonance imaging of

myocardium at risk: distinction between reversible and irreversible injury throughout infarct healing. J Am Coll Cardiol 2000;36:1985–91.
[70] Barkhausen J, Ebert W, Debatin JF, et al. Imaging of myocardial infarction: comparison of magnevist and gadophrin-3 in rabbits. J Am Coll Cardiol 2002;39:1392–8.
[71] Amado LC, Gerber BL, Gupta SN, et al. Accurate and objective infarct sizing by contrast-enhanced magnetic resonance imaging in a canine myocardial infarction model. J Am Coll Cardiol 2004;44: 2383–9.
[72] Mahrholdt H, Wagner A, Holly TA, et al. Reproducibility of chronic infarct size measurement by contrast-enhanced magnetic resonance imaging. Circulation 2002;106:2322–7.
[73] Wagner A, Mahrholdt H, Thomson L, et al. Effects of time, dose, and inversion time for acute myocardial infarct size measurements based on magnetic resonance imaging-delayed contrast enhancement. J Am Coll Cardiol 2006;47:2027–33.
[74] Christian TF, Gibbons RJ, Gersh BJ. Effect of infarct location on myocardial salvage assessed by technetium-99m isonitrile. J Am Coll Cardiol 1991;17:1303–8.
[75] Gruppo Italiano per lo Studio della Streptochinasi nell'Infarto Miocardico (GISSI). Effectiveness of intravenous thrombolytic treatment in acute myocardial infarction. Lancet 1986;1: 397–402.
[76] ISIS-2 (Second International Study of Infarct Survival) Collaborative Group. Randomized trial of intravenous streptokinase, oral aspirin, both, or neither among 17,187 cases of suspected acute myocardial infarction: ISIS-2. J Am Coll Cardiol 1988; 12:3A–13A.
[77] Grines CL, Browne KF, Marco J, et al. A comparison of immediate angioplasty with thrombolytic therapy for acute myocardial infarction. The Primary Angioplasty in Myocardial Infarction Study Group. N Engl J Med 1993;328:673–9.
[78] Zijlstra F, de Boer MJ, Hoorntje JC, et al. A comparison of immediate coronary angioplasty with intravenous streptokinase in acute myocardial infarction. N Engl J Med 1993;328:680–4.
[79] Choi KM, Kim RJ, Gubernikoff G, et al. Transmural extent of acute myocardial infarction predicts long-term improvement in contractile function. Circulation 2001;104:1101–7.
[80] Tarantini G, Razzolini R, Cacciavillani L, et al. Influence of transmurality, infarct size, and severe microvascular obstruction on left ventricular remodeling and function after primary coronary angioplasty. Am J Cardiol 2006;98:1033–40.
[81] Beek AM, Kuhl HP, Bondarenko O, et al. Delayed contrast-enhanced magnetic resonance imaging for the prediction of regional functional improvement after acute myocardial infarction. J Am Coll Cardiol 2003;42:895–901.
[82] Kim RJ, Wu E, Rafael A, et al. The use of contrast-enhanced magnetic resonance imaging to identify reversible myocardial dysfunction. N Engl J Med 2000;343:1445–53.
[83] Schvartzman PR, Srichai MB, Grimm RA, et al. Nonstress delayed-enhancement magnetic resonance imaging of the myocardium predicts improvement of function after revascularization for chronic ischemic heart disease with left ventricular dysfunction. Am Heart J 2003;146:535–41.
[84] Bonow RO. Identification of viable myocardium. Circulation 1996;94:2674–80.
[85] Bello D, Shah DJ, Farah GM, et al. Gadolinium cardiovascular magnetic resonance predicts reversible myocardial dysfunction and remodeling in patients with heart failure undergoing beta-blocker therapy. Circulation 2003;108:1945–53.
[86] Kim RJ, Shah DJ. Fundamental concepts in myocardial viability assessment revisited: when knowing how much is "alive" is not enough. Heart 2004;90:137–40.
[87] Gerber BL, Garot J, Bluemke DA, et al. Accuracy of contrast-enhanced magnetic resonance imaging in predicting improvement of regional myocardial function in patients after acute myocardial infarction. Circulation 2002;106:1083–9.
[88] Hombach V, Grebe O, Merkle N, et al. Sequelae of acute myocardial infarction regarding cardiac structure and function and their prognostic significance as assessed by magnetic resonance imaging. Eur Heart J 2005;26:549–57.
[89] Vanoverschelde JL, D'Hondt AM, Marwick T, et al. Head-to-head comparison of exercise-redistribution-reinjection thallium single-photon emission computed tomography and low dose dobutamine echocardiography for prediction of reversibility of chronic left ventricular ischemic dysfunction. J Am Coll Cardiol 1996;28:432–42.
[90] Perrone-Filardi P, Pace L, Prastaro M, et al. Assessment of myocardial viability in patients with chronic coronary artery disease. Rest-4-hour-24-hour 201Tl tomography versus dobutamine echocardiography. Circulation 1996;94:2712–9.
[91] Bax JJ, Wijns W, Cornel JH, et al. Accuracy of currently available techniques for prediction of functional recovery after revascularization in patients with left ventricular dysfunction due to chronic coronary artery disease: comparison of pooled data. J Am Coll Cardiol 1997;30:1451–60.
[92] Nelson C, McCrohon J, Khafagi F, et al. Impact of scar thickness on the assessment of viability using dobutamine echocardiography and thallium single-photon emission computed tomography: a comparison with contrast-enhanced magnetic resonance imaging. J Am Coll Cardiol 2004;43: 1248–56.
[93] Thiele H, Nagel E, Paetsch I, et al. Functional cardiac MR imaging with steady-state free precession (SSFP) significantly improves endocardial border

delineation without contrast agents. J Magn Reson Imaging 2001;14:362–7.
[94] Grothues F, Smith GC, Moon JC, et al. Comparison of interstudy reproducibility of cardiovascular magnetic resonance with two-dimensional echocardiography in normal subjects and in patients with heart failure or left ventricular hypertrophy. Am J Cardiol 2002;90:29–34.
[95] Kim RJ, Manning WJ. Viability assessment by delayed enhancement cardiovascular magnetic resonance: will low-dose dobutamine dull the shine? Circulation 2004;109:2476–9.
[96] Klein C, Nekolla SG, Bengel FM, et al. Assessment of myocardial viability with contrast-enhanced magnetic resonance imaging: comparison with positron emission tomography. Circulation 2002;105: 162–7.
[97] Kuhl HP, Beek AM, van der Weerdt AP, et al. Myocardial viability in chronic ischemic heart disease: comparison of contrast-enhanced magnetic resonance imaging with (18)F-fluorodeoxyglucose positron emission tomography. J Am Coll Cardiol 2003;41:1341–8.
[98] Lee VS, Resnick D, Tiu SS, et al. MR imaging evaluation of myocardial viability in the setting of equivocal SPECT results with (99m)Tc sestamibi. Radiology 2004;230:191–7.
[99] Kitagawa K, Sakuma H, Hirano T, et al. Acute myocardial infarction: myocardial viability assessment in patients early thereafter comparison of contrast-enhanced MR imaging with resting (201)Tl SPECT. Single photon emission computed tomography. Radiology 2003;226:138–44.
[100] Baks T, Cademartiri F, Moelker AD, et al. Multislice computed tomography and magnetic resonance imaging for the assessment of reperfused acute myocardial infarction. J Am Coll Cardiol 2006;48:144–52.
[101] Mahnken AH, Koos R, Katoh M, et al. Assessment of myocardial viability in reperfused acute myocardial infarction using 16-slice computed tomography in comparison to magnetic resonance imaging. J Am Coll Cardiol 2005;45:2042–7.
[102] Lardo AC, Cordeiro MA, Silva C, et al. Contrast-enhanced multidetector computed tomography viability imaging after myocardial infarction: characterization of myocyte death, microvascular obstruction, and chronic scar. Circulation 2006;113: 394–404.
[103] Felker GM, Shaw LK, O'Connor CM. A standardized definition of ischemic cardiomyopathy for use in clinical research. J Am Coll Cardiol 2002; 39:210–8.
[104] Uretsky BF, Thygesen K, Armstrong PW, et al. Acute coronary findings at autopsy in heart failure patients with sudden death: results from the Assessment of Treatment with Lisinopril and Survival (ATLAS) trial. Circulation 2000;102:611–6.
[105] Roberts WC, Siegel RJ, McManus BM. Idiopathic dilated cardiomyopathy: analysis of 152 necropsy patients. Am J Cardiol 1987;60:1340–55.
[106] Kubo N, Morimoto S, Hiramitsu S, et al. Feasibility of diagnosing chronic myocarditis by endomyocardial biopsy. Heart Vessels 1997;12:167–70.
[107] McCrohon JA, Moon JC, Prasad SK, et al. Differentiation of heart failure related to dilated cardiomyopathy and coronary artery disease using gadolinium-enhanced cardiovascular magnetic resonance. Circulation 2003;108:54–9.
[108] Patel MR, Heitner JF, Klem I. Presence and pattern of scar on delayed-enhancement MRI differentiates ischemic from non-ischemic cardiomyopathy. Circulation 2004;108(Suppl):755.
[109] Felker GM, Thompson RE, Hare JM, et al. Underlying causes and long-term survival in patients with initially unexplained cardiomyopathy. N Engl J Med 2000;342:1077–84.
[110] Kyle RA, Gertz MA, Greipp PR, et al. A trial of three regimens for primary amyloidosis: colchicine alone, melphalan and prednisone, and melphalan, prednisone, and colchicine. N Engl J Med 1997; 336:1202–7.
[111] Mahrholdt H, Wagner A, Deluigi CC, et al. Presentation, patterns of myocardial damage, and clinical course of viral myocarditis. Circulation 2006;114: 1581–90.
[112] Mahrholdt H, Goedecke C, Wagner A, et al. Cardiovascular magnetic resonance assessment of human myocarditis: a comparison to histology and molecular pathology. Circulation 2004;109:1250–8.
[113] Patel MR, Cawley PJ, Heitner JF, et al. Delayed enhancement MRI improves the ability to detect cardiac involvement in patients with sarcoidosis. Circulation 2004;110:II-645.
[114] Smedema JP, Snoep G, van Kroonenburgh MP, et al. Evaluation of the accuracy of gadolinium-enhanced cardiovascular magnetic resonance in the diagnosis of cardiac sarcoidosis. J Am Coll Cardiol 2005;45:1683–90.
[115] Schulz-Menger J, Wassmuth R, Abdel-Aty H, et al. Patterns of myocardial inflammation and scarring in sarcoidosis as assessed by cardiovascular magnetic resonance. Heart 2006;92:399–400.
[116] Maceira AM, Joshi J, Prasad SK, et al. Cardiovascular magnetic resonance in cardiac amyloidosis. Circulation 2005;111:186–93.
[117] Rochitte CE, Oliveira PF, Andrade JM, et al. Myocardial delayed enhancement by magnetic resonance imaging in patients with Chagas' disease: a marker of disease severity. J Am Coll Cardiol 2005;46:1553–8.
[118] Moon JC, McKenna WJ, McCrohon JA, et al. Toward clinical risk assessment in hypertrophic cardiomyopathy with gadolinium cardiovascular magnetic resonance. J Am Coll Cardiol 2003;41: 1561–7.

[119] Choudhury L, Mahrholdt H, Wagner A, et al. Myocardial scarring in asymptomatic or mildly symptomatic patients with hypertrophic cardiomyopathy. J Am Coll Cardiol 2002;40:2156–64.

[120] Beer M, Weidemann F, Breunig F, et al. Impact of enzyme replacement therapy on cardiac morphology and function and late enhancement in Fabry's cardiomyopathy. Am J Cardiol 2006;97:1515–8.

[121] Weidemann F, Breunig F, Beer M, et al. The variation of morphological and functional cardiac manifestation in Fabry disease: potential implications for the time course of the disease. Eur Heart J 2005;26:1221–7.

[122] Moon JC, Sachdev B, Elkington AG, et al. Gadolinium enhanced cardiovascular magnetic resonance in Anderson-Fabry disease. Evidence for a disease specific abnormality of the myocardial interstitium. Eur Heart J 2003;24:2151–5.

[123] Basso C, Thiene G, Corrado D, et al. Hypertrophic cardiomyopathy and sudden death in the young: pathologic evidence of myocardial ischemia. Hum Pathol 2000;31:988–98.

[124] Maron BJ, Epstein SE, Roberts WC. Hypertrophic cardiomyopathy and transmural myocardial infarction without significant atherosclerosis of the extramural coronary arteries. Am J Cardiol 1979; 43:1086–102.

[125] Varnava AM, Elliott PM, Sharma S, et al. Hypertrophic cardiomyopathy: the interrelation of disarray, fibrosis, and small vessel disease. Heart 2000; 84:476–82.

[126] Tanaka M, Fujiwara H, Onodera T, et al. Quantitative analysis of myocardial fibrosis in normals, hypertensive hearts, and hypertrophic cardiomyopathy. Br Heart J 1986;55:575–81.

[127] Mahrholdt H, Choudhury L, Wagner A, et al. Relation of myocardial scarring to clinical risk factors for sudden cardiac death in hypertrophic cardiomyopathy. Circulation 2002;106:II-652.

[128] Gradel C, Jain D, Batsford WP, et al. Relationship of scar and ischemia to the results of programmed electrophysiological stimulation in patients with coronary artery disease. J Nucl Cardiol 1997;4: 379–86.

[129] Buxton AE, Hafley GE, Lehmann MH, et al. Prediction of sustained ventricular tachycardia inducible by programmed stimulation in patients with coronary artery disease. Utility of clinical variables. Circulation 1999;99:1843–50.

[130] De Sutter J, Tavernier R, Van de Wiele C, et al. Infarct size and recurrence of ventricular arrhythmias after defibrillator implantation. Eur J Nucl Med 2000;27:807–15.

[131] van der Burg A, Bax JJ, Boersma E, et al. Impact of viability, ischemia, scar tissue, and revascularization on outcome after aborted sudden death. Circulation 2003;108:1954–9.

[132] Gioia G, Bagheri B, Gottlieb CD, et al. Prediction of outcome of patients with life-threatening ventricular arrhythmias treated with automatic implantable cardioverter-defibrillators using SPECT perfusion imaging. Circulation 1997;95: 390–4.

[133] Wetstein L, Mark R, Kaplinsky E, et al. Histopathologic correlates of inducible ventricular tachycardia in two experimental canine models of myocardial infarction. Am J Med Sci 1986;291: 222–31.

[134] Bello D, Fieno DS, Kim RJ, et al. Infarct morphology identifies patients with substrate for sustained ventricular tachycardia. J Am Coll Cardiol 2005; 45:1104–8.

[135] Klem I, Weinsaft J, Heitner JF, et al. The utility of contrast enhanced MRI for screening patients at risk for malignant ventricular tachyarrhythmias. J Cardiovasc Magn Reson 2004;6:84.

[136] Nazarian S, Bluemke DA, Lardo AC, et al. Magnetic resonance assessment of the substrate for inducible ventricular tachycardia in nonischemic cardiomyopathy. Circulation 2005;112: 2821–5.

[137] Kwong RY, Chan A, Brown K, et al. Impact of unrecognized myocardial scar detected by cardiac magnetic resonance imaging on event-free survival in patients presenting with signs or symptoms of coronary artery disease. Circulation 2006;113: 2733–43.

[138] Yan AT, Shayne AJ, Brown KA, et al. Characterization of the per-infarct zone by contrast-enhanced magnetic resonance imaging is a powerful predictor of post-myocardial infarction mortality. Circulation 2006;114:32–9.

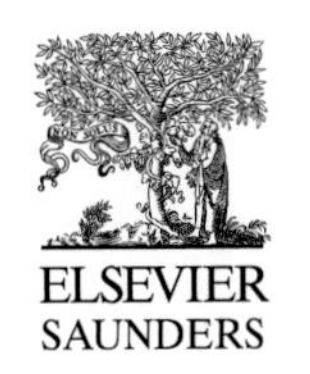
ELSEVIER
SAUNDERS

Cardiol Clin 25 (2007) 57–70

CARDIOLOGY
CLINICS

Detection of Myocardial Ischemia by Stress Perfusion Cardiovascular Magnetic Resonance

Han W. Kim, MD*, Igor Klem, MD, Raymond J. Kim, MD

Duke Cardiovascular Magnetic Resonance Center, Duke University Health Systems, Durham, NC 27710, USA

With recent technical and clinical advances, adenosine stress perfusion MRI has evolved from a promising research tool to an everyday clinical test. In part because of the transition, cardiovascular magnetic resonance imaging (CMR) itself has changed from a modality that was used nearly exclusively for rare clinical indications such as cardiac neoplasms and arrhythmogenic right ventricular cardiomyopathy to one that is considered a competitive first-line test for common indications such as the evaluation of ischemic heart disease. In 2006, a consensus panel from the American College of Cardiology Foundation (ACCF) deemed the following indications as appropriate uses of stress perfusion MRI: evaluating chest pain syndromes in patients who have intermediate probability of coronary artery disease (CAD) and ascertaining the physiologic significance of indeterminate coronary artery lesions [1]. In part, ACCF report reflects the growing clinical experience with stress perfusion MRI. In dedicated CMR clinical centers, perfusion stress testing is often the fastest growing component of the clinical volume and can comprise nearly half of all referrals [2]. The purpose of this article is to review the current state of stress perfusion MRI and addresses the following topics: validation of stress perfusion MRI in preclinical studies, diagnostic performance in patients, imaging protocol, and image interpretation.

Overview

The goal of perfusion MRI is to create a movie of the transit of contrast media (typically gadolinium-based) with the blood during its initial pass through the left ventricular (LV) myocardium (first-pass contrast enhancement). Myocardial perfusion by MRI may be assessed quantitatively or semiquantitatively by measuring dynamic signal intensities within the myocardium in consecutive images (Fig. 1). During pharmacological vasodilation (eg, adenosine), myocardial blood flow increases fourfold to fivefold downstream of normal coronary arteries, but does not increase downstream of severely diseased arteries, because the arteriolar beds already are vasodilated maximally. These physiological differences result in lower peak myocardial signal intensity and lengthening in the measures of myocardial contrast transit time (eg, signal upslope, arrival time, time-to-peak signal, and mean transit time) in regions supplied by diseased vessels (see Fig. 1) [3]. Signal intensity parameters can be plotted with respect to time and, with some assumptions, quantitatively modeled to provide absolute tissue blood flow in milliliters per minutes per gram or used in a semiquantitative fashion to index relative differences in regional flow [3]. Alternatively, the images can be interpreted visually for the presence or absence of perfusion defects.

Compared with competing technologies such as radionuclide imaging, perfusion MRI has many potential advantages: more than an order of magnitude improvement in spatial resolution (typical voxel dimensions, MRI $3.0 \times 1.8 \times 8$ mm = 43 mm^3 versus single photon emission computed tomography (SPECT) $10 \times 10 \times 10$ mm = 1000 mm^3), the ability to identify regional differences in flow over the full range of coronary vasodilation (ie, no plateau in signal at high flow rates, as seen with radionuclide tracers) [4,5], the lack of ionizing

* Corresponding author.
E-mail address: kim00050@notes.duke.edu (H.W. Kim).

doi:10.1016/j.ccl.2007.02.002

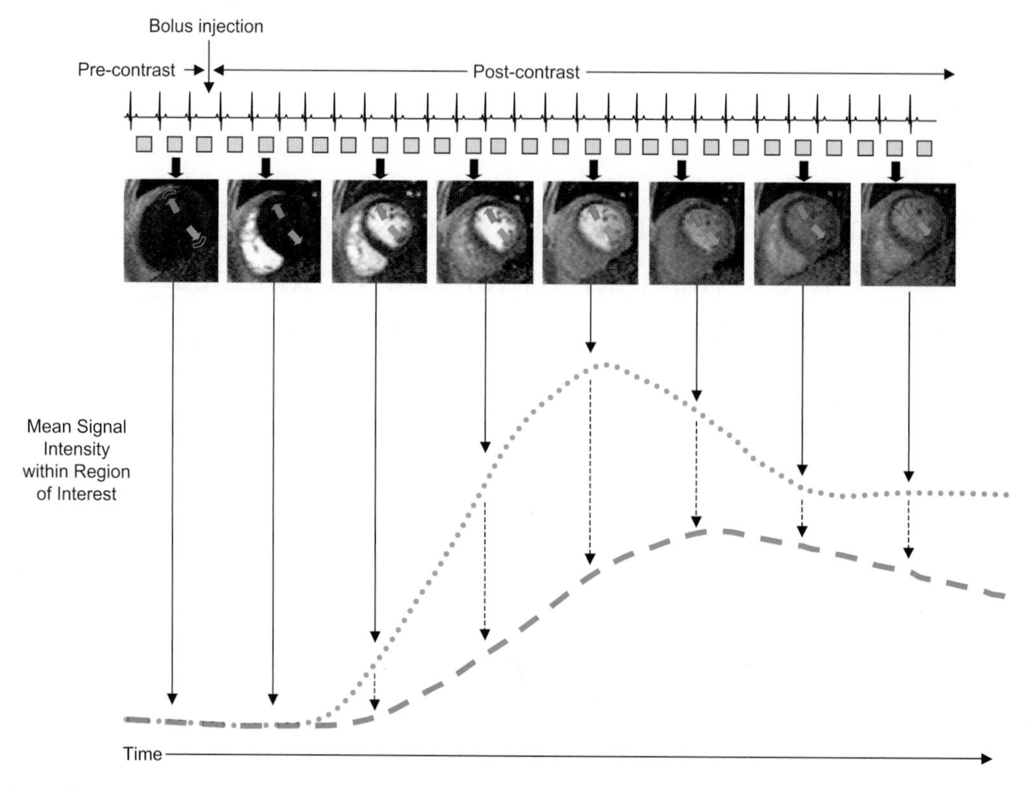

Fig. 1. Signal intensity time curves from two myocardial regions. In this example, there is hypoperfusion of the anterior wall (*red arrow and dashed red line*), while the perfusion of the inferior wall (*blue arrow and dotted blue line*) is normal. From these curves, various parameters can be extracted to derive quantitative measures of blood flow.

radiation, and an examination time of 30 to 45 minutes versus 2 to 3 hours.

Preclinical validation

Several studies have shown a good correlation between semiquantitative and quantitative MRI indices of perfusion with tissue perfusion in animal models [6–10]. In a porcine model with ligation of the left circumflex coronary (LCx) artery, Wilke and colleagues [6] performed MR perfusion studies both at rest and during vasodilation with adenosine. The authors found a linear correlation between relative MRI perfusion indices and true perfusion as measured by radioactive microspheres. Similarly, in a chronically instrumented canine model, Klocke and colleagues [8] produced regional differences in flow with selective LCx infusion of graded doses of adenosine or partial LCx obstruction using a hydraulic occlusion device. Regional differences in the area under the upslope of the MRI signal intensity curve linearly correlated with flow differences measured by fluorescent microspheres (Fig. 2). Moreover, regional flow differences of at least twofold were discerned consistently by perfusion MRI, suggesting that clinically relevant coronary stenoses of 70% or greater could be detected reliably.

Extending these observations are the findings from Lee and colleagues [9]. In this study, perfusion MRI was compared with technetium-99m (^{99m}Tc) sestamibi and 201-Thallium (^{201}Tl) SPECT imaging in the quantification of regional differences in vasodilated blood flow in viable myocardium. The authors used a canine model, where a hydraulic occluder was placed in the left circumflex coronary artery to produce graded reductions in regional flows. When circumflex microsphere flow was reduced by at least 50%, perfusion defects were apparent on the MR images by visual inspection and analysis of the signal intensity curves. Moreover, flows derived from the initial areas under the MRI signal intensity time curves were related linearly to reference microsphere flows

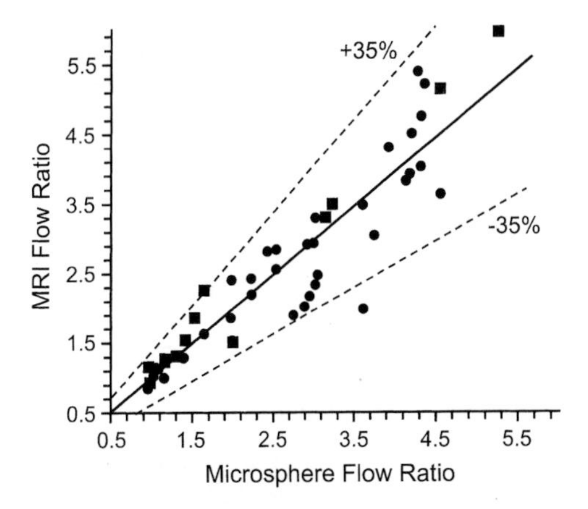

Fig. 2. MRI versus microsphere flow ratios in a canine model. Solid line is linear regression (MRI ratio = 0.96 microsphere +0.07); dotted lines indicate 95% confidence limits for individual values. ●, ratios of LCx to remote MRI areas and relative microsphere flows during LCx adenosine infusion; ■, ratios of remote to LCx MRI areas and relative microsphere flows during LCx constriction in the presence of global LV vasodilation. (*From* Klocke FJ, Simonetti OP, Judd RM, et al. Limits of detection of regional differences in vasodilated flow in viable myocardium by first-pass magnetic resonance perfusion imaging. Circulation 2001;104:2414; with permission.)

over the full range of vasodilation. In contrast, with SPECT imaging, perfusion defects were not evident until flow was reduced by at least 85%, and the relationships between both ^{99m}Tc and ^{201}Tl activity and microsphere flows were curvilinear, plateauing as flows increased (Fig. 3).

More recently, Christian and colleagues [10] used a Fermi function deconvolution method to quantify absolute perfusion in a canine model of coronary artery stenosis. Vessel occluders or intracoronary adenosine infusion catheters were used to produce a wide range of coronary flows. These authors derived myocardial flow in the endocardial and epicardial layers of the heart by perfusion MRI. They showed that quantitative coronary flow by MRI in both layers was linearly related to flow by fluorescent microspheres (without plateauing at higher flow rates) in the corresponding locations. These findings and those from others [7] demonstrate that perfusion MRI, with its advantage of high spatial resolution, has the potential to discern differences in endocardial and epicardial flow.

Diagnostic performance in patients

The diagnostic performance of stress perfusion MRI has been evaluated in numerous studies in people [11–29]. Overall, these studies have shown good correlations with radionuclide imaging and x-ray coronary angiography, although there have been some variable results. Table 1 summarizes the published stress perfusion MRI studies in humans with coronary angiography comparison. A total of 20 studies have been completed, consisting of 1086 patients who had known or suspected CAD. On average, the sensitivity and specificity of perfusion MRI for detecting obstructive CAD were 83% (range, 44% to 93%) and 82% (range, 60% to 100%), respectively. Likely on the basis of these studies, the most recent consensus report on clinical indications for CMR classified perfusion imaging as a class II indication for the assessment of CAD (provides clinically relevant information and is frequently useful) [30].

Despite the mostly favorable results of these studies, numerous issues should be considered. Some studies are of limited clinical applicability, because they required central venous catheters [15,19], imaged only one slice per heartbeat [15], or excluded patients who had diabetes [24]. Many studies had small sample sizes; eight had 30 or fewer patients. Most included patients already known to have CAD or known to have prior myocardial infarction (MI). In these studies, there is pretest referral or spectrum bias, which can raise test sensitivity and/or specificity artificially [31,32]. Importantly, in many studies, after the data were collected, several methods of analysis were tested, and different thresholds for test abnormality were appraised. For these studies, the reported sensitivity and specificity values are optimistic, because the endpoints were chosen retrospectively, and they represent optimized values.

Two practical issues also limit clinical applicability. First, there is no consensus regarding the optimal pulse sequence or imaging protocol. The studies in Table 1 are very heterogeneous in terms of the techniques and methods employed. For example, the dose of gadolinium contrast administered varied sixfold, with doses ranging from 0.025 to 0.15 mmol/kg. The inconsistent results in the literature likely reflect the lack of a standard method for performing perfusion MRI. Second, many of the studies used a quantitative approach for diagnostic assessment. Although a quantitative approach has the advantage, potentially, of allowing absolute blood flow to be measured or parametric maps of perfusion to be generated, the approach is laborious and requires extensive interactive postprocessing. At present, a quantitative approach is not feasible for everyday clinical use.

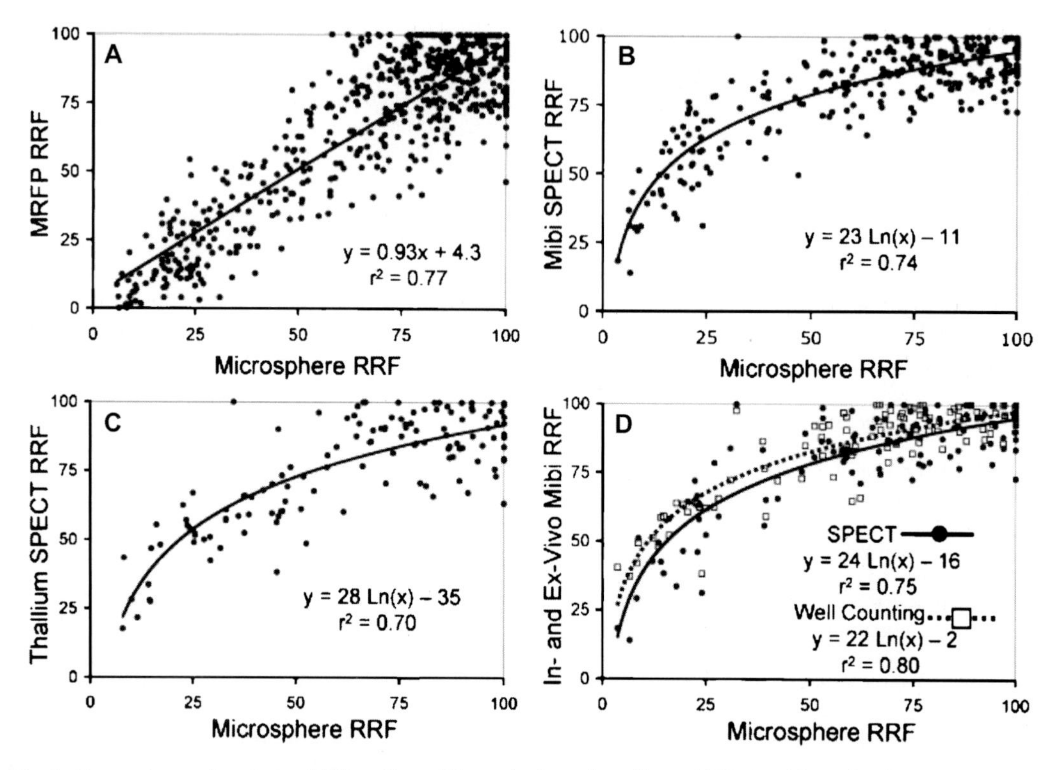

Fig. 3. Comparisons of perfusion MRI, radionuclide, and microsphere flows. MRI signal intensity time curves were related linearly to reference microsphere flows over the full range of vasodilation. Relationships between ^{99m}Tc-sestamibi and ^{201}thallium activity and microsphere flows were curvilinear, plateauing as flows increased. Data suggest that perfusion MRI, unlike radionuclide imaging, has the potential for detecting stenoses producing only moderate limitations in flow reserve. (*A*) Normalized magnetic resonance first-pass perfusion (MRFP) imaging and full-thickness microsphere relative regional flows (RRF). (*B*) Normalized ^{99m}Tc-sestamibi and full-thickness microsphere RRFs. (*C*) Normalized ^{201}Tl and full-thickness microsphere RRFs. (*D*) In vivo SPECT and ex vivo well counting values of ^{99m}Tc-sestamibi versus microsphere RRFs. (*From* Lee DC, Simonetti OP, Harris KR. Magnetic resonance versus radionuclide pharmacological stress perfusion imaging for flow-limiting stenoses of varying severity. Circulation 2004;110:62; with permission.)

In contrast, image interpretation by simple visual assessment would be a realistic approach for a clinical CMR practice. Unfortunately, the results in the literature regarding visual assessment of perfusion MRI are mixed, generally demonstrating adequate sensitivity but relatively poor specificity for the detection of CAD. In large part, image artifacts are responsible for reduced specificity. In this context, it is noteworthy that recently an interpretation algorithm that combines data from perfusion MRI and delayed enhancement MRI (DE-MRI) has been introduced that substantially improves the specificity and accuracy of rapid visual assessment for the detection of CAD [29,33]. Based on these data, the authors have adopted a multicomponent approach to stress testing, which permits rapid visual image interpretation with high diagnostic accuracy.

Multicomponent CMR stress testing protocol

The multicomponent approach to CMR stress testing includes the following:

1. Cine MRI for the assessment of cardiac morphology and regional and global systolic function at baseline
2. Stress perfusion MRI to visualize regions of myocardial hypoperfusion during vasodilation (eg, with adenosine infusion)
3. Rest perfusion MRI to aid in distinguishing true perfusion defects from image artifacts
4. DE-MRI for the determination of myocardial infarction (MI) (Fig. 4)

The timeline of the multicomponent CMR stress test is displayed in Fig. 5. Details regarding

Table 1
Stress perfusion MRI studies in humans with coronary angiography comparison

Year	Author	Reference	n	Pts with known CAD excluded	Protocol			X-ray angiography (CAD definition)	Analysis method[2]	Sens	Spec
					MRI perfusion protocol[1]	Gadolinium dose (mmol/kg)	Pulse-sequence				
1993	Klein	AJR 161(2):257–63	5	no	Stress only	0.05	IR-GRE	>50	Prospective	81*	100*
1994	Hartnell	AJR 163(5):1061–7	18	no	Rest/Stress	0.04	IR-GRE	≥ 70	Prospective	83	100
1994	Eichenberger	JMRI 4(3):425–31	10	no	Rest/Stress	0.05	GRE	>75	Retrospective	44*	80*
2000	Al-Saadi	Circ 101(12):1379–83	34	yes	Rest/Stress	0.025	IR-GRE	≥ 75	Prospective[3]	90	83
2001	Bertschinger	JMRI 14(5):556–62	14	no	Stress only	0.1	SR-EPI	≥ 50	Retrospective	85	81
2001	Schwitter	Circ 103(18):2230–5	48	yes	Stress only	0.1	SR-GRE-EPI	≥ 50	Retrospective	87	85
2001	Panting	JMRI 13(2):192–200	22	no	Rest/Stress	0.05	IR Spin Echo-EPI	>50	Retrospective	79	83
2002	Sensky	Int J CV Imaging 18(5):373–83	30	no	Rest/Stress	0.025	IR-GRE	>50	Prospective	93*	60*
2002	Ibrahim	JACC 39(5):864–70	25	no	Rest/Stress	0.05	SR-GRE-EPI	>75	Retrospective	69*	89*
2003	Chiu	Radiology 226(3):717–22	13	no[4]	Rest/Stress	0.05	IR-SSFP	>50	NS	92*	92*
2003	Ishida	Radiology 229(l):209–16	104	no	Stress/Rest	0.075	SR-GRE-EPI	≥ 70	Prospective	90	85
2003	Nagel	Circ 108(4):432–7	84	no	Rest/Stress	0.025	SR-GRE-EPI	≥ 75	Retrospective	88	90
2003	Doyle	JCMR 5(3):475–85	138	no	Rest/Stress	0.04	SR-GRE	≥ 70	Prospective[3]	57	85
2004	Wolff	Circ 110(6):732–7	75	no	Stress/Rest	0.05–0.15	SR-GRE-EPI	≥ 70	Prospective[5]	93	75
2004	Giang	EHJ 25(18):1657–65	80	no	Stress only	0.05–0.15	SR-GRE-EPI	≥ 50	Retrospective[5]	93	75
2004	Paetsch	Circ 110(7):835–42	79	no	Stress/Rest	0.05	SR-GRE-EPI	>50	Prospective	91	62
2004	Plein	JACC 44(11):2173–81	68	no[4]	Rest/Stress	0.05	SR-GRE[6]	≥ 70	Prospective	88	83
2005	Plein	Radiology 235(2):423–30	92	no	Rest/Stress	0.05	SR-GRE[6]	>70	Retrospective	88	82
2006	Klem	JACC 47(8):1630–8	100	yes	Stress/Rest	0.063	SR-GRE[6]	≥ 70	Prospective	84†	58†
2006	Cury	Radiology 240(l):39–45	47	no	Stress/Rest	0.1	SR-GRE-EPI	≥ 70	Prospective	81§	87§
Total		20	1086								
Average										83	82

Abbreviations: MRI, magnetic resonance imaging; CAD, coronary artery disease; n, number of patients; IR, inversion recovery pre-pulse; SR, saturation recovery pre-pulse; GRE, gradient-recalled echo; EPI, echo-planar imaging; SSFP, steady-state free precession; DE-MRI, delayed enhancement MRI; Sens, sensitivity; Spec, specificity; NS, not stated.

* Numbers based on a regional rather than per patient analysis.

[1] When both rest and stress imaging were performed the order is as listed.

[2] Prospective studies were those in which the criteria for test abnormality were prespecified before data analysis.

[3] Pilot study performed first to determine the best threshold for test abnormality.

[4] At enrollment all patients had the clinical diagnosis of non-ST elevation MI or acute coronary syndrome.

[5] Reported sensitivity and specificity are from a fraction of the total cohort, a subgroup with the best results.

[6] With parallel imaging acceleration.

† Sensitivity/specificity were higher after incorporating DE-MRI (89% and 87%, respectively).

§ Sensitivity/specificity were higher after incorporating DE-MRI (87% and 89%, respectively).

From Kim HW, Rehwald W, White JA, et al. Magnetic Resonance Imaging of the Heart. In: Fuster V, O'Rourke RA. editors. Hurst's The Heart. New York: McGraw-Hill Medical, in press.

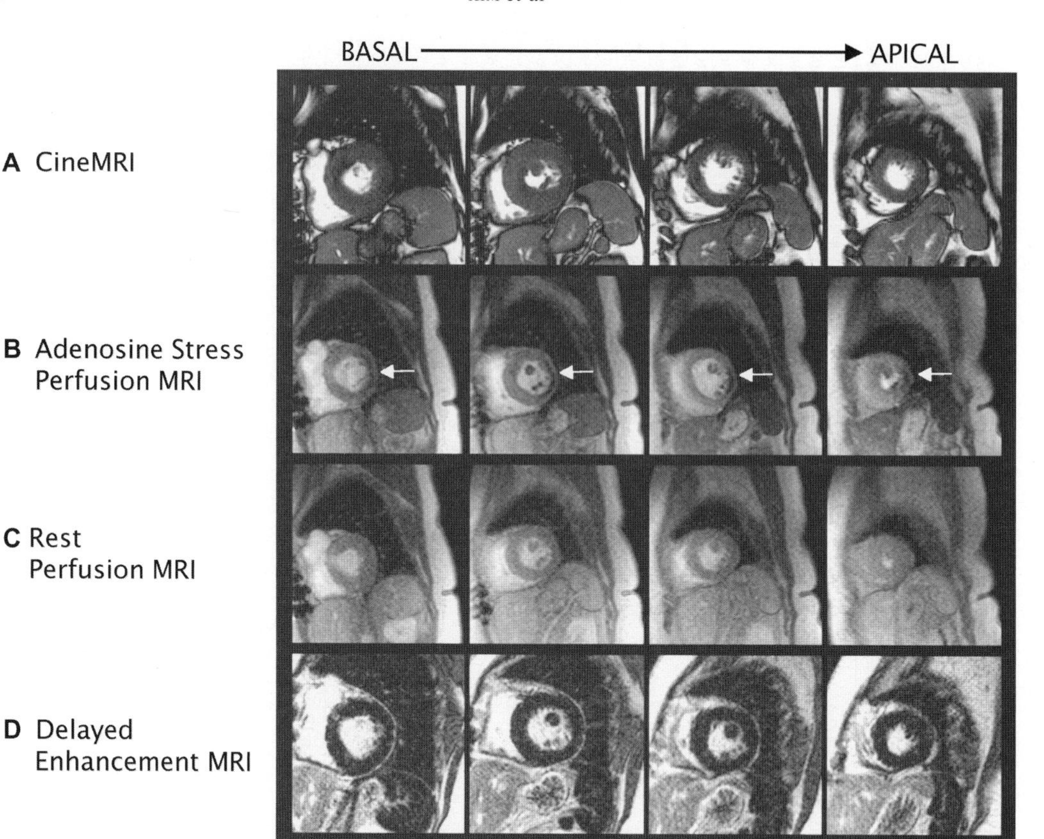

Fig. 4. Components of the multicomponent CMR stress test. Cine MRI (*A*), stress (*B*), and rest perfusion (*C*) MRI, and delayed-enhancement MRI (*D*) are performed at identical short axis locations. During image interpretation, the different components are analyzed side by side to facilitate differentiation of perfusion defects due to infarction, ischemia, or artifact. Arrows points to perfusion defects seen during adenosine infusion, but not at rest consistent with the presence of ischemic heart disease.

cine MRI and DE-MRI are discussed elsewhere in this issue of *Clinical Cardiology*.

Stress perfusion imaging is performed after scouting and cine imaging. Typically, before adenosine administration, the patient table is pulled partially out of bore of the magnet to allow direct observation and full access to the patient. Adenosine (140 μg/kg/min) then is infused under continuous electrocardiography and blood pressure monitoring for at least 2 minutes. The perfusion sequence then is applied by the scanner operator, which automatically recenters the patient back in the scanner bore and commences imaging. Gadolinium contrast (0.075 to 0.10 mmol/kg body weight) then is administered, followed by a saline flush (approximately 50 mL) at a rate of at least 3 mL/s by means of an antecubital vein. On the console, the perfusion images are observed as they are acquired, with breath holding starting from the appearance of contrast in the right ventricular cavity. If the scanner software does not provide real-time image display, breath holding should be started no more than 5 to 6 seconds after beginning gadolinium injection. Breath holding is performed to ensure the best possible image quality (ie, no artifacts caused by respiratory motion) during the initial wash-in of contrast into the LV myocardium. Once the contrast bolus has transited the LV myocardium, adenosine is stopped, and imaging is completed 5 to 10 seconds later. Typically, the total imaging time is 40 to 50 seconds, and the total time of adenosine infusion is 3 to 3.5 minutes. During vasodilation, direct access to the patient is limited only during imaging of the first pass.

Before the rest perfusion scan, a waiting period of about 15 minutes is required for gadolinium to sufficiently clear from the blood pool. During this time, additional cine scans and or velocity/flow

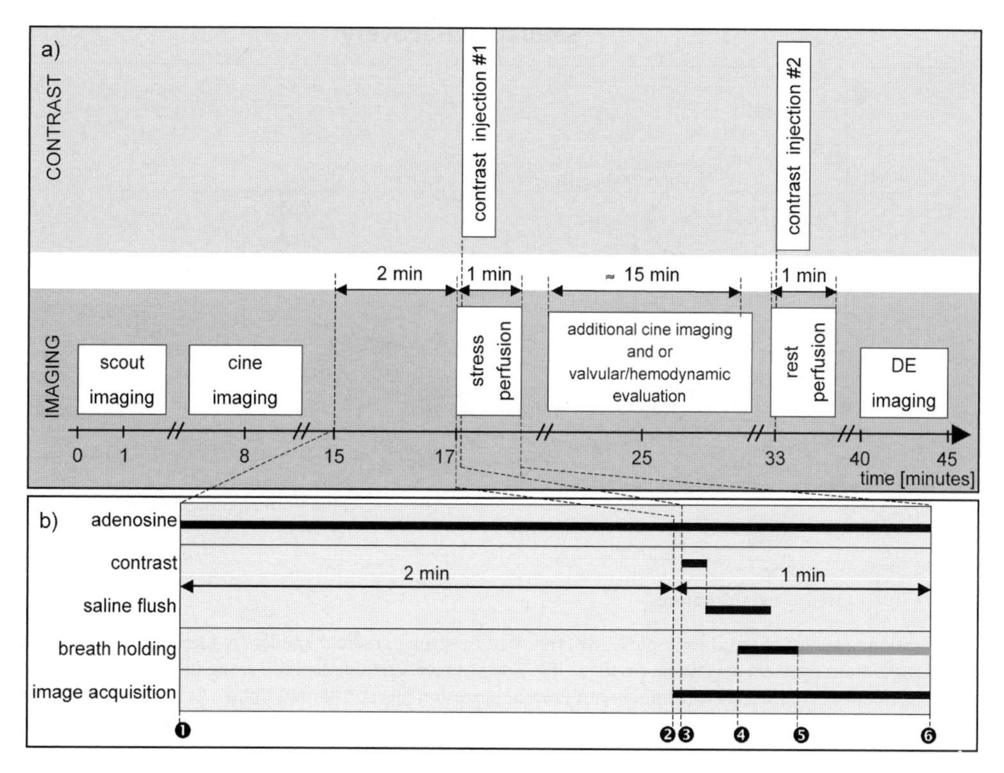

Fig. 5. Timeline for the multicomponent cardiovascular magnetic resonance imaging (CMR) stress test. See text for details.

imaging for valvular or hemodynamic evaluation can be performed. For the rest perfusion scan, an additional dose of 0.075 to 0.10 mmol/kg gadolinium is given, and the imaging parameters are identical to the stress scan. Approximately 5 minutes after rest perfusion, delayed enhancement imaging can be performed. The total scan time for a comprehensive CMR stress test, including cine imaging, stress and rest perfusion, and delayed enhancement, is usually well under 45 minutes.

Unlike vasodilator radionuclide imaging, in which adenosine typically is infused for 6 minutes (tracer injection at 3 minutes), stress perfusion MRI is performed using an abbreviated adenosine protocol ($\leq$3.5 minutes total), because the requirements for imaging are different [29]. With radionuclide imaging, maintaining a vasodilated state for 2 to 3 minutes after tracer injection is necessary to allow time for tracer uptake into myocytes. In contradistinction with MRI, currently available gadolinium media are inert, extracellular agents that do not cross sarcolemmal membranes [34], and vasodilation needs to be maintained only for the initial first pass through the myocardium. Although severe reactions to adenosine are rare, a shortened protocol is relevant, because moderate reactions that affect patient tolerability are relatively commonplace [35]. A minimum 2-minute infusion duration was chosen on the basis of physiological studies in humans demonstrating that maximum coronary blood flow is reached, on average, 1 minute after the start of intravenous adenosine infusion (140 μg/kg/min) and in nearly everyone by 2 minutes [36].

Various pulse sequences are in use for perfusion MRI, and the pace of development is rapid. Common imaging engines are steady-state free precession (SSFP), gradient recalled echo, and gradient recalled echo-echo planar imaging hybrid sequences (for details see earlier article by Kim and colleagues, A Clinical CMR Service). Virtually all sequences include a saturation prepulse modifier to provide T1 weighting and to accentuate regional differences in myocardial gadolinium concentration (Fig. 6). Because images are acquired in single-shot mode, a parallel imaging modifier is essential to speed imaging [37,38] and allow adequate LV coverage and reduce motion artifacts [39]. In general, image readout times more than 120 to130 milliseconds can lead to

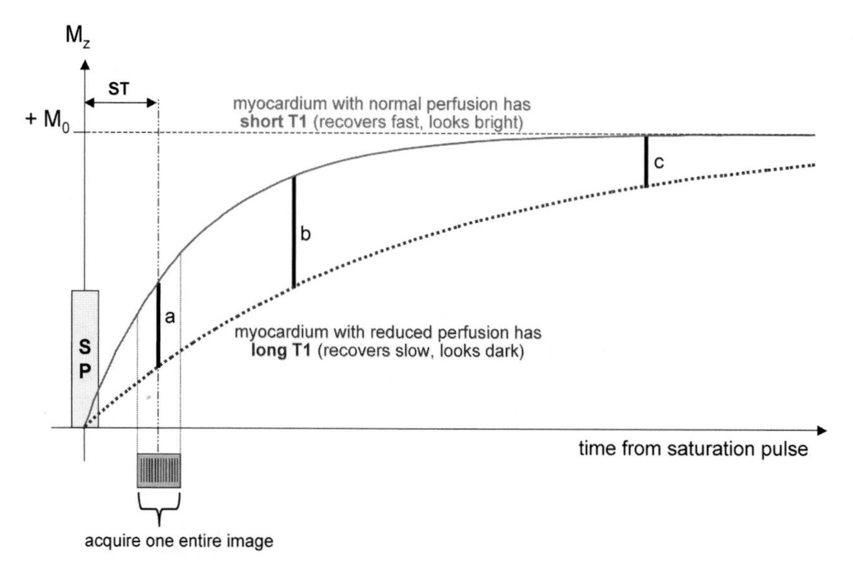

Fig. 6. Saturation recovery. A saturation pulse (SP) followed by strong gradient spoilers reduces the net magnetization to zero. Magnetization recovers depending on tissue T1. For instance, immediately following intravenous bolus administration of gadolinium contrast, myocardium with normal perfusion has substantial uptake of gadolinium; thus it has short T1, and appears bright on saturation recovery perfusion MRI. In comparison, myocardium with reduced perfusion has diminished uptake of gadolinium, longer T1, and appears dark. Ideally, data readout should follow the saturation pulse at a specific saturation recovery time (time point b rather than time point a or c) to achieve maximum separation between the T1 relaxation curves of normal and abnormal myocardium. To perform multi-slice imaging for every heartbeat during the first pass, however, a shorter saturation recovery time is employed where the separation between the two curves is less (time point a). ST, saturation recovery time; SP, saturation pulse.

substantial motion artifacts in images acquired during periods of the cardiac cycle in which there is rapid LV motion. Usually four to five short-axis views are obtained every heartbeat with a total of 40 to 60 heartbeats consisting of the entire first pass. Although more views could be obtained every two heartbeats, this is not recommended unless tachycardia is present, because clinically, the benefit of improving LV coverage does not outweigh the detriment of halving the sampling frequency of the dynamic first-pass process.

Additionally, an important parameter to consider in stress perfusion MRI is the delay between the saturation recovery prepulse modifier and image readout (saturation recovery time or ST). The purpose of the saturation prepulse modifier is to provide strong T1 weighting and accentuate regional differences in myocardial gadolinium concentration during the first pass (see Fig. 6). Ideally, the ST would be relatively long (at point B in Fig. 6) so that the difference in the T1 relaxation curves and signal intensities of normal and hypoperfused myocardium would be maximal. In clinical practice, however, to image four to five short axis slices per cardiac cycle, a shorter ST (point a in Fig. 6) is used by necessity, which results in overall reduced image signal-to-noise ratio (SNR) and smaller differences in signal intensities between normal and hypoperfused myocardium. Despite this constraint in timing, image quality is usually sufficient for visual interpretation. When heart rates exceed 100 beats per minute, however, the authors prefer to use a higher dose of gadolinium contrast (a total dose of 0.20 mmol/kg divided equally for stress and rest imaging) to compensate for the reduction in ST needed to obtain complete ventricular coverage every heartbeat.

Image interpretation

Interpretation algorithm for coronary artery disease

An overview of the interpretation algorithm that facilitates rapid visual interpretation for a multicomponent CMR stress test is presented with examples in Fig. 7. Using this stepwise

A Interpretation Algorithm

START

DE-MRI

\+ → CAD[1]

− → Stress Perfusion

\+ → Rest Perfusion

− → No CAD[2]

"Reversible" defect → CAD[3]

"Matched" defect → No CAD[4]

B Examples

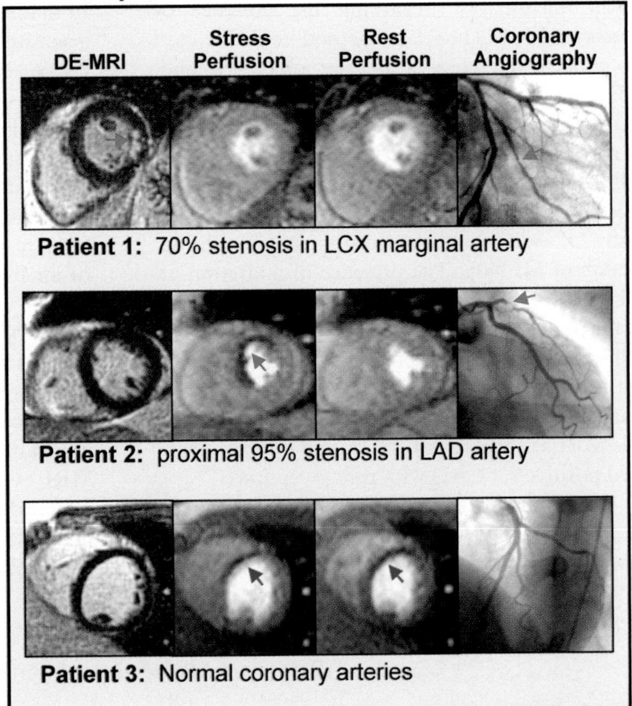

Fig. 7. Interpretation algorithm for incorporating delayed-enhancement MRI with stress and rest perfusion MRI for the detection of coronary disease. (*A*) Schema of the interpretation algorithm. (*1*) Positive delayed-enhancement MRI (DE-MRI) study. Hyperenhanced myocardium consistent with a prior myocardial infarction (MI) is detected. Does not include isolated midwall or epicardial hyperenhancement, which can occur in nonischemic disorders. (*2*) Standard negative stress study. No evidence of prior MI or inducible perfusion defects. (*3*) Standard positive stress study. No evidence of prior MI, but perfusion defects are present with adenosine that are absent or reduced at rest. (*4*) Artifactual perfusion defect. Matched stress and rest perfusion defects without evidence of prior MI on DE-MRI. (*B*) Patient examples. *Top row*. Patient with a positive DE-MRI study demonstrating an infarct in the inferolateral wall (*red arrow*), although perfusion MRI is negative. The interpretation algorithm (*step 1*) classified this patient as positive for CAD. Coronary angiography verified disease in a circumflex marginal artery. Cine MRI demonstrated normal contractility. *Middle row*. Patient with a negative DE-MRI study but with a prominent reversible defect in the anteroseptal wall on perfusion MRI (*red arrow*). The interpretation algorithm (*step 3*) classified this patient as positive for CAD. Coronary angiography demonstrated a proximal 95% left anterior descending coronary artery stenosis. *Bottom row*. Patient with a matched stress–rest perfusion defect (*blue arrows*) but without evidence of prior MI on DE-MRI. The interpretation algorithm (*step 4*) classified the perfusion defects as artifactual. Coronary angiography demonstrated normal coronary arteries. CAD, coronary artery disease. (*Adapted from* Klem I, Heitner JF, Shah DJ, et al. Improved detection of coronary artery disease by stress perfusion cardiovascular magnetic resonance with the use of delayed enhancement infarction imaging. Circulation 2006;47:1630–8.)

algorithm, a CMR stress test is deemed positive for CAD if myocardial infarction is present on DE-MRI or if perfusion defects are present during stress imaging, but absent at rest (reversible defect) in the absence of infarction. Conversely, the test is deemed negative for CAD if no abnormalities are found (eg, no MI and no stress/rest perfusion defects) or if perfusion defects are seen at both stress and rest imaging (matched defect) in the absence of infarction. In the latter, matched defects are regarded as artifacts and not suggestive of CAD with rare exceptions (see next section). When both DE-MRI and stress perfusion MRI are abnormal, the test is scored positive for ischemia if the perfusion defect is larger than the area of infarction.

The interpretation algorithm is based on two simple principles. First, with perfusion MRI and

DE-MRI, there are two independent methods to obtain information regarding the presence or absence of MI. Thus, one method could be used to confirm the results of the other. Second, DE-MRI image quality (eg, SNR) is far better than perfusion MRI, because it is less demanding in terms of scanner hardware (DE-MRI images can be built up over several seconds rather than in 0.1 seconds as is required for first-pass perfusion) [40]. Thus, DE-MRI should be more accurate for the detection of MI [40]. The presence of infarction on DE-MRI favors the presence of CAD, irrespective of the perfusion MRI results. Conceptually, it then follows that perfusion defects that have similar intensity and extent during both stress and rest (matched defect) but do not have infarction on DE-MRI are artifactual and should not be considered positive for CAD with rare exceptions.

Klem and colleagues [29] reported that the determination of CAD using the multicomponent CMR stress test and interpretation algorithm significantly improved diagnostic performance. In that study, the interpretation algorithm yielded a sensitivity of 89%, specificity of 87%, and diagnostic accuracy of 88% for the detection of CAD (major coronary artery with stenosis $\geq$70% or left main stenosis $\geq$50%). In comparison, when stress and rest perfusion were considered alone (without DE-MRI), the sensitivity, specificity, and diagnostic accuracy were 84%, 58%, and 68% respectively. Thus, the interpretation algorithm had markedly higher specificity and diagnostic accuracy than perfusion MRI alone ($P<.0001$ for both). Notably, the higher specificity with the interpretation algorithm was primarily the result of correctly changing the diagnosis from positive to negative for CAD in 12 patients in whom infarction was not observed on DE-MRI even though perfusion MRI demonstrated matched stress–rest perfusion defects. Importantly, in this study, the imaging protocol and interpretation algorithm was prespecified, and all

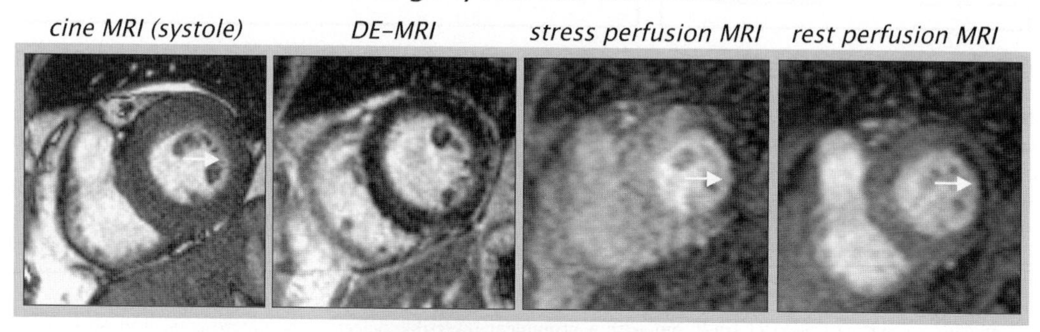

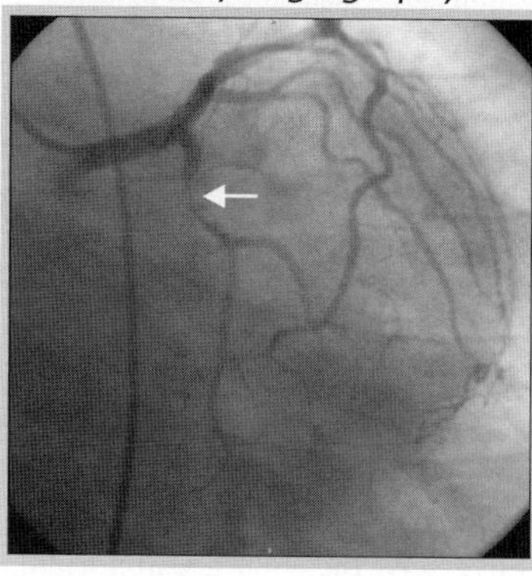

Fig. 8. Example of resting myocardial ischemia. Cine MRI demonstrates hypokinesis of the lateral wall without evidence of myocardial infarction on delayed-enhancement MRI. Dense, nearly transmural perfusion defects are present at stress and rest (although larger with stress). Coronary angiography demonstrates a high-grade lesion in the proximal left circumflex coronary artery. Red arrows point to the abnormalities.

patients were consecutively recruited prospectively from a pool referred for elective coronary angiography. Patients who had known CAD (eg, prior MI or revascularization) were excluded to reduce pretest referral or spectrum bias. Moreover, to avoid post-test referral bias, all patients underwent angiography within 24 hours of CMR without regard to the CMR findings. Thus, it is likely that these results reflect the actual real-world performance of a multicomponent CMR stress test with appropriate image interpretation.

Artifacts

Image artifacts often occur at the interface between the LV cavity and the endocardium (arising from susceptibility effects or rapid cardiac motion) and may mimic true perfusion defects [41]. Characteristics that may be useful in distinguishing between artifact and true perfusion defects include the following:

1. Artifacts are more common in the phase–encode direction; true perfusion defects should follow coronary artery distribution territories.
2. Artifacts are transitory, varying in signal intensity in consecutive images during the transit of contrast media through the myocardium; true perfusion defects often linger for multiple image frames and should follow smooth image intensity trajectories.
3. Artifacts are present at both stress and rest imaging; true perfusion defects generally appear only during vasodilator stress.

Concerning this latter point, it is important to recognize that the interpretation of stress–rest perfusion MRI is not analogous to stress–rest SPECT imaging. For instance, matched perfusion defects on perfusion MRI are more far likely to represent artifact than prior MI. Additionally, the authors also have observed that severe, but matched perfusion defects can occur in the setting of critical resting ischemia (Fig. 8). Unlike artifacts, these perfusion defects are transmural (or nearly transmural) and persist for nearly the entire first pass and are associated with wall motion abnormalities in the same location as the perfusion defects. Although extremely rare, recognition of true perfusion defects occurring at both stress and rest with limited or absent MI on DE-MRI is important, as they are associated with total or subtotal occlusions and are potentially reversible following revascularization.

Perfusion defects caused by microvascular dysfunction

Data regarding the use of multicomponent CMR stress testing in patients with microvascular dysfunction are limited. However, the high spatial resolution of perfusion MRI, which allows the identification of perfusion defects that primarily affect the subendocardium, may be useful in

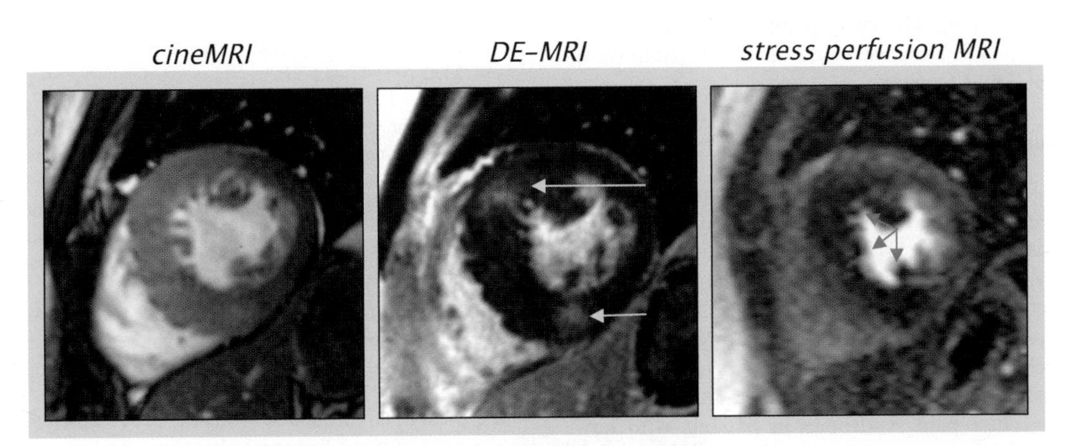

Fig. 9. Evaluation of hypertrophic cardiomyopathy by cardiovascular magnetic resonance imaging. Cine MRI demonstrates asymmetric septal hypertrophy. On delayed-enhancement MRI (DE-MRI), there is evidence of scarring in the ventricular septum at the right ventricular insertion sites. The stress perfusion MR images show a dense perfusion defect in the septum also, although the region of ischemia is larger than the area of scarring on DE-MRI. This patient had normal epicardial coronary arteries on angiography. (*Adapted from* Shah DJ, Judd RM, Kim RJ. Technology insight: MRI of the myocardium. Nat Clin Pract Cardiovasc Med 2005;2:602; with permission.)

patients with potential microvascular dysfunction, such as cardiac syndrome X [42], hypertrophic cardiomyopathy (HCM) [43], or aortic stenosis. For example, in patients who have HCM, the authors have observed stress-induced perfusion defects in the absence of epicardial coronary disease (Fig. 9). These perfusion defects are most apparent in the more hypertrophied portions of the myocardium and colocalize with regions of scarring on DE-MRI (presented elsewhere in this issue of *Clinical Cardiology*). The clinical significance of these MRI findings has yet to be determined. Nonetheless, since both scarring and ischemia are likely to have prognostic implications, multicomponent CMR testing may have utility in risk stratification.

Reporting

At the authors' institution, CMR stress tests are scored regionally using the American Heart Association 17 segment model [44]. For the determination of the presence of CAD, the components are scored while viewing the images side by side (see Fig. 4). MI is scored from DE-MRI when hyperenhancement is present, unless the hyperenhancement is isolated to the midwall or subepicardium [29,45,46]. As previously described, these latter patterns are found in nonischemic rather than ischemic disorders [47,48]. Stress and rest perfusion images are scored for perfusion defects in 16 segments (segment 17 at the apex usually is not visualized) using the interpretation algorithm on a four-point scale: 0, normal; 1, probably normal; 2, probably abnormal; and 3, definitely abnormal [29]. The corresponding coronary artery territory is assigned based on the distribution of abnormal segments.

Summary

Perfusion MRI stress testing is emerging as an improved method for detecting CAD. When combined with DE-MRI, the sensitivity, specificity, and diagnostic accuracy of the multicomponent stress CMR exam rival other currently available modalities for evaluating myocardial ischemia. Importantly, CMR perfusion stress testing has been deemed appropriate for evaluating chest pain syndromes in patients who have intermediate probability of CAD and for ascertaining the physiologic significance of indeterminate coronary artery lesions. In the future, improvements in parallel imaging and pulse sequence technology, use of higher magnetic field strengths, and protocol optimizations will continue the rapid advance in image quality. Currently ongoing multicenter clinical trials will soon be available and will establish the diagnostic accuracy and prognostic value of CMR perfusion stress testing in a broad population of patients.

References

[1] Hendel RC, Patel MR, Kramer CM, et al. ACCF/ACR/SCCT/SCMR/ASNC/NASCI/SCAI/SIR 2006 appropriateness criteria for cardiac computed tomography and cardiac magnetic resonance imaging: a report of the American College of Cardiology Foundation Quality Strategic Directions Committee Appropriateness Criteria Working Group. J Am Coll Cardiol 2006;48:1475–97.

[2] Rehwald WG, Wagner A, Albert TSE, et al. Clinical CMR imaging techniques. In: Manning WJ, Pennell DJ, editors. Cardiovascular magnetic resonance. New York: Churchill Livingstone; in press.

[3] Jerosch-Herold M, Seethamraju RT, Swingen CM, et al. Analysis of myocardial perfusion MRI. J Magn Reson Imaging 2004;19:758–70.

[4] Beller GA, Holzgrefe HH, Watson DD. Effects of dipyridamole-induced vasodilation on myocardial uptake and clearance kinetics of thallium-201. Circulation 1983;68:1328–38.

[5] Glover DK, Okada RD. Myocardial kinetics of Tc-MIBI in canine myocardium after dipyridamole. Circulation 1990;81:628–37.

[6] Wilke N, Jerosch-Herold M, Wang Y, et al. Myocardial perfusion reserve: assessment with multisection, quantitative, first-pass MR imaging. Radiology 1997;204:373–84.

[7] Epstein FH, London JF, Peters DC, et al. Multislice first-pass cardiac perfusion MRI: validation in a model of myocardial infarction. Magn Reson Med 2002;47:482–91.

[8] Klocke FJ, Simonetti OP, Judd RM, et al. Limits of detection of regional differences in vasodilated flow in viable myocardium by first-pass magnetic resonance perfusion imaging. Circulation 2001;104:2412–6.

[9] Lee DC, Simonetti OP, Harris KR, et al. Magnetic resonance versus radionuclide pharmacological stress perfusion imaging for flow-limiting stenoses of varying severity. Circulation 2004;110:58–65.

[10] Christian TF, Rettmann DW, Aletras AH, et al. Absolute myocardial perfusion in canines measured by using dual-bolus first-pass MR imaging. Radiology 2004;232:677–84.

[11] Plein S, Greenwood JP, Ridgway JP, et al. Assessment of non-ST-segment elevation acute coronary syndromes with cardiac magnetic resonance imaging. J Am Coll Cardiol 2004;44:2173–81.

[12] Plein S, Radjenovic A, Ridgway JP, et al. Coronary artery disease: myocardial perfusion MR imaging with sensitivity encoding versus conventional angiography. Radiology 2005;235:423–30.

[13] Klein MA, Collier BD, Hellman RS, et al. Detection of chronic coronary artery disease: value of pharmacologically stressed, dynamically enhanced turbo-fast low-angle shot MR images. AJR Am J Roentgenol 1993;161:257–63.

[14] Hartnell G, Cerel A, Kamalesh M, et al. Detection of myocardial ischemia: value of combined myocardial perfusion and cineangiographic MR imaging. AJR Am J Roentgenol 1994;163:1061–7.

[15] Al-Saadi N, Nagel E, Gross M, et al. Noninvasive detection of myocardial ischemia from perfusion reserve based on cardiovascular magnetic resonance. Circulation 2000;101:1379–83.

[16] Eichenberger AC, Schuiki E, Kochli VD, et al. Ischemic heart disease: assessment with gadolinium-enhanced ultrafast MR imaging and dipyridamole stress. J Magn Reson Imaging 1994;4:425–31.

[17] Bertschinger KM, Nanz D, Buechi M, et al. Magnetic resonance myocardial first-pass perfusion imaging: parameter optimization for signal response and cardiac coverage. J Magn Reson Imaging 2001;14:556–62.

[18] Schwitter J, Nanz D, Kneifel S, et al. Assessment of myocardial perfusion in coronary artery disease by magnetic resonance: a comparison with positron emission tomography and coronary angiography. Circulation 2001;103:2230–5.

[19] Panting JR, Gatehouse PD, Yang GZ, et al. Echo-planar magnetic resonance myocardial perfusion imaging: parametric map analysis and comparison with thallium SPECT. J Magn Reson Imaging 2001;13:192–200.

[20] Sensky PR, Samani NJ, Reek C, et al. Magnetic resonance perfusion imaging in patients with coronary artery disease: a qualitative approach. Int J Cardiovasc Imaging 2002;18:373–83.

[21] Ibrahim T, Nekolla SG, Schreiber K, et al. Assessment of coronary flow reserve: comparison between contrast-enhanced magnetic resonance imaging and positron emission tomography. J Am Coll Cardiol 2002;39:864–70.

[22] Chiu CW, So NM, Lam WW, et al. Combined first-pass perfusion and viability study at MR imaging in patients with non-ST segment-elevation acute coronary syndromes: feasibility study. Radiology 2003;226:717–22.

[23] Ishida N, Sakuma H, Motoyasu M, et al. Noninfarcted myocardium: correlation between dynamic first-pass contrast-enhanced myocardial MR imaging and quantitative coronary angiography. Radiology 2003;229:209–16.

[24] Nagel E, Klein C, Paetsch I, et al. Magnetic resonance perfusion measurements for the noninvasive detection of coronary artery disease. Circulation 2003;108:432–7.

[25] Doyle M, Fuisz A, Kortright E, et al. The impact of myocardial flow reserve on the detection of coronary artery disease by perfusion imaging methods: an NHLBI WISE study. J Cardiovasc Magn Reson 2003;5:475–85.

[26] Wolff SD, Schwitter J, Coulden R, et al. Myocardial first-pass perfusion magnetic resonance imaging: a multicenter dose-ranging study. Circulation 2004;110:732–7.

[27] Giang TH, Nanz D, Coulden R, et al. Detection of coronary artery disease by magnetic resonance myocardial perfusion imaging with various contrast medium doses: first European multicentre experience. Eur Heart J 2004;25:1657–65.

[28] Paetsch I, Jahnke C, Wahl A, et al. Comparison of dobutamine stress magnetic resonance, adenosine stress magnetic resonance, and adenosine stress magnetic resonance perfusion. Circulation 2004;110:835–42.

[29] Klem I, Heitner JF, Shah DJ, et al. Improved detection of coronary artery disease by stress perfusion cardiovascular magnetic resonance with the use of delayed-enhancement infarction imaging. J Am Coll Cardiol 2006;47:1630–8.

[30] Pennell DJ, Sechtem UP, Higgins CB, et al. Clinical indications for cardiovascular magnetic resonance (CMR): consensus panel report. Eur Heart J 2004;25:1940–65.

[31] Cecil MP, Kosinski AS, Jones MT, et al. The importance of work-up (verification) bias correction in assessing the accuracy of SPECT thallium-201 testing for the diagnosis of coronary artery disease. J Clin Epidemiol 1996;49:735–42.

[32] Detrano R, Janosi A, Lyons KP, et al. Factors affecting sensitivity and specificity of a diagnostic test: the exercise thallium scintigram. Am J Med 1988;84:699–710.

[33] Cury RC, Cattani CA, Gabure LA, et al. Diagnostic performance of stress perfusion and delayed-enhancement MR imaging in patients with coronary artery disease. Radiology 2006;240:39–45.

[34] Weinmann HJ, Brasch RC, Press WR, et al. Characteristics of gadolinium-DTPA complex: a potential NMR contrast agent. AJR Am J Roentgenol 1984;142:619–24.

[35] Cerqueira MD, Verani MS, Schwaiger M, et al. Safety profile of adenosine stress perfusion imaging: results from the Adenoscan Multicenter Trial Registry. J Am Coll Cardiol 1994;23:384–9.

[36] Rossen JD, Quillen JE, Lopez AG, et al. Comparison of coronary vasodilation with intravenous dipyridamole and adenosine. J Am Coll Cardiol 1991;18:485–91.

[37] Sodickson DK, Manning WJ. Simultaneous acquisition of spatial harmonics (SMASH): fast imaging with radiofrequency coil arrays. Magn Reson Med 1997;38:591–603.

[38] Pruessmann KP, Weiger M, Scheidegger MB, et al. SENSE: sensitivity encoding for fast MRI. Magn Reson Med 1999;42:952–62.

[39] Storey P, Chen Q, Li W, et al. Band artifacts due to bulk motion. Magn Reson Med 2002;48:1028–36.

[40] Fuster V, Kim RJ. Frontiers in cardiovascular magnetic resonance. Circulation 2005;112:135–44.
[41] Di Bella EV, Parker DL, Sinusas AJ. On the dark rim artifact in dynamic contrast-enhanced MRI myocardial perfusion studies. Magn Reson Med 2005;54:1295–9.
[42] Panting JR, Gatehouse PD, Yang GZ, et al. Abnormal subendocardial perfusion in cardiac syndrome X detected by cardiovascular magnetic resonance imaging. N Engl J Med 2002;346:1948–53.
[43] Shah DJ, Judd RM, Kim RJ. Technology insight: MRI of the myocardium. Nat Clin Pract Cardiovasc Med 2005;2:597–605.
[44] Cerqueira MD, Weissman NJ, Dilsizian V, et al. Standardized myocardial segmentation and nomenclature for tomographic imaging of the heart: a statement for healthcare professionals from the Cardiac Imaging Committee of the Council on Clinical Cardiology of the American Heart Association. Circulation 2002;105:539–42.
[45] Kim RJ, Wu E, Rafael A, et al. The use of contrast-enhanced magnetic resonance imaging to identify reversible myocardial dysfunction. N Engl J Med 2000;343:1445–53.
[46] Mahrholdt H, Wagner A, Judd RM, et al. Delayed enhancement cardiovascular magnetic resonance assessment of nonischaemic cardiomyopathies. Eur Heart J 2005;26:1461–74.
[47] Choudhury L, Mahrholdt H, Wagner A, et al. Myocardial scarring in asymptomatic or mildly symptomatic patients with hypertrophic cardiomyopathy. J Am Coll Cardiol 2002;40:2156–64.
[48] McCrohon JA, Moon JC, Prasad SK, et al. Differentiation of heart failure related to dilated cardiomyopathy and coronary artery disease using gadolinium-enhanced cardiovascular magnetic resonance. Circulation 2003;108:54–9.

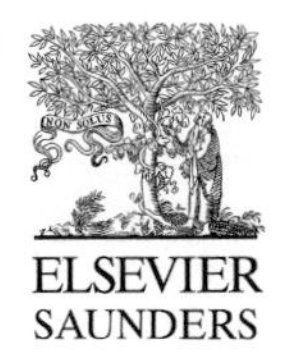
ELSEVIER
SAUNDERS

Cardiol Clin 25 (2007) 71–95

CARDIOLOGY
CLINICS

The Role of Cardiovascular MRI in Heart Failure and the Cardiomyopathies

James A. White, MD[a,b,*], Manesh R. Patel, MD[c]

[a]*Department of Medicine, Division of Cardiology, University of Western Ontario, 1151 Richmond Street, Suite 2, London, Ontario, Canada N6A 5B8*
[b]*London Health Sciences Center, 800 Commissioners Road East, PO Box 5010, London, Ontario, Canada N6A 5W9*
[c]*Department of Medicine, Division of Cardiology, Duke University Medical Center 3934, Durham, NC 27710, USA*

Heart failure represents a complex physiologic state characterized by a reduced cardiac output that is insufficient to meet systemic demands. The pathophysiology of this syndrome is complex due to the wide spectrum of underlying etiologic processes including ischemic heart disease, myocarditits, primary myocardial disease, hypertension, valvular heart disease, and acquired infiltrative and pericardial disorders. The differentiation of these conditions is paramount to the appropriate prescription of care within this population. Current guidelines for the management of heart failure [1] identify three general evaluation steps; (1) characterization of the myocardial and valvular structures and their function; (2) differentiation of ischemic versus nonischemic causes, including the identification of potentially modifiable substrate; and (3) risk stratification for therapeutic management, such as revascularization benefit. This process typically requires multiple investigations both noninvasive and invasive. The use of modern cardiovascular MRI (CMR) techniques provides the potential to address all three of these critical steps, centralizing diagnostic testing into a single imaging modality. The assessment of cardiac morphology, function, flow, perfusion, tissue injury, and fibrosis in a single imaging test offers the potential for a paradigm shift in the noninvasive diagnosis and monitoring of patients with congestive heart failure. In this review, the authors outline a diagnostic approach for the primary use of CMR in the phenotypic characterization, risk stratification, and therapeutic management of patients with congestive heart failure.

The cardiovascular MRI toolbox

A brief review of the repertoire of pulse sequences commercially available for CMR is crucial in understanding its ability to comprehensively evaluate patients with heart failure. These pulse sequences can be considered the CMR clinician's "toolbox" and include cine imaging using segmented, breath-held steady-state free precession (SSFP) or real-time pulse sequences; morphologic imaging using turbo spin-echo (TSE)-based sequences; perfusion imaging; inversion-recovery delayed-enhancement imaging; phase-contrast flow imaging; and more recently, three-dimensional SSFP coronary angiography. In addition, pulse sequences for the assessment of specific myocardial tissue characteristics such as iron overload and tissue edema are also under investigation. Overall, this expanding collection of available pulse sequences should be considered clinical instruments used to arrive at a diagnostic end point. They are to be dynamically selected by the CMR clinician based on the evolving phenotypic picture during the examination, highlighting the interactive role of the clinician and the technologist in the performance of high-quality CMR.

* Corresponding author.
E-mail address: white191@mc.duke.edu (J.A. White).

doi:10.1016/j.ccl.2007.02.003

A stepwise approach to the undifferentiated heart failure patient using cardiovascular MRI

A standardized, stepwise approach to the performance and interpretation of CMR offers the potential for a rapid and cost-effective diagnostic algorithm for patients who have undifferentiated heart failure. The steps outlined in the following sections illustrate how the information provided within the comprehensive CMR study affords not only differentiation of heart failure etiology but also risk stratification and optimal prescription of medical and invasive care.

Step 1: Assess morphology and function

The CMR heart failure evaluation should begin with the simultaneous assessment of myocardial structure and function using standard segmented, breath-held cine imaging. This imaging is typically performed in, although not limited to, the conventional serial short-axis views and the three cardinal long-axis views, as is the convention in echocardiography (Fig. 1). The ability of CMR to image in any plane without the need for optimal transthoracic imaging windows allows for unprecedented flexibility for the interrogation of abnormal heart structures. This characteristic can be exploited for the evaluation of specific structural or functional abnormalities that may not be best represented by conventional imaging planes, such as arrhythmogenic right ventricular cardiomyopathy (ARVC). Visual inspection of the left ventricular (LV) and right ventricular (RV) architecture identifies patterns of regional or diffuse wall thinning and concentric or asymmetric hypertrophy, and provide clues to other myopathic processes such as noncompaction. The atria and cardiac valves are similarly assessed for primary or secondary structural abnormalities, whereas the pericardium is assessed for thickness and calcification. Functional consequences of these morphologic changes are simultaneously evaluated through looped playback of the segmented cine image, making note of regional and global systolic function and valvular flow abnormalities.

The exceptional delineation of the blood–myocardium interface using SSFP pulse sequences allows for accurate and reproducible quantitative assessment of chamber dimensions and systolic function using manual or semiautomated planimetry techniques. Additional pulse sequences for the qualitative and quantitative assessment of ventricular function may be employed during the study. For example, tagged cine imaging can be performed to assist in the evaluation of tissue mechanics—a potentially valuable tool in patients being considered for cardiac resynchronization

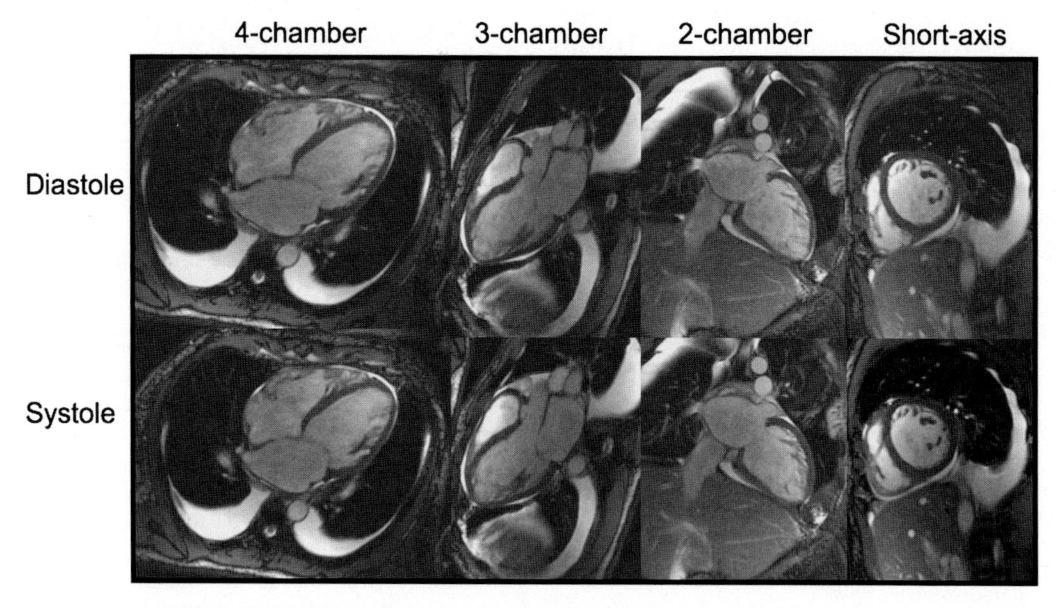

Fig. 1. Example of SSFP cineMRI in a patient who has idiopathic dilated cardiomyopathy. Four-chamber enlargement is accompanied by severe systolic dysfunction. A small pericardial effusion and a moderate-sized pleural effusion are also seen.

therapy (CRT). Systolic and diastolic performance indices can also be assessed through flow imaging of aortic outflow (stroke volume and cardiac output) and transmitral inflow patterns (E:A ratio, peak filling rate, and deceleration slope), respectively.

Step 2: Characterize the cardiomyopathy

As mentioned previously, the CMR clinician has a comprehensive toolbox of imaging techniques at his or her disposal to characterize the etiology of cardiomyopathy and to identify modifiable components in the disease process. Although frequently suspected on cine imaging, the etiology and severity of the underlying disease is frequently best characterized using specific pulse sequences designed for tissue characterization or perfusion. Certain cardiomyopathies may also require specialized imaging such as customized imaging planes or dedicated pulse sequences.

Tissue characterization—pattern of fibrosis

One of the most important advancements in CMR has been the development of delayed-enhancement MRI (DE-MRI), a technique that has dramatically expanded the role of CMR in the evaluation of heart failure patients. Highly specific patterns of fibrosis and scarring have been identified in many of the cardiomyopathy states [2,3] and are summarized in Fig. 2. Ischemic cardiomyopathy is characterized by subendocardial-based areas of late enhancement that correlate to irreversible myocardial necrosis on histopathology, a pattern consistent with the "wave front phenomenon" originally described by Reimer and colleagues [4]. Patients who have nonischemic dilated cardiomyopathy may also have DE-MRI evidence of scarring in up to 28% of cases; however, this is typically in a noncoronary distribution and frequently appears as a midwall striae [5]. Many of the remaining nonischemic cardiomyopathies similarly have distinctive patterns of late enhancement, including myocarditis, sarcoidosis, amyloidoisis, Anderson-Fabry's disease, Chagas' disease, ARVC, and myocardial noncompaction. Therefore, based on the presence and pattern of myocardial fibrosis, the etiology of the cardiomyopathy can be accurately ascertained.

Delineation of the underlying etiology is of clinical value for patients who have heart failure.

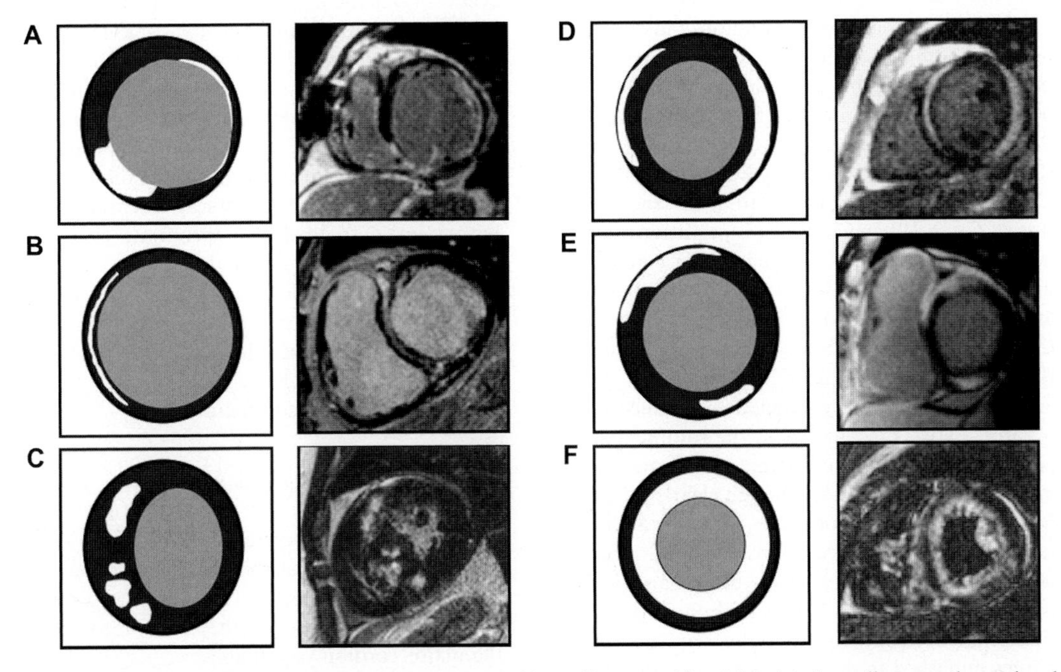

Fig. 2. Characteristic patterns of late enhancement in specific cardiomyopathies. (*A*) Ischemic cardiomyopathy: regional thinning with 50% transmural scar in lateral wall and 100% transmural scar in inferoseptal wall. (*B*) Idiopathic dilated cardiomyopathy: midwall late enhancement in the basal septum. (*C*) HCM: patchy late enhancement within septum. (*D*) Myocarditis: epicardial-zone late enhancement in inferolateral and anteroseptal walls. (*E*) Sarcoidosis: dense epicardial-zone late enhancement. (*F*) Amyloidosis: diffuse late enhancement progressing from subendocardium to epicardium (pattern may also be seen in uremic cardiomyopathy and post heart transplantation).

Further diagnostic and therapeutic strategies are highly dependent on this determination, as is the patient's long-term prognosis. Felker and colleagues [6] showed that survival is markedly different for etiologic subgroups of patients who had initially unexplained heart failure. Further, it has been recently appreciated that within these subgroups, the burden of myocardial fibrosis as seen on DE-MRI can identify higher-risk populations that have increased rates of mortality and cardiovascular events.

Identification of modifiable substrate

Cardiomyopathy patients frequently have varying degrees of myocardial fibrosis based on the subtype and the severity of their disease. Areas of myocardium free of significant fibrosis offer an important opportunity to modify this disease process, provided that a modifiable substrate can be identified. One of the most frequently sought modifiable substrates is myocardial ischemia, an evaluation effectively performed using CMR stress perfusion.

Current CMR first-pass stress perfusion techniques offer up to a 30-fold improvement in voxel resolution (2.8 × 1.8 × 8 mm) compared with conventional nuclear single-photon emission CT (SPECT) techniques. Studies to date have demonstrated comparable accuracy of CMR stress perfusion to that of nuclear SPECT imaging for the detection of coronary artery disease (CAD) [7–13]. Many of these studies, however, evaluated CMR stress perfusion in isolation for the detection of CAD. When CMR stress perfusion is evaluated in concert with delayed enhancement, an improvement in sensitivity and specificity (89% and 87%, respectively) is realized [14]. Overall, CMR stress perfusion is an accurate and valuable tool for the detection of underlying CAD.

The role of coronary magnetic resonance angiography (MRA) techniques in the routine assessment of patients with undifferentiated heart failure has not been examined. Although clearly valuable for the detection of anomalous coronary architecture [15,16], a wide range in sensitivity and specificity for the detection of obstructive coronary disease has been reported [17]. This variability represents significant heterogeneity in pulse sequence techniques published to date. The recent introduction of three-dimensional whole-heart SSFP techniques has reignited interest in coronary MRA, with improved signal-to-noise ratio and reduced complexity of scanning protocols. With the ongoing refinement of these three-dimensional MRA techniques, coronary imaging may become a valuable addition to the comprehensive CMR examination for patients with heart failure.

The modification of mechanical dyssynchrony has now become an important therapeutic target for heart failure patients with intraventricular dyssynchrony. The identification of dyssynchrony is routinely performed using tissue Doppler echocardiography techniques; however, the incorporation of such an evaluation into the CMR examination is also feasible. Tagged cine imaging, a process of delivering linear or grid-oriented saturation prepulses within the tissue imaging plane, creates a set of anatomic tissue landmarks that deform with ventricular contraction (Fig. 3). These landmarks can be used to track tissue mechanics such as time to peak contraction and regional strain [18]. Similarly, phase contrast imaging has been used to characterize ventricular dyssynchrony [19]. In a recently published head-to-head study, comparable estimations of ventricular dyssynchrony were seen with this technique versus tissue Doppler imaging in a population of patients referred for CRT [19]. Other techniques such as displacement encoding with stimulated echoes (DENSE) can also be used that offer high-resolution mapping of myocardial displacement with intrinsic black-blood T1 contrast, allowing clear separation of myocardium from blood pool [20]. Therefore, for patients being considered for CRT, a CMR study incorporating the accurate assessment of ejection fraction, intraventricular dyssynchrony, and scar distribution can be employed to identify appropriate candidates for this invasive and costly therapy.

Other modifiable, nonischemic etiologies include pericardial constriction, valvular heart disease, cardiac sarcoidosis, hemochromatosis, and Fabry's disease. The characterization of these conditions is discussed separately.

Characterization of specific nonischemic cardiomyopathies

The nonischemic cardiomyopathies are distinguished by unique morphologic, functional, and tissue characteristics. The following is a review of the important features as they pertain to each of the major cardiomyopathies.

Idiopathic dilated cardiomyopathy. Idiopathic dilated cardiomyopathy (IDC) is a diagnosis of exclusion. The term is applied following a systematic exclusion of all obvious or detectable causes of cardiomyopathy [21], including CAD, peripartum

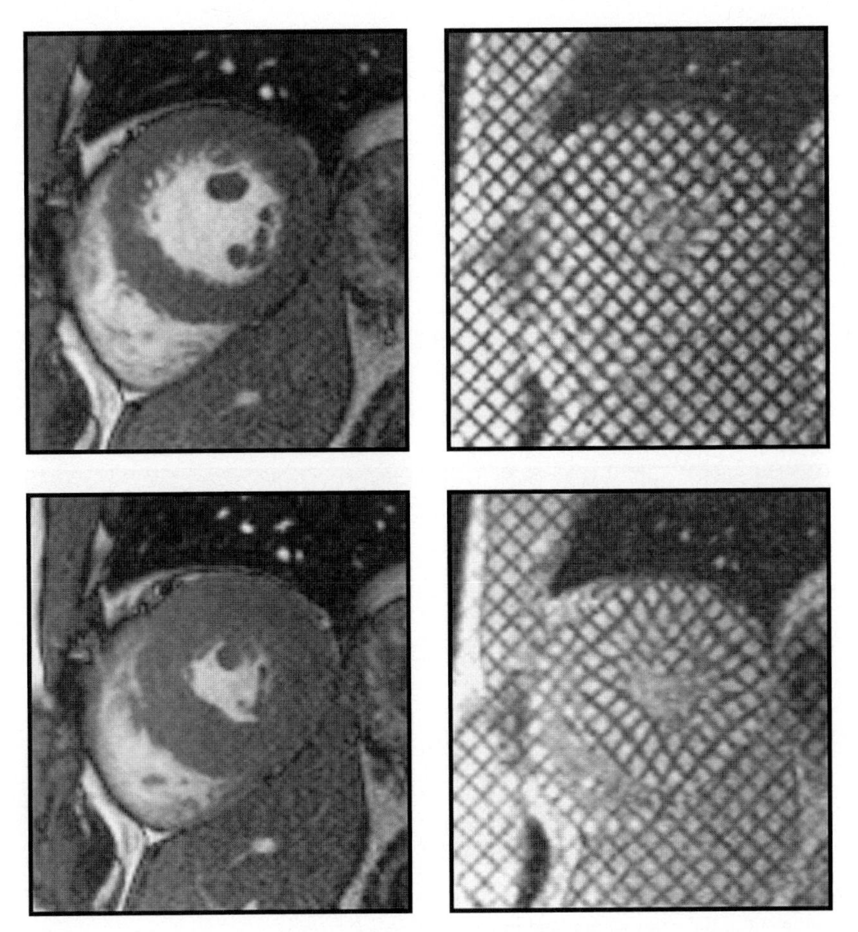

Fig. 3. Example of functional assessment using tagged cine imaging (*right images*). Corresponding nontagged cine images are shown (*left images*).

cardiomyopathy, toxin or chemotherapy exposure, tachycardia-induced cardiomyopathy, and certain endocrinopathies. Exclusion of these causes leaves a group of more elusive conditions that are frequently implicated in discussions of IDC, including infectious or autoimmune myocarditis, decompensated hypertensive heart disease, excessive alcohol exposure, and the familial myocardial diseases [21].

Several studies have demonstrated the high sensitivity (81%–100%) of DE-MRI for the detection of underlying CAD in patients who have poor LV function [5,22]. In contrast, patients who have IDC exhibit non–CAD-type scarring in approximately 10% to 28% of cases [5,22]. This scarring is typically midwall, predominantly involves the basal or mid portions of the interventricular septum (Fig. 4), and is more frequent in patients who have long-standing LV dysfunction.

Recently, McCrohon and colleagues [22] performed DE-MRI in patients who had ischemic cardiomyopathy and IDC diagnosed on the basis of coronary angiography findings. They reported that all patients (n = 27) who had ischemic cardiomyopathy displayed DE-MRI findings consistent with myocardial infarction. In patients who had IDC (n = 63), 41% were found to have scarring −13% in an ischemic pattern and 28% in a midwall nonischemic pattern. Other investigators have found similar data [23,24] that support that a diagnosis of IDC should be strongly considered when no scar or a midwall nonischemic scar pattern is seen in patients who have LV dysfunction. The mechanism of subendocardial scarring in patients who have normal coronary anatomy likely represents coronary artery embolism, vasospasm, or the spontaneous lysis of thrombus with minimal residual stenosis.

The presence of scarring in patients who have IDC has significant prognostic value. The presence of scarring on DE-MRI identifies patients who

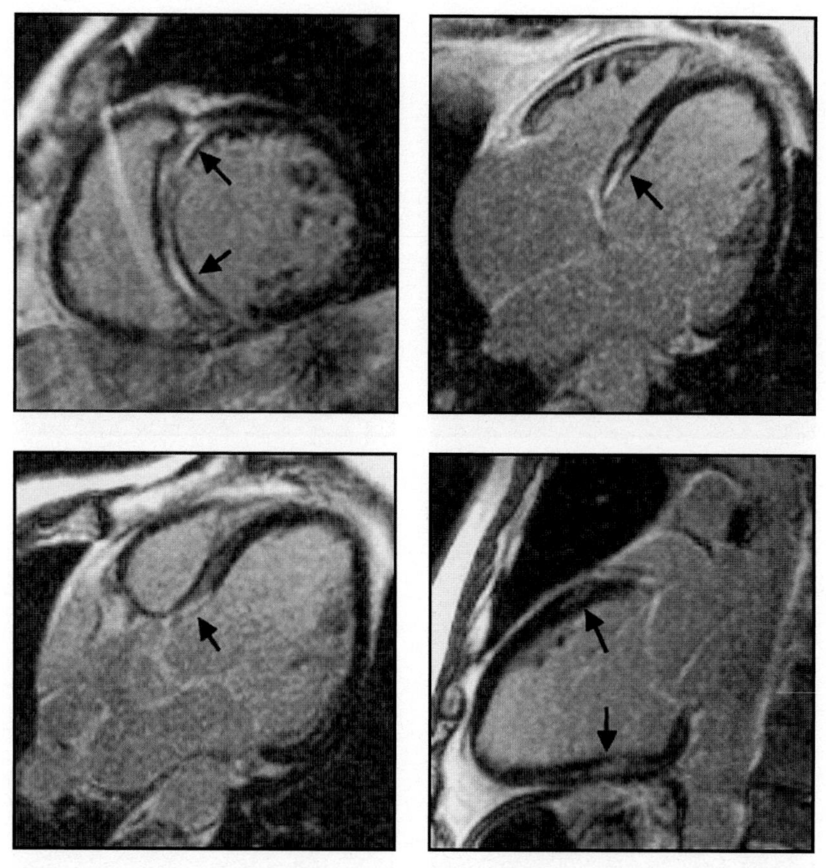

Fig. 4. Example of delayed enhancement MR images in a patient with idiopathic dilated cardiomyopathy. There is midwall hyperenhancement in the basal septum and inferior wall (*black arrows*).

have an elevated likelihood of inducible ventricular arrhythmias on electrophysiologic study [25] and those less likely to have recovery of systolic function during optimal medical therapy [26]. A recent study also supported the utility of DE-MRI in determining the future risk of cardiovascular events in patients who have IDC. In this study, the presence of midwall fibrosis, a finding seen in 35% of patients, was the single independent predictor of death or hospitalization (hazards ratio 3.4, $P = .01$), and predicted the occurrence of sudden cardiac death (SCD) or ventricular tachycardia (hazards ratio 5.2, $P = .03$) [27].

Myocarditis. In acute or fulminate cases of heart failure, the diagnosis of acute myocarditis should be considered. During the acute and subacute phases of myocarditis, CMR may aid in diagnosis and may differentiate this condition from ischemia-related disease [28]. Friedrich and colleagues [29] were the first to systematically evaluate myocardial hyperenhancement in patients who had myocarditis. Using a non–breath-held T1-weighted spin-echo pulse sequence, the investigators showed that hyperenhancement is present in patients who have acute myocarditis and evolves during the first 2 weeks after symptom onset. These techniques, however, produced regions of hyperenhancement that were on average 40% to 50% higher in signal intensity than normal regions. Current inversion-recovery DE-MRI techniques produce signal intensities over 400% higher than normal myocardium and have been similarly investigated in this population [30]. With the improved sensitivity of this technique, hyperenhancement was found to be a frequent finding, occurring in 28 of 32 patients (88%). Fig. 5 demonstrates an example of a patient who has acute myocarditis and a characteristic distribution of hyperenhancement. The epicardial

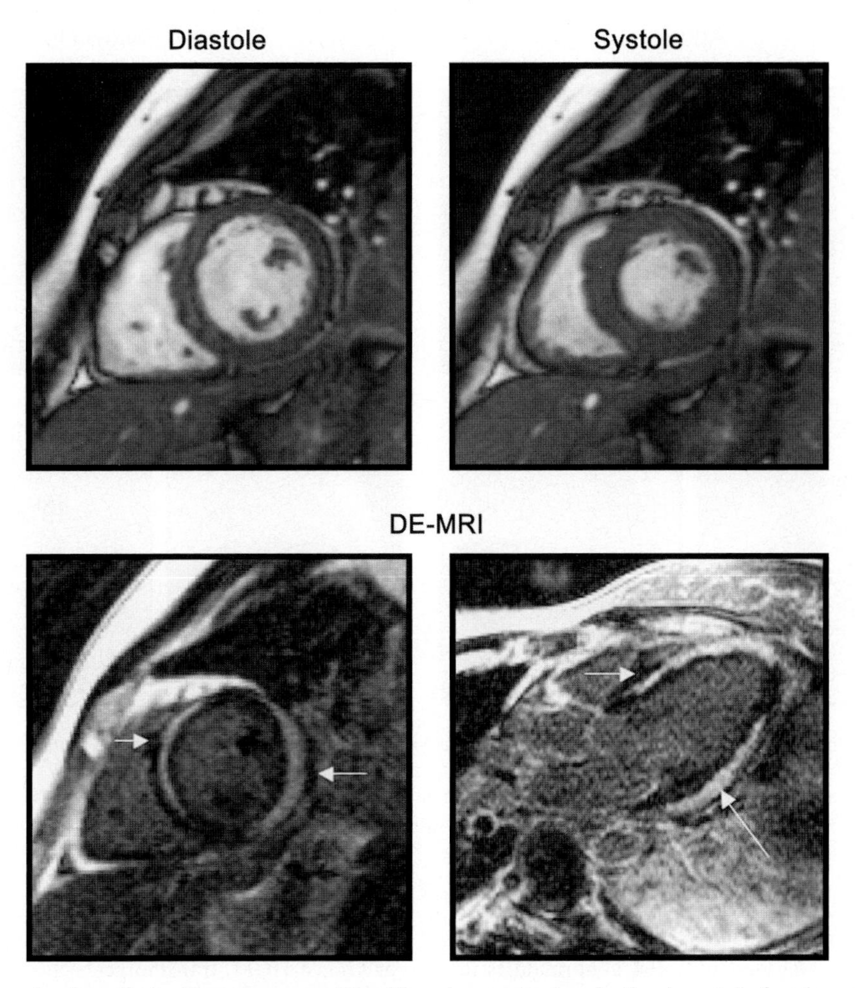

Fig. 5. Example of a patient with acute myocarditis. There is a moderate reduction in systolic function with marked epicardial zone hyperenhancement on delayed enhancement imaging (*white arrows*).

zone is typically affected, with varying degrees of progression toward the endocardium and sparring of the subendocardium. Involvement frequently localizes to the lateral and inferolateral walls. The anteroseptal wall may also be involved, in isolation and in combination, as is shown in this example. A recent article by Mahrholdt and colleagues [31] also suggested a potential relationship between pattern of hyperenhancement, etiologic viral agent, and disease course.

T2-weighted, black-blood fast spin-echo images may also demonstrate areas of increased signal in patients who have acute myocarditis (Fig. 6). The clinical utility of this finding has been investigated by Abdel-Aty and colleagues [32], who reported a sensitivity of 84% and a specificity of 74% for acute myocarditis, as defined by clinical criteria. Sensitivities as low as 45%, however, have also been reported [33], suggesting that this technique requires further investigation.

Patients who have chronic myocarditis, typically defined as the presence of chronic heart failure with no obstructive coronary disease and histologic evidence of myocarditis, may also demonstrate abnormalities on DE-MRI. De Cobelli and colleagues [34] showed that midwall hyperenhancement was present in 84% of patients who had chronic active myocarditis and in 44% who had borderline myocarditis by histologic criteria (N = 23). The pattern of hyperenhancement seen in these patients was identical to that typically seen with IDC, supporting the theory that a significant number of patients who have IDC may have myocarditis as a component of their

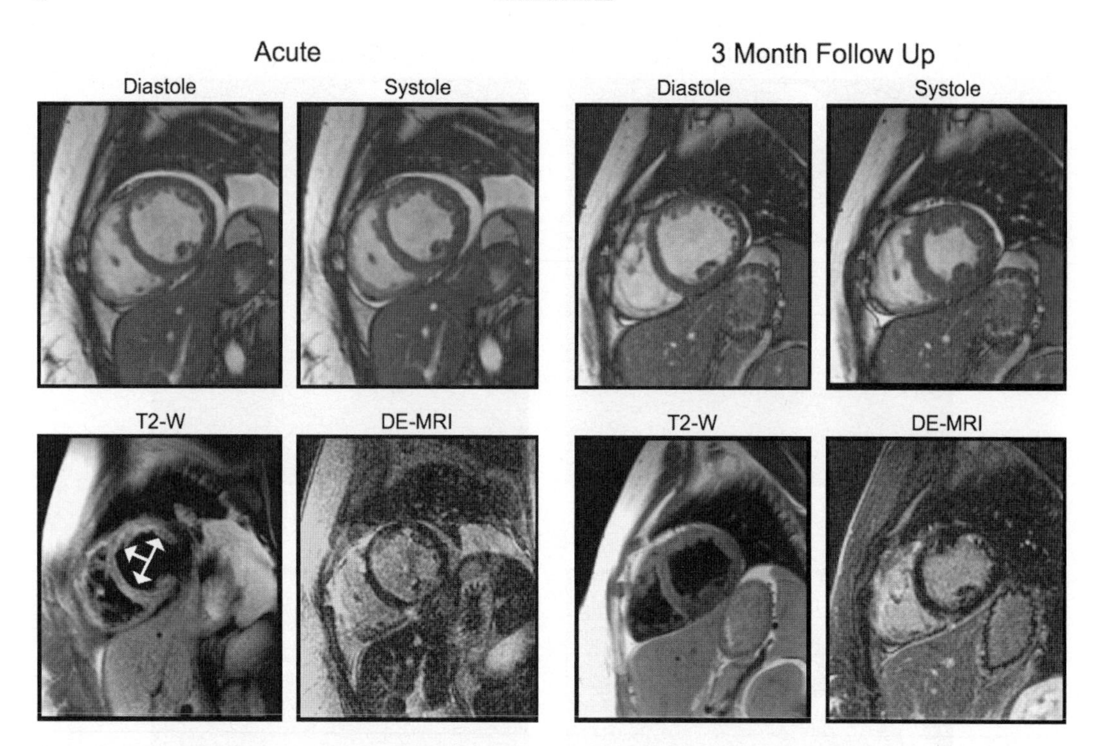

Fig. 6. Example of a patient presenting with fulminant myocarditis. Initial CMR assessment ("Acute") demonstrates severe systolic dysfunction with relative sparing of the lateral wall (*white arrows*). T2-weighted (T2-W) imaging shows marked increase in signal in myocardium with exception of lateral wall. Delayed-enhancement imaging (DE-MRI) shows minimal areas of necrosis. CMR performed 3 months later ("3 Month Follow Up") shows resolution of LV dysfunction, reduced T2 signal, and persistence of hyperenhancement.

pathophysiology. This study also reported that T2-weighted imaging demonstrated abnormalities in 36% of patients who had active myocarditis but in none who had borderline myocarditis.

Hypertrophic cardiomyopathy. HCM is a genetically transmitted disorder of the myocardium that affects approximately 2 per 1000 individuals [35]. The abnormal myocyte architecture seen in this condition has been linked to a myriad of genetic mutations involving contractile proteins, each leading to abnormal thickening of the myocardium in varying phenotypic patterns. Depending on the location and severity of this thickening, obstruction to LV blood flow can occur at the outflow tract or midventricular level. The ability of CMR to assessing myocardial architecture, tissue characteristics, function, and hemodynamics in these patients is unmatched.

The identification and quantification of myocardial hypertrophy in patients with HCM has been shown to be superior using cineMRI imaging versus echocardiography techniques [36,37]. In approximately 6% of patients who have suspected or known HCM, transthoracic echocardiography fails to detect the presence of hypertrophy compared with cineMRI evaluation [37]. This limitation is especially true for apical disease [38], for which CMR evaluation is now considered a class I indication (class II for other phenotypes) [39]. The extent of LV hypertrophy may also be significantly underestimated using echocardiographic techniques (maximal wall thickness 24 ± 3 mm by echocardiography versus 32 ± 1 mm with cineMRI, $P < .001$) [37]. Given that a maximal wall thickness of 30 mm or more is a predictor of SCD [40], these findings are of clinical significance. SSFP cine imaging is also of benefit for the visualization of systolic anterior motion of the mitral valve leaflet and the resultant flow disturbances from LV outflow tract obstruction and mitral insufficiency. These findings can be further interrogated using phase-contrast flow imaging (Fig. 7).

The recognition of increased wall thickness as a risk factor for SCD in HCM, independent of

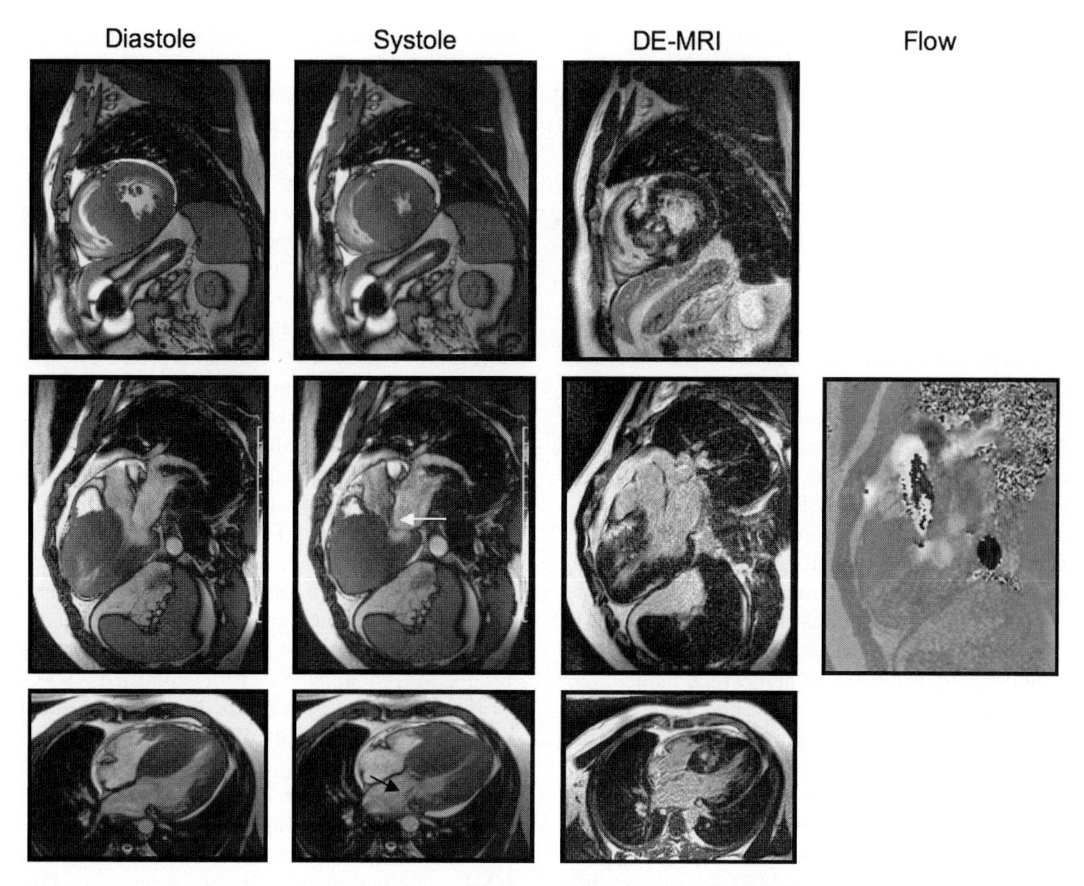

Fig. 7. Example of patient who has severe hypertrophic obstructive cardiomyopathy, shown in the mid–short-axis (*top row*), three-chamber (*middle row*), and four-chamber (*bottom row*) views. There is systolic anterior motion of the anterior mitral valve leaflet with resultant turbulent flow in the LV outflow tract (*white arrow*) and mitral insufficiency (*black arrow*). Delayed-enhancement imaging (DE-MRI) demonstrates marked fibrosis within the thickened portions of the interventricular septum. Phase contrast flow imaging (Flow) performed in the three-chamber view confirms flow acceleration originating within the LV outflow tract (image coregistered with cine image).

outflow tract obstruction, raises questions regarding the pathophysiologic mechanism of events in these patients. A study by Choudhury and colleagues [41] recognized that these regions of severely hypertrophied myocardium were more likely to contain scarring (as evidenced by DE-MRI)—a potential substrate for ventricular arrhythmias. The pattern of scarring seen is typically patchy, midmyocardial, and found at the junction of the interventricular septum and RV free walls (see Fig. 7) [41–44]. Scarring may also be apical in patients who have the apical variant of this disease [45]. Hyperenhancement in these patients correlates to areas of increased collagen deposition on histopathology [36]; however, the mechanism for this deposition remains to be elucidated. One pathologic study identified abnormal intramural arteries in regions of scarring, suggesting a potential ischemic mechanism [46]. Regardless of mechanism, it appears that the extent of scarring is related to disease progression, being more prevalent and extensive in patients who have more advanced structural disease [47].

The prognostic utility of delayed enhancement in patients who have HCM is currently under investigation. The burden of scarring has been shown to be inversely related to ejection fraction and is increased in patients who have recognized risk factors for SCD [48], suggesting that DE-MRI may be an important part of the evaluation of patients who have known or suspected HCM. Given its additional capabilities to view abnormal myocardial architecture in any imaging plane and assess flow gradients or associated valvular pathology, CMR is already an invaluable tool in the diagnosis and monitoring of patients with HCM. Further, it offers the ability to accurately assess therapeutic interventions such as alcohol septal ablation both with respect to the success of targeted therapy [49] and resultant ventricular remodeling [50].

Arrhythmogenic right ventricular cardiomyopathy. Arrhythmogenic right ventricular cardiomyopathy (ARVC) is a progressive cardiomyopathy characterized by fibro-fatty replacement of the myocardium and is associated with an elevated risk of arrhythmogenic death and right heart failure. Typically occurring in younger individuals, this cardiomyopathy is challenging to diagnose, drawing on clinical, morphologic, functional, and electrophysiologic parameters to meet current diagnostic criteria [51]. CMR is considered the diagnostic imaging test of choice in this population because it offers exceptional RV morphologic and functional characterization and may demonstrate abnormal characteristics of myocardial tissue.

Morphologically, the right ventricle may have regional wall thinning, hypertrophy, or dilation. Therefore, any architectural abnormality of the right ventricle in the absence of an explained cause should provoke a thorough examination of other functional and tissue abnormalities supportive of the diagnosis of ARVC. CineMRI is currently the most reproducible and valuable component of the ARVC CMR examination, carrying a 90% positive predictive value for ARVC [52]. Functional abnormalities may be global or segmental and range in severity depending on disease phenotype and stage. Particular attention should be given to the examination of the RV infundibulum extending to the RV apex and the inferior wall below the tricuspid valve annulus, known as the "triangle of dysplasia." Functional assessment should be performed in serial imaging planes in the short-axis and four-chamber views to provide full visualization of RV morphology and function. In addition, the authors recommend dedicated views of the RV outflow tract (right-sided three-chamber view) to assess for size and wall motion abnormalities in this region. Fig. 8 shows an example of a patient who has ARVC and characteristic regional RV dysfunction.

Two abnormal tissue types have been targeted for CMR evaluation in this population: fat and fibrous collagen deposition. Fatty replacement of RV and LV myocardium can be demonstrated using T1-weighted turbo spin-echo techniques. Interpretation of these findings is challenging, however, because the RV wall is a thin structure and adjacent pericardial fat frequently produces partial-volume effects leading to false-positive reports. Indeed, a recent report suggested a high rate of false-positive reporting for intramyocardial fat, leading to the erroneous diagnosis of ARVC [53]. Diagnostic accuracy is improved, however, when interpreted by experienced investigators [52,54], and this technique has been shown to predict arrhythmia inducibility in experienced hands [55]. Therefore, although potentially valuable, it is important for these images to be interpreted by experienced investigators and not used in isolation for establishing an "MRI diagnosis" of ARVC.

A role of delayed-enhancement imaging for the detection of fibrous collagen within the RV wall has also recently been proposed [56,57]. Optimally performed in concert with a fat-saturation prepulse to minimize adjacent pericardial fat signal, investigators have shown that delayed-enhancement imaging may demonstrate areas of increased gadolinium uptake within the RV free wall and interventricular septum in patients with confirmed ARVC. In one study, the presence of hyperenhancement predicted the inducibility of ventricular tachycardia at electrophysiologic testing [57]. This technique requires further investigation before it is routinely used in the evaluation of ARVC.

The diagnostic accuracy of the comprehensive CMR examination, inclusive of cine imaging, DE-MRI, and TSE imaging, is likely to be high in experienced hands for the detection of ARVC. A study including these components has recently reported a high sensitivity for the identification of task force–positive ARVC in a population being screened for familial disease [56]. Due to the rarity of this condition, however, there is an ongoing need for standardization of imaging protocols and registry networks to further evaluate diagnostic biomarkers for this disease.

The restrictive cardiomyopathies. The restrictive cardiomyopathies encompass primary and secondary diseases of the myocardium and pericardium, primarily limiting diastolic ventricular filling, although systolic function may also be impaired. The systematic CMR evalutation of myocardial function, tissue morphology, pericardial thickness, and transvalvular flow can reliably separate the various restrictive processes and differentiate them from common mimickers such as pulmonary vascular disease and pericardial effusion.

Constrictive pericarditis. The diagnosis of constrictive pericarditis requires morphologic

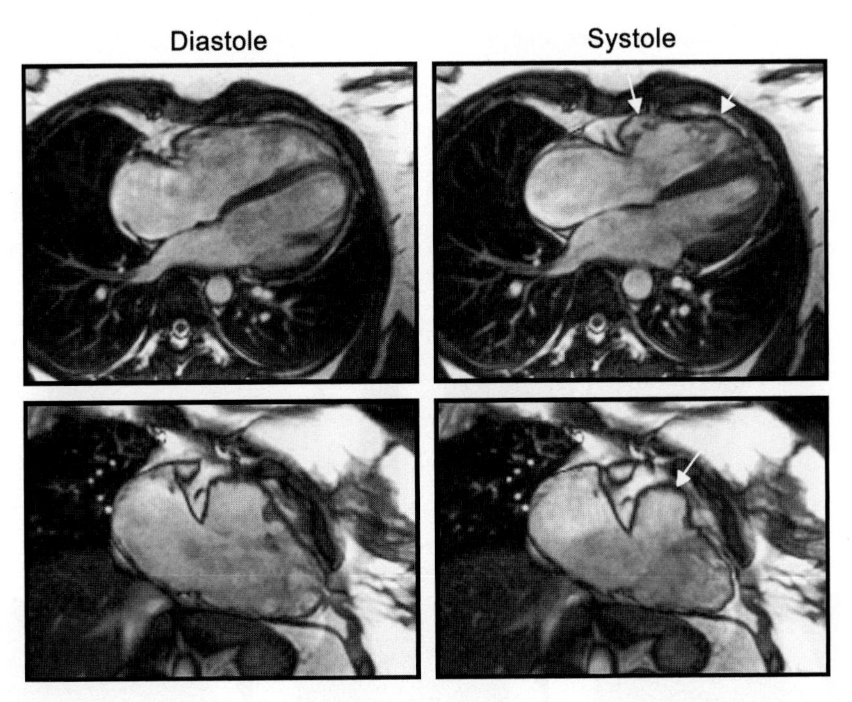

Fig. 8. Example of a patient with confirmed ARVC. Cine (SSFP) imaging of the four-chamber (*top row*) and right-sided two-chamber (*bottom row*) views demonstrates regional akinesis of the right ventricular wall (*arrows*).

confirmation of an abnormally thickened pericardium and demonstration of constrictive physiology. CMR may be the only imaging modality to reliably perform both of these evaluations. Short- and long-axis imaging is performed using the segmented SSFP cine pulse sequence to assess pericardial thickness and biventricular function. This methodology frequently identifies the characteristic diastolic septal "bounce" indicative of ventricular interdependence, a sign of constrictive physiology. Observation of this finding on cine-MRI has been shown to have a sensitivity of 81% and a specificity of 100% for the detection of surgically confirmed constriction among patients suspected of the disease [58]. The use of real-time cine imaging to confirm constrictive physiology should be employed whenever possible. By asking the patient to take slow, deep breaths during a 5- to 10-second short-axis, real-time cine acquisition in the midventricle, the early inspiratory flattening and inversion of the interventricular septum can be provoked [59]. An illustrative example of this is shown in Fig. 9.

Morphologic black-blood TSE pulse sequences may also be employed to confirm the presence of pericardial thickening (see Fig. 9). Using older, nongated versions of this technique (standard spin-echo pulse sequences), a pericardial thickness of more than 4 mm was found to be useful in identifying patients who had constriction, whereas a thickness less than 2 mm was found in normal individuals [60]. The normal parietal pericardium should appear as a faint or thin dark line layered between intrapericardial and extrapericardial fat. Calcification, if present, appears dark on all pulse sequences (see Fig. 9), although it is most clearly appreciated on proton density–weighted images. One particular advantage to performing TSE imaging in addition to SSFP cine imaging for the evaluation of pericardial thickening is related to the SSFP-related chemical shift artifact. This black line occurs frequently at the junction between fat and pericardial fluid (if present) and may be prominent in some cases and mistaken for pericardial thickening.

Finally, the use of tagged cine imaging can aid in identifying nondisjunction of the visceral and parietal pericardium throughout the cardiac cycle. Although patients may have a adherent pericardium without true constriction, such as post-pericardiotomy, this technique may be useful in select cases.

Sarcoidosis. Approximately 5% to 7% of patients who have sarcoidosis develop clinical

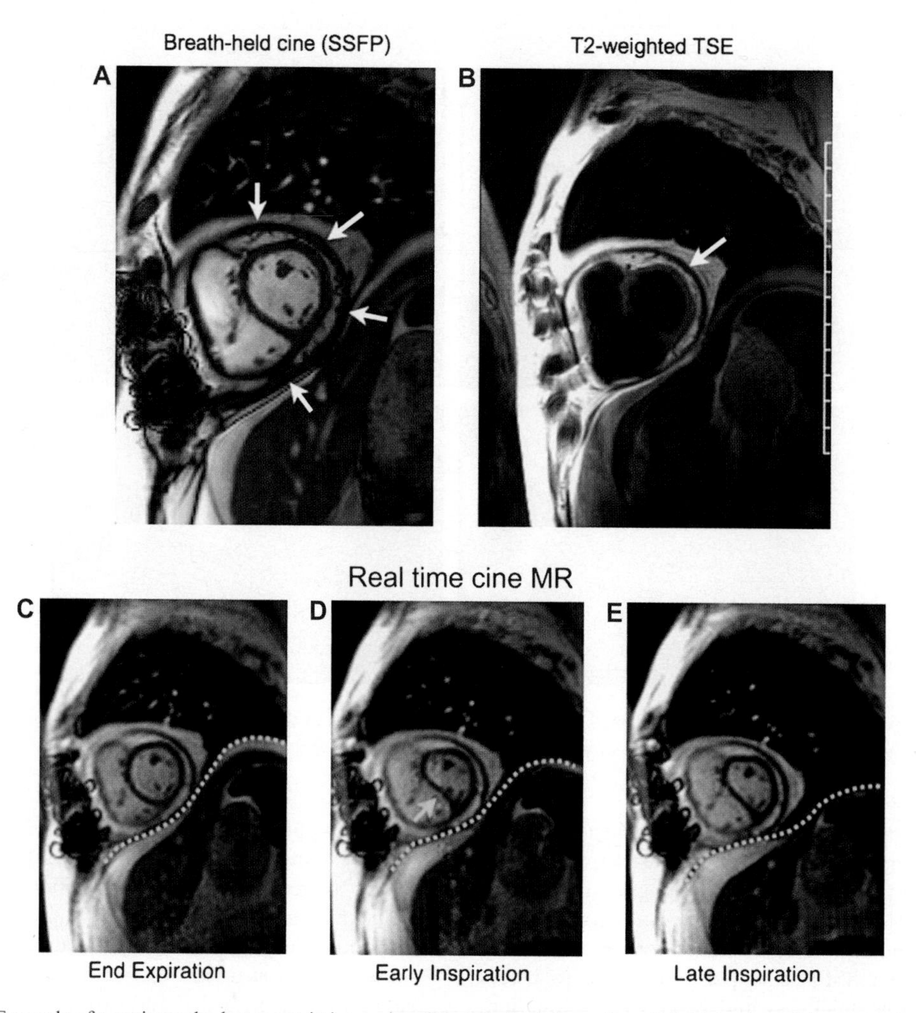

Fig. 9. Example of a patient who has constrictive pericarditis. Marked circumferential thickening of the parietal pericardium (*white arrows*) is demonstrated on (*A*) breath-held, segmented cineMRI and (*B*) T2-weighted, double inversion-recovery black-blood imaging. (*C–E*) Real-time cineMRI performed during free breathing. There is flattening and inversion of the interventricular septum (*yellow arrow*) during early inspiration (*diaphragm marked by dotted yellow line*).

evidence of cardiac involvement [61–64]; however, 20% to 30% will have pathologic evidence of such at autopsy [65–67]. Sudden cardiac death (SCD) is a leading cause of death in this patient population [68], suggesting that screening for cardiac involvement in patients who do not have cardiac symptoms is of potential value. Recent studies have demonstrated the ability of DE-MRI to detect cardiacs, a finding that frequently occurs in the absence of LV dysfunction [69,70]. The characteristic pattern of late enhancement in these patients is similar to other causes of myocarditis and is predominantly seen in the epicardial zone (Fig. 10). Although the anteroseptal and inferolateral walls are commonly involved, it is not uncommon to see enhancement in other territories, including the right ventricle. Until recently, the clinical relevance of this finding was unclear; however, in a study by Patel and colleagues [71], 81 patients who had biopsy-proven extracardiac sarcoidosis were found to have a relatively high prevalence of delayed enhancement. In comparison to the current Japan Ministry of Health Consensus Criteria for cardiac involvement, DE-MRI was twice as sensitive for the detection of cardiac involvement (26% versus 12%) and was the only independent predictor of adverse clinical events including cardiac death.

Amyloid cardiomyopathy. Cardiac involvement in systemic amyloidosis is common, occurring in up

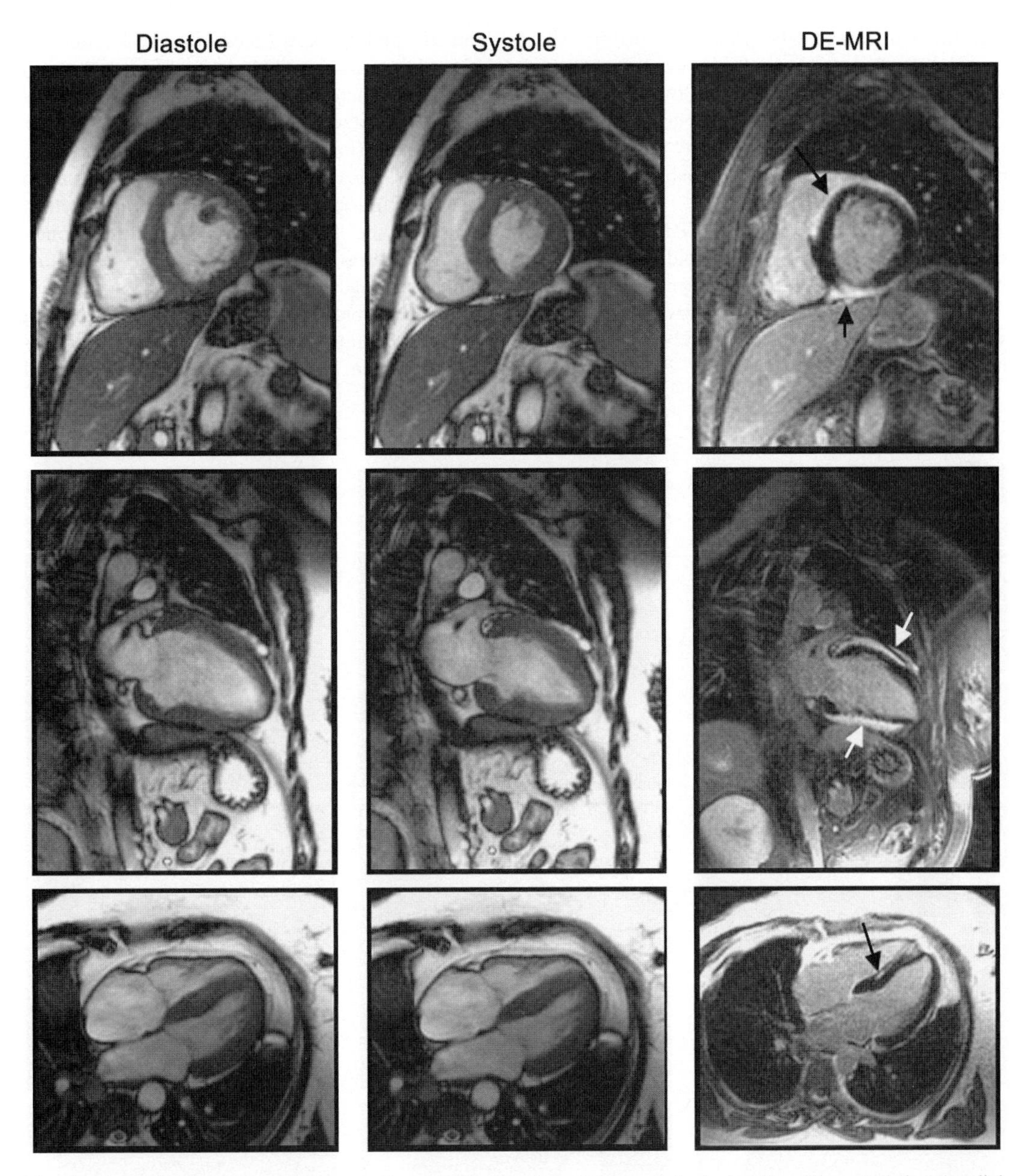

Fig. 10. Example of a patient who has cardiac sarcoidosis and moderate systolic dysfunction. Characteristic epicardial-zone dense fibrosis is seen on delayed-contrast imaging (DE-MRI) in the anteroseptal and inferior walls, with extension into the septum (*arrows*).

to 50% of patients with the most common form of this disease, AL or "primary" amyloidosis [72]. Amyloid infiltration of the myocardium is associated with a poor prognosis, with a median survival of only 6 months [72–74]. Confirmation of cardiac involvement requires pathologic examination of multiple endomyocardial tissue samples, with each sample having a 55% sensitivity for the detection of amyloid protein [75]. The ability to noninvasively document tissue involvement is therefore highly attractive for the diagnosis, risk stratification, and appropriate prescription of care in this population.

Several studies have reported a characteristic diffuse hyperenhancement pattern on DE-MRI, typically more prominent in the subendocardium and the basal segments (Fig. 11) [76,77]. Although varying degrees of myocyte apoptosis and fibrosis are seen histologically, the expansion of the mural interstitial space secondary to amyloid protein deposition likely plays a dominant role in the diffuse hyperenhancement pattern seen on DE-MRI.

A prognostic role for DE-MRI in patients suspected of having cardiac amyloid has recently been reported [78]. Among 46 patients with pathologically confirmed systemic amyloidosis and suspected cardiac involvement, 65% had diffuse hyperenhancement on DE-MRI. Patients who had this finding experienced a fourfold reduction in median survival (144 days versus 600 days) and had an increased rate of death or heart transplantation (hazard ratio 6.7).

The performance of DE-MRI in patients who have amyloidosis requires particular attention to the prescription of pulse sequence parameters, primarily the time from inversion (TI time). Fig. 12 demonstrates that tissues with an abnormally increased gadolinium volume of distribution have rapid T1 relaxation curves, allowing for clear separation of abnormal and normal myocardium when a TI time that nulls the normal

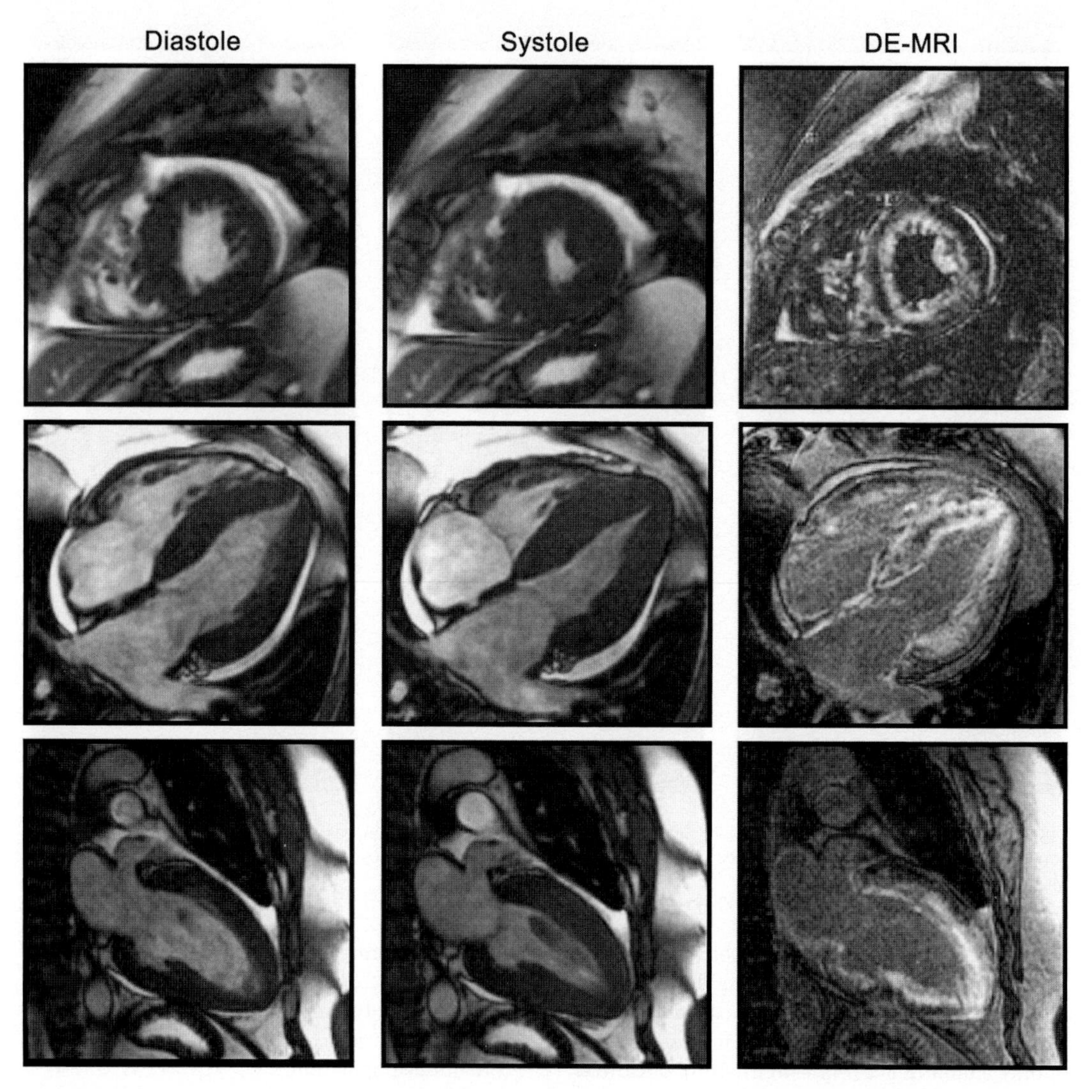

Fig. 11. Example of a patient who has systemic amyloidosis and cardiac involvement. Cine imaging shows thickened LV walls with preserved systolic function. Delayed-enhancement imaging (DE-MRI) demonstrates diffuse subendocardial gadolinium uptake in the LV and RV myocardium and interatrial septum.

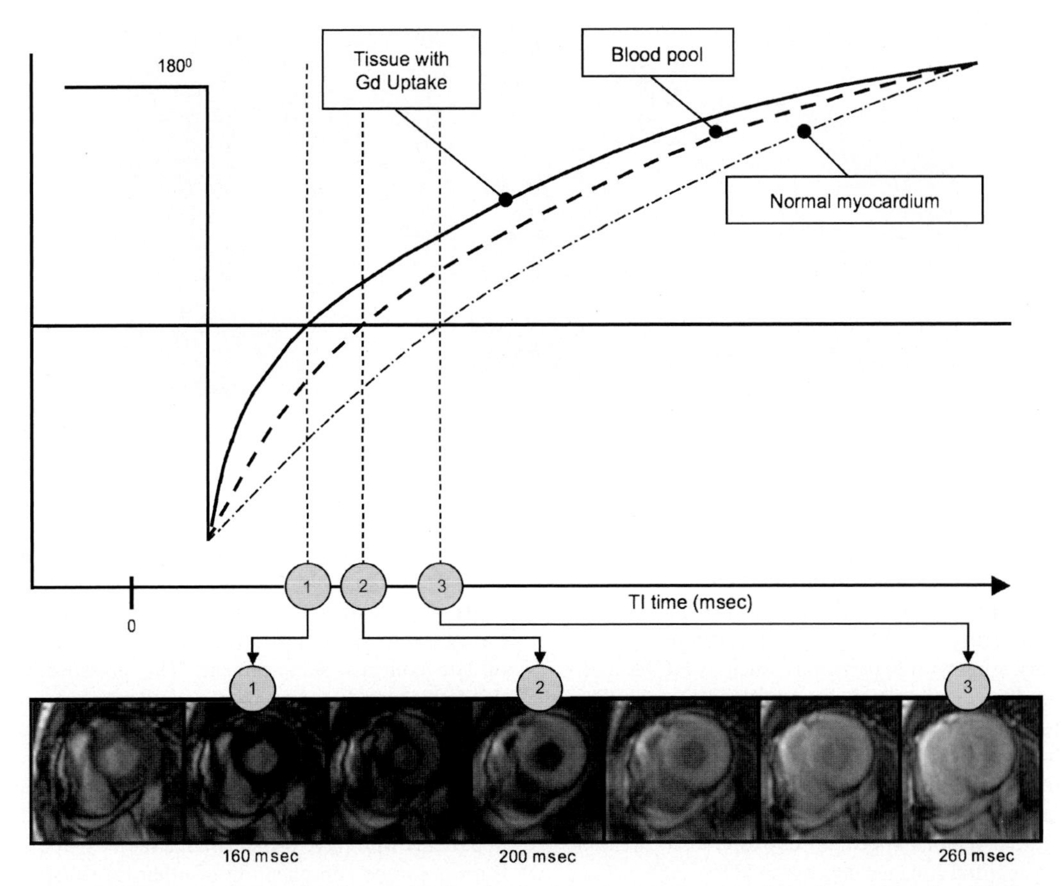

Fig. 12. Schematic diagram (*top*) of longitudinal magnetization recovery over time following an inversion (180°) prepulse. Normal myocardium reaches null point at time point 3, whereas blood pool reaches null point at time point 2. Myocardium with diffuse uptake of gadolinium (Gd) crosses at time point 1. TI scout images (*bottom*) demonstrate corresponding postcontrast image at given time points in a patient with cardiac amyloidosis and diffuse enhancement. Clearest delineation of abnormal tissue seen at time point 2. *Abbreviation:* msec, milliseconds.

myocardium is selected. However, when diffuse myocardial gadolinium uptake is present, however, the inability to null the myocardium inherently leads to difficulty in differentiating abnormal from normal tissue. By using a TI scout sequence (serial images using a range of TI times) to identify the TI times corresponding to the null point of the blood pool and the myocardium, the longer of these two values can be used to prescribe segmented imaging. This method ensures that abnormal tissue has an elevated signal compared with adjacent myocardium or blood pool. If the null point of blood is used one must confirm that myocardial T1 relaxation is abnormally shorter than that of blood (ie; the myocardium crosses the null point prior to blood pool on TI scout images [see Fig. 12]).

Anderson-Fabry's disease. Fabry's disease is an X-linked metabolic storage disorder caused by the genetic deficiency of lysosomal α-galactosidase A and results in the accumulation of glycosphingolipids in a variety of organs [79]. The classic Fabry's disease complex includes pain and hypohidrosis due to peripheral and autonomic nervous system involvement starting in adolescence. These symptoms are frequently followed by cardiac and renal involvement, which are the largest contributors of morbidity and mortality in this population [79]. Cardiac disease includes infiltration of the myocardium, conduction system, vascular endothelium, and cardiac valves. These complications occur more frequently in heterozygote female patients and, most notably, in a cardiac variant occurring in male patients.

CMR can be used to assess LV mass, function, and characteristic patterns of myocardial fibrosis. Moon and colleagues [80] reported that 50% of patients with genetically confirmed Fabry's disease

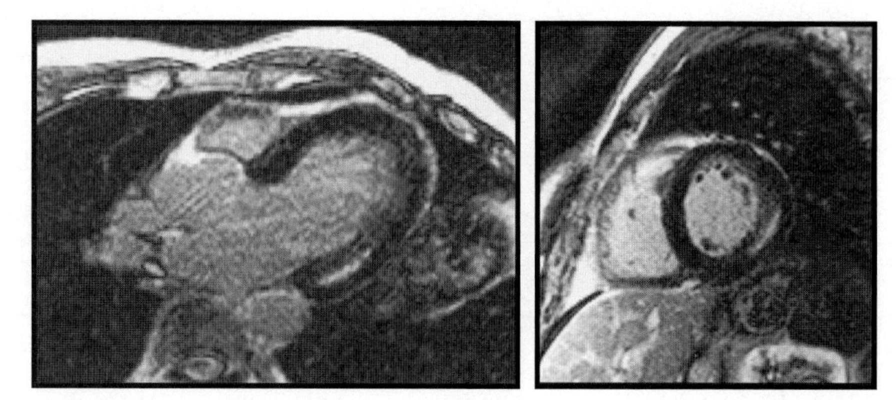

Fig. 13. Example of delayed enhancement images in a patient who has known Fabry's disease demonstrating typical midwall hyperenhancement in the posterolateral wall.

have midmyocardial hyperenhancement. In these patients, hyperenhancement was most frequently observed in the basal inferolateral wall, with sparing of the subendocardium (Fig. 13). This pattern of scarring is unique to other cardiomyopathies presenting with hypertrophy, such as HCM, making this an important distinguishing feature. This is clinically valuable as up to 5% of patients who have the diagnosis of HCM are subsequently found to have Fabry's disease [81], the treatment of which may be very different. Histologically, hyperenhanced regions appear to correspond to areas of myocardial collagen deposition [82].

With developing interest in the use of enzyme replacement therapy in this population [83], the accurate detection and monitoring of myocardial function and fibrosis in these patients may be of great importance. In support of this is a recent study of 35 patients who had genetically proven Fabry's disease that showed a 50% prevalence of late contrast enhancement. The presence of this finding predicted a lack of response to enzyme therapy as measured by regression of LV hypertrophy [84].

Iron overload cardiomyopathy. Heart failure due to iron overload is the leading cause of death in patients who have β-thalassemia major [85] and is a recognized complication of other transfusion-dependent anemias and hereditary hemochromatosis [86]. Because intensive chelation therapy

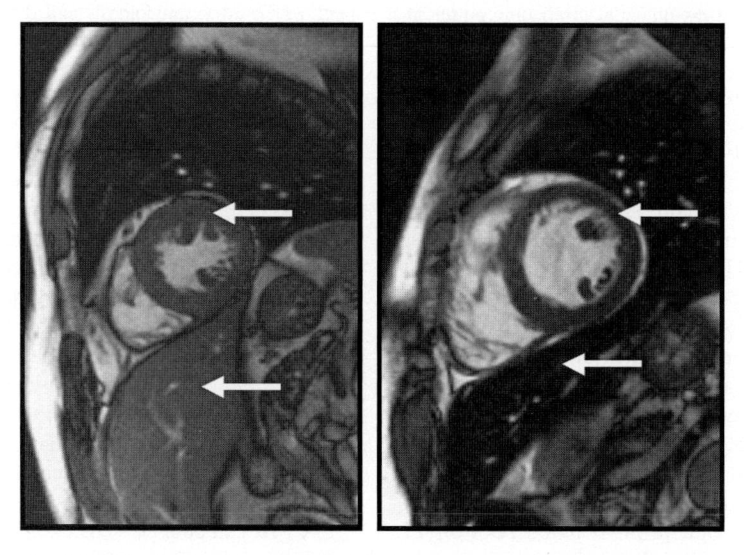

Fig. 14. Examples of an SSFP cine image of a normal patient (*left*) and a patient who has Beta thallasemia major (*right*). Observe the reduction in signal of the myocardium and liver, indicative of the rapid dephasing (T2*) effects consistent with iron overload.

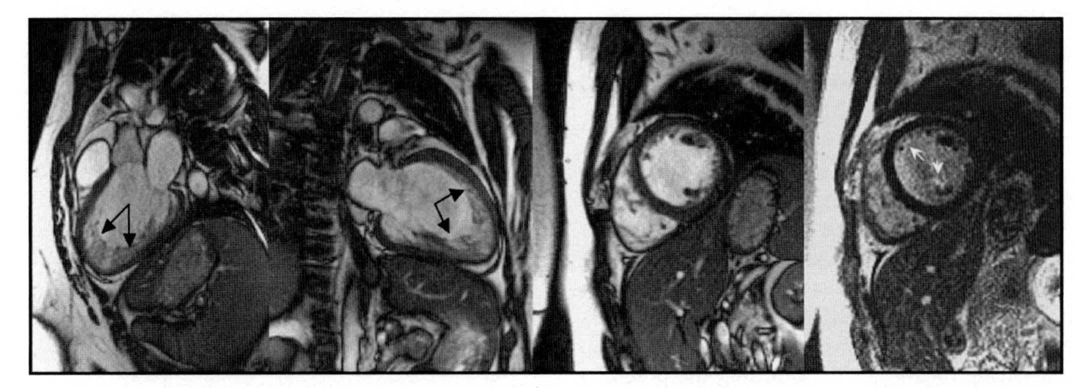

Fig. 15. Example of myocardial noncompaction. Delamination of myocardial architecture in the apical and mid segments seen on SSFP imaging (*black arrows*). Fibrosis may be seen within or surrounding abnormal papillary muscle bundles on delayed-contrast imaging (*white arrows*).

may attenuate or reverse ventricular dysfunction in these patients [87–89], the ability to identify and monitor myocardial iron overload is of clinical interest.

Routine cine imaging may suggest iron overload in moderate to severe cases. Rapid dephasing of proton spins occurs in tissues that have high ferrous content due an inherent inhomogeneity of local magnetic fields. This results in a loss of signal that translates into a darkening of involved organs on MRI (Fig. 14). The rate of intrinsic spin dephasing, known as T2*, can be quantified and used as a surrogate marker of tissue iron content. Studies have assessed the quantification of T2* as a tool for the assessment of iron overload cardiomyopathy in patients with β-thallasemia [90,91]. Once a time consuming process, a recent study has introduced a single breath-hold pulse sequence that varies the time to echo (TE time) sequentially on consecutive heartbeats, allowing for a more rapid determination [91]. Overall, these studies have shown that shortened myocardial T2* times correlate directly with increasing tissue iron levels, the occurrence of systolic and diastolic dysfunction, and clinical heart failure [90,92]. In addition, T2* lengthens in patients receiving aggressive chelation therapy and heralds improvements in LV function [93,94]. CMR is potentially the only imaging modality that currently provides a diagnostic and a prognostic evaluation of patients who have iron overload cardiomyopathy.

Endomyocardial fibroelastosis. Endomyocardial fibroelastosis can be seen early in life as a primary disorder or can present at any age secondary to disorders related to hypereosinophilia and leukemia [95]. Characterized by diffuse fibrosis and thickening of the endocardium with adherent thrombus, this condition may present with symptoms related to myocardial dysfunction, thromboembolism, or SCD [96]. Although little has been published on the role of CMR in evaluating patients suspected of this condition [97,98], the ability of CMR to accurately identify fibrosis and thrombus using inversion-recovery delayed-enhancement techniques makes this modality ideal for the identification and monitoring of such patients.

Myocardial noncompaction. Characterized by an abnormal architecture of the mid and distal LV segments and typically referred to as "noncompaction," this cardiomyopathy has an estimated prevalence of 0.05% in the general population. Morphologically, these patients have exaggerated areas of noncompacted myocardium. Delamination of the myocardium is a normal finding and is seen, to some degree, in over 90% of healthy subjects [99]. In this population, however, excessive separation of endocardial muscle bundles is associated with progressive systolic dysfunction in addition to ventricular arrhythmias and embolic events from LV thrombus [100,101]. Due to its apical predominance, MRI has been used to provide optimal imaging and evaluation of ventricular architecture and function. A study by Petersen and colleagues [99] showed that a maximal diastolic ratio of noncompacted to compact myocardium of 2.3:1 had a sensitivity of 86% and a specificity of 99% for the identification of myocardial noncompaction cardiomyopathy. The authors have also observed a characteristic pattern of hyperenhancement within the abnormal, noncompacted myocardium and related papillary muscles on DE-MRI, suggesting that myocardial fibrosis may be part of the disease's natural history (Fig. 15).

Chagas' disease. Chagas' disease is an inflammatory disease caused by the parasitic protozoan *Trypanosoma cruzi.* Heart failure is a late manifestation of chronic infection, occurring in approximately 20% of patients, and is typically preceded by a long asymptomatic phase. DE-MRI can identify cardiac involvement during this asymptomatic phase, affording the potential for therapy before the development of overt heart failure. It can also characterize the severity of cardiac involvement, showing a close correlation with ECG abnormalities, LV dysfunction, and ventricular arrhythmias. In a study by Rochitte and colleagues [102], the prevalence of scarring by DE-MRI progressively increased from 20% in asymptomatic patients who did not have evidence of structural heart disease to 100% in patients who had LV dysfunction and ventricular tachycardia. Another study by Bocchi and colleagues [103] showed a similar 100% prevalence of hyperenhancement in patients who had biopsy-proven Chagas' disease. In comparison, only 70% of these patients were shown to have abnormalities by gallium 67 imaging. Hyperenhancement typically occurs in the epicardial portions of the LV apex and inferolateral wall, although transmural scarring and patterns mimicking subendocardial myocardial infarction have also been seen.

Uremic cardiomyopathy. Patients who have end-stage renal disease (ESRD) are known to have an elevated prevalence of myocardial dysfunction, LV hypertrophy, and cardiovascular mortality [104]. Although this population's demographics reflect an increased prevalence of conventional risk factors for heart failure, such as hypertension and diabetes, a pleotropic mechanism of the uremic milieu on the myocardium has also been proposed that leads to interstitial fibrosis and LV dysfunction [105,106]. A study by Mark and colleagues [107] was recently published that demonstrated a high prevalence (28%) of hyperenhancement on DE-MRI in 134 patients who had ESRD. Half of these patients had a nonischemic pattern that was described as diffuse. In this report, however, the scarring appeared to be regional and did not involve all segments. In the authors' experience, a delayed-enhancement pattern phenotypically similar to amyloid cardiomyopathy may also be seen in patients who have ESRD. This finding is typically associated with marked concentric hypertrophy. These patients frequently demonstrate increased precontrast tissue signal on T1-weighted imaging sequences such as gradient-echo perfusion sequences. Although pathologic examination of endomyocardial biopsies yields no evidence of amyloid deposition in these patients, they are burdened by a similarly poor prognosis (unpublished data).

Step 3: Risk stratification and therapeutic management

Implications of myocardial scar: prognosis and patient risk stratification

The role of scar determination in the risk stratification of heart failure patients is rapidly expanding. As discussed in the prior sections related to specific cardiomyopathies, the presence of myocardial scar identifies subgroups at high risk of clinical cardiac events in patients with IDC [27], HCM [48], Chagas' disease [102], sarcoidosis [71], and amyloidosis [78]. The presence of scarring on DE-MRI has also been shown to identify arrhythmic substrate in patients who have ischemic cardiomyopathy [108,109], IDC [25,27], chronic myocarditis [34], and ARVC [57]. DE-MRI, therefore, has the potential to assist in the prescription of care aimed at high-risk individuals, for example, the use of implantable cardiac defibrillators for the prevention of SCD.

Implications of myocardial scar: response to therapy

Therapy aimed at modifying the course of disease relies on this disease's substrate being modifiable. This concept is being increasingly supported as the literature demonstrating the relationship between myocardial scar burden and response to medical and invasive therapy expands, offering a physiologic explanation for recognized disparities in response rates between ischemic and nonischemic heart failure patients [110]. Myocardial scar burden by DE-MRI is a strong predictor of functional or clinical improvement in heart failure patients undergoing medical therapy, surgical and percutaneous revascularization therapy, as well as device therapy for the purpose of resynchronization.

Bello and colleagues [24] showed that functional recovery in patients undergoing β-blocker therapy for chronic heart failure is strongly related to the transmural extent of myocardial scarring. Contractility improved in 56% of segments with no scarring versus only 3% of segments with 75% or more scarring. Similarly, in patients undergoing surgical revascularization, the probability of improvement in contractile function in dysfunctional segments is inversely related to the transmural extent of scarring (Fig. 16). In patients who had ventricular dysfunction undergoing bypass surgery, 78% of patients with no scar showed evidence for functional recovery versus only 2% patients with 75% or more transmural scar [111]. Further, in segments with akinesia or dyskinesia, this relationship is even stronger, with 86% improving when there is no scar and 0% improving when there is more than 75% scar (see Fig. 16). These results have since been reproduced by other investigators [112]. A recent study by Baks and colleagues [113] demonstrated that functional recovery following recanalization of chronic total occlusions using a drug-eluting stent is also predicted by DE-MRI. Therefore, decisions regarding therapy for dysfunctional myocardium by way of medical or any invasive revascularization technique may be best accomplished through the advanced use of DE-MRI.

The use of device therapy is a rapidly expanding therapy in patients who have systolic heart failure. CRT is recognized for its ability to improve heart failure symptoms, mitral insufficiency, and mortality in select patients who have LV dyssynchrony [114]. Approximately 30% of heart failure patients, however, do not respond to this invasive and costly therapy. Two recent, independent studies by Bleeker and colleagues [115] and White and colleagues [116] showed that posterolateral wall scar and septal wall scar, respectively, negate the benefits of CRT. It is therefore apparent that regional viability is critical for targeted dysnchronous myocardial segments to respond to and to propagate electrical stimulation from biventricular pacing therapy [116]. The use of DE-MRI offers a novel concept in defining the appropriateness of pacing therapy in patients otherwise meeting current inclusion criteria.

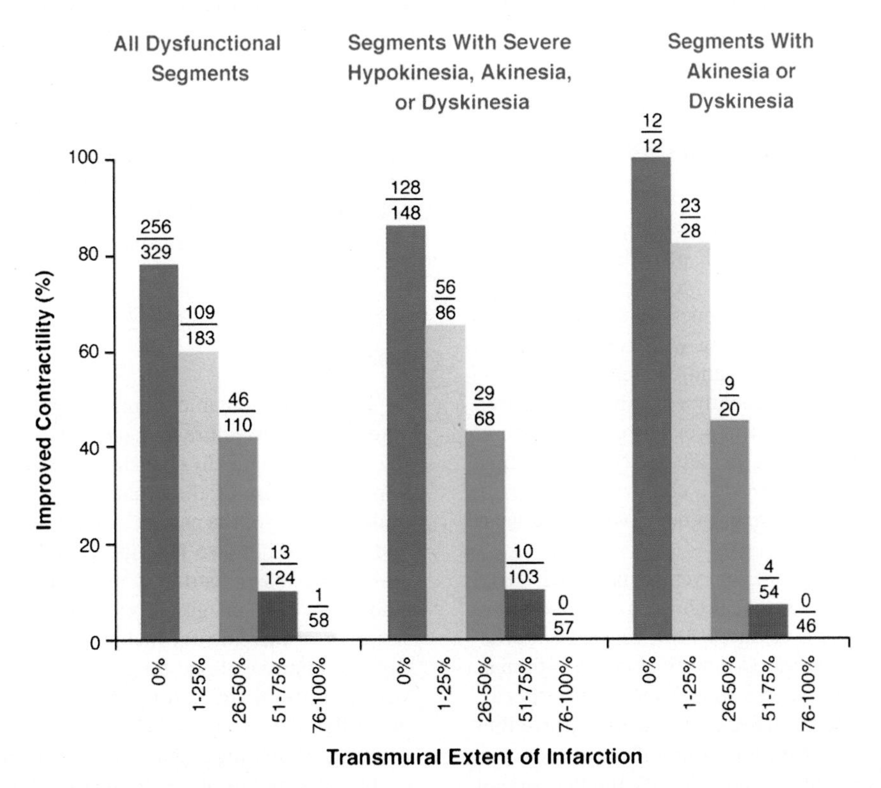

Fig. 16. Relationship between infarction transmurality and likelihood of functional improvement following surgical revascularization. (*From* Kim RJ, Wu E, Rafael A, et al. The use of contrast-enhanced magnetic resonance imaging to identify reversible myocardial dysfunction. N Engl J Med 2000;343(20):1445–53; with permission.)

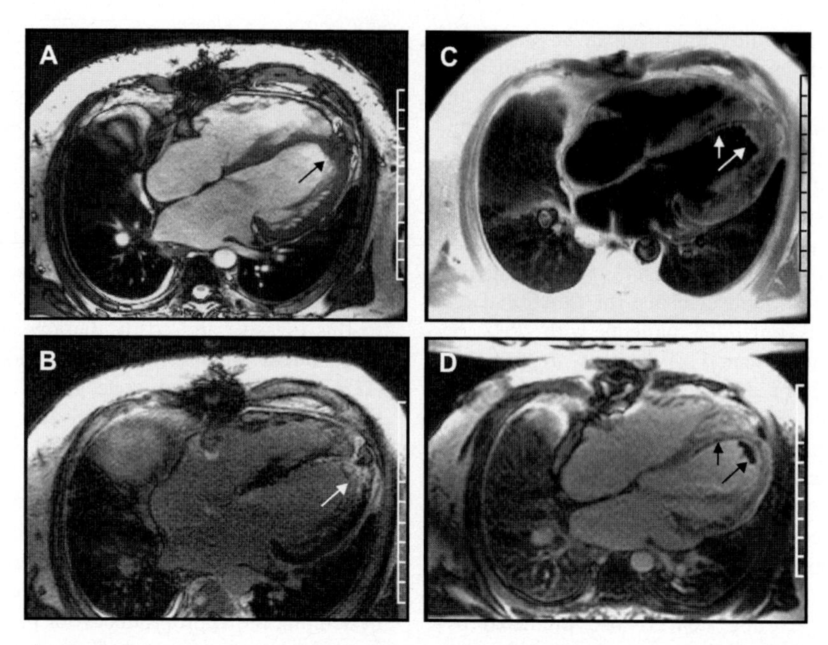

Fig. 17. Example of apical thrombus in a patient who had prior myocardial infarction. (*A*) SSFP imaging shows and akinetic, thickened segment (*black arrow*) in apex of left ventricle. (*B*) Double inversion-recovery TSE (black-blood) imaging delineates an endoluminal structure (*white arrow*) separate from the LV wall. (*C*) Late enhancement identifies myocardial infarction as substrate for thrombus formation (*white arrows*) but poorly differentiates thrombus. (*D*) "Long-TI" delayed enhancement image accurately depicts apical thrombus and thrombus extending along septal wall (*black arrows*).

Supplemental information provided by cardiovascular MRI

In addition to the assessment of myocardial disease and function, CMR provides valuable and detailed assessments of valvular morphology, function, and hemodynamics. A significant portion of patients presenting with congestive heart failure have primary and/or secondary valve dysfunction that frequently contributes to deteriorating cardiac performance. The combination of routine cine imaging planes and phase contrast flow imaging can provide a comprehensive evaluation of valve disease in patients who have heart failure.

The development of ventricular and atrial thrombi is also a frequent concern in heart failure patients owing to reduced flow, scarred endothelium, and an increased rate of atrial arrhythmias. CMR has been shown to be superior to echocardiography for the detection of cardiac thrombus [117]. The application of a modified inversion-recovery postcontrast imaging technique, similar to that used in scar imaging, allows for clear identification of luminal thrombus (Fig. 17). By prescribing a TI time equivalent to the null point of tissue with no gadolinium uptake (typically 600–650 milliseconds), thrombus appears black, whereas all other tissues appear gray or bright.

Summary

The evaluation and management of patients who have heart failure and specific cardiomyopathies remains clinically challenging. Essential to the appropriate care of these patients is not only an understanding of the patient's cardiac morphology and function but also identification of pathologic and modifiable substrate. Current care often includes multiple imaging studies during the prescription of incremental therapeutic interventions such as pharmacologic therapies, myocardial revascularization, and cardiac resynchronization or defibrillator therapy. CMR represents a single evolving technology that potentially addresses each of these points of care for heart failure patients through the application of commercially available techniques. Careful application of this technology provides an opportunity to improve diagnostic efficiency and care in these patients.

References

[1] Hunt SA, Baker DW, Chin MH, et al. ACC/AHA guidelines for the evaluation and management of chronic heart failure in the adult: executive summary a report of the American College of Cardiology/American Heart Association Task Force on Practice Guidelines (Committee to Revise the 1995 Guidelines for the Evaluation and Management of Heart Failure): developed in collaboration with the International Society for Heart and Lung Transplantation; Endorsed by the Heart Failure Society of America. Circulation 2001;104(24): 2996–3007.

[2] Mahrholdt H, Wagner A, Judd RM, et al. Delayed enhancement cardiovascular magnetic resonance assessment of non-ischaemic cardiomyopathies. Eur Heart J 2005;26(15):1461–74.

[3] Shah DJ, Judd RM, Kim R, et al. In: Edelman RR, Hesselink JR, Zlatkin MB, editors. Clinical magnetic resonance imaging. 3rd edition. New York: Elsevier; 2006.

[4] Reimer KA, Lowe JE, Rasmussen MM, et al. The wavefront phenomenon of ischemic cell death. 1. Myocardial infarct size vs duration of coronary occlusion in dogs. Circulation 1977;56(5):786–94.

[5] Soriano CJ, Ridocci F, Estornell J, et al. Noninvasive diagnosis of coronary artery disease in patients with heart failure and systolic dysfunction of uncertain etiology, using late gadolinium-enhanced cardiovascular magnetic resonance. J Am Coll Cardiol 2005;45(5):743–8.

[6] Felker GM, Thompson RE, Hare JM, et al. Underlying causes and long-term survival in patients with initially unexplained cardiomyopathy. N Engl J Med 2000;342(15):1077–84.

[7] Cury RC, Cattani CA, Gabure LA, et al. Diagnostic performance of stress perfusion and delayed-enhancement MR imaging in patients with coronary artery disease. Radiology 2006;240(1):39–45.

[8] Plein S, Greenwood JP, Ridgway JP, et al. Assessment of non-ST-segment elevation acute coronary syndromes with cardiac magnetic resonance imaging. J Am Coll Cardiol 2004;44(11):2173–81.

[9] Paetsch I, Jahnke C, Wahl A, et al. Comparison of dobutamine stress magnetic resonance, adenosine stress magnetic resonance, and adenosine stress magnetic resonance perfusion. Circulation 2004; 110(7):835–42.

[10] Wolff SD, Schwitter J, Coulden R, et al. Myocardial first-pass perfusion magnetic resonance imaging: a multicenter dose-ranging study. Circulation 2004;110(6):732–7.

[11] Ishida N, Sakuma H, Motoyasu M, et al. Noninfarcted myocardium: correlation between dynamic first-pass contrast-enhanced myocardial MR imaging and quantitative coronary angiography. Radiology 2003;229(1):209–16.

[12] Sensky PR, Samani NJ, Reek C, et al. Magnetic resonance perfusion imaging in patients with coronary artery disease: a qualitative approach. Int J Cardiovasc Imaging 2002;18(5):373–83 [discussion: 385–376].

[13] Al-Saadi N, Nagel E, Gross M, et al. Noninvasive detection of myocardial ischemia from perfusion reserve based on cardiovascular magnetic resonance. Circulation 2000;101(12):1379–83.

[14] Klem I, Heitner JF, Shah DJ, et al. Improved detection of coronary artery disease by stress perfusion cardiovascular magnetic resonance with the use of delayed enhancement infarction imaging. J Am Coll Cardiol 2006;47(8):1630–8.

[15] Bunce NH, Lorenz CH, Keegan J, et al. Coronary artery anomalies: assessment with free-breathing three-dimensional coronary MR angiography. Radiology 2003;227(1):201–8.

[16] Casolo G, Del Meglio J, Rega L, et al. Detection and assessment of coronary artery anomalies by three-dimensional magnetic resonance coronary angiography. Int J Cardiol 2005;103(3):317–22.

[17] Budoff MJ, Achenbach S, Duerinckx A. Clinical utility of computed tomography and magnetic resonance techniques for noninvasive coronary angiography. J Am Coll Cardiol 2003;42(11): 1867–78.

[18] Lardo AC, Abraham TP, Kass DA. Magnetic resonance imaging assessment of ventricular dyssynchrony: current and emerging concepts. J Am Coll Cardiol 2005;46(12):2223–8.

[19] Westenberg JJ, Lamb HJ, van der Geest RJ, et al. Assessment of left ventricular dyssynchrony in patients with conduction delay and idiopathic dilated cardiomyopathy: head-to-head comparison between tissue Doppler imaging and velocity-encoded magnetic resonance imaging. J Am Coll Cardiol 2006;47(10):2042–8.

[20] Aletras AH, Wen H. Mixed echo train acquisition displacement encoding with stimulated echoes: an optimized DENSE method for in vivo functional imaging of the human heart. Magn Reson Med 2001;46(3):523–34.

[21] Burkett EL, Hershberger RE. Clinical and genetic issues in familial dilated cardiomyopathy. J Am Coll Cardiol 2005;45(7):969–81.

[22] McCrohon JA, Moon JC, Prasad SK, et al. Differentiation of heart failure related to dilated cardiomyopathy and coronary artery disease using gadolinium-enhanced cardiovascular magnetic resonance. Circulation 2003;108(1):54–9.

[23] Wu E, Judd RM, Vargas JD, et al. Visualisation of presence, location, and transmural extent of healed Q-wave and non-Q-wave myocardial infarction. Lancet 2001;357(9249):21–8.

[24] Bello D, Shah DJ, Farah GM, et al. Gadolinium cardiovascular magnetic resonance predicts

reversible myocardial dysfunction and remodeling in patients with heart failure undergoing beta-blocker therapy. Circulation 2003;108(16): 1945–53.
[25] Nazarian S, Bluemke DA, Lardo AC, et al. Magnetic resonance assessment of the substrate for inducible ventricular tachycardia in nonischemic cardiomyopathy. Circulation 2005;112(18): 2821–5.
[26] Park S, Choi BW, Rim SJ, et al. Delayed hyperenhancement magnetic resonance imaging is useful in predicting functional recovery of nonischemic left ventricular systolic dysfunction. J Card Fail 2006; 12(2):93–9.
[27] Assomull RG, Prasad SK, Lyne J, et al. Cardiovascular magnetic resonance, fibrosis, and prognosis in dilated cardiomyopathy. J Am Coll Cardiol 2006; 48:1977–85.
[28] Laissy JP, Hyafil F, Feldman LJ, et al. Differentiating acute myocardial infarction from myocarditis: diagnostic value of early- and delayed-perfusion cardiac MR imaging. Radiology 2005;237(1): 75–82.
[29] Friedrich MG, Strohm O, Schulz-Menger J, et al. Contrast media-enhanced magnetic resonance imaging visualizes myocardial changes in the course of viral myocarditis. Circulation 1998;97(18): 1802–9.
[30] Mahrholdt H, Goedecke C, Wagner A, et al. Cardiovascular magnetic resonance assessment of human myocarditis: a comparison to histology and molecular pathology. Circulation 2004;109(10):1250–8.
[31] Mahrholdt H, Wagner A, Deluigi CC, et al. Presentation, patterns of myocardial damage, and clinical course of viral myocarditis. Circulation 2006; 114(15):1581–90.
[32] Abdel-Aty H, Boye P, Zagrosek A, et al. Diagnostic performance of cardiovascular magnetic resonance in patients with suspected acute myocarditis: comparison of different approaches. J Am Coll Cardiol 2005;45(11):1815–22.
[33] Laissy JP, Messin B, Varenne O, et al. MRI of acute myocarditis: a comprehensive approach based on various imaging sequences. Chest 2002;122(5): 1638–48.
[34] De Cobelli F, Pieroni M, Esposito A, et al. Delayed gadolinium-enhanced cardiac magnetic resonance in patients with chronic myocarditis presenting with heart failure or recurrent arrhythmias. J Am Coll Cardiol 2006;47(8):1649–54.
[35] Maron BJ, Gardin JM, Flack JM, et al. Prevalence of hypertrophic cardiomyopathy in a general population of young adults. Echocardiographic analysis of 4111 subjects in the CARDIA Study. Coronary artery risk development in (young) adults. Circulation 1995;92(4):785–9.
[36] Moon JC, Reed E, Sheppard MN, et al. The histologic basis of late gadolinium enhancement cardiovascular magnetic resonance in hypertrophic cardiomyopathy. J Am Coll Cardiol 2004;43(12): 2260–4.
[37] Rickers C, Wilke NM, Jerosch-Herold M, et al. Utility of cardiac magnetic resonance imaging in the diagnosis of hypertrophic cardiomyopathy. Circulation 2005;112(6):855–61.
[38] Moon JC, Fisher NG, McKenna WJ, et al. Detection of apical hypertrophic cardiomyopathy by cardiovascular magnetic resonance in patients with non-diagnostic echocardiography. Heart 2004; 90(6):645–9.
[39] Pennell DJ, Sechtem UP, Higgins CB, et al. Clinical indications for cardiovascular magnetic resonance (CMR): consensus panel report. Eur Heart J 2004;25(21):1940–65.
[40] Sorajja P, Nishimura RA, Ommen SR, et al. Use of echocardiography in patients with hypertrophic cardiomyopathy: clinical implications of massive hypertrophy. J Am Soc Echocardiogr 2006;19(6): 788–95.
[41] Choudhury L, Mahrholdt H, Wagner A, et al. Myocardial scarring in asymptomatic or mildly symptomatic patients with hypertrophic cardiomyopathy. J Am Coll Cardiol 2002;40(12):2156–64.
[42] Soler R, Rodriguez E, Monserrat L, et al. Magnetic resonance imaging of delayed enhancement in hypertrophic cardiomyopathy: relationship with left ventricular perfusion and contractile function. J Comput Assist Tomogr 2006;30(3):412–20.
[43] Teraoka K, Hirano M, Ookubo H, et al. Delayed contrast enhancement of MRI in hypertrophic cardiomyopathy. Magn Reson Imaging 2004;22(2): 155–61.
[44] Amano Y, Takayama M, Takahama K, et al. Delayed hyper-enhancement of myocardium in hypertrophic cardiomyopathy with asymmetrical septal hypertrophy: comparison with global and regional cardiac MR imaging appearances. J Magn Reson Imaging 2004;20(4):595–600.
[45] Jassal DS, Chaithiraphan V, Neilan TG, et al. Delayed contrast enhancement CMR imaging in apical hypertrophic cardiomyopathy. Int J Cardiol 2006;113(2):e56–7.
[46] Maron BJ, Wolfson JK, Epstein SE, et al. Intramural ("small vessel") coronary artery disease in hypertrophic cardiomyopathy. J Am Coll Cardiol 1986;8(3):545–57.
[47] Moon JC, Mogensen J, Elliott PM, et al. Myocardial late gadolinium enhancement cardiovascular magnetic resonance in hypertrophic cardiomyopathy caused by mutations in troponin I. Heart 2005;91(8):1036–40.
[48] Moon JC, McKenna WJ, McCrohon JA, et al. Toward clinical risk assessment in hypertrophic cardiomyopathy with gadolinium cardiovascular magnetic resonance. J Am Coll Cardiol 2003;41(9):1561–7.
[49] van Dockum WG, ten Cate FJ, ten Berg JM, et al. Myocardial infarction after percutaneous transluminal septal myocardial ablation in hypertrophic

obstructive cardiomyopathy: evaluation by contrast-enhanced magnetic resonance imaging. J Am Coll Cardiol 2004;43(1):27–34.
[50] van Dockum WG, Beek AM, ten Cate FJ, et al. Early onset and progression of left ventricular remodeling after alcohol septal ablation in hypertrophic obstructive cardiomyopathy. Circulation 2005;111(19):2503–8.
[51] McKenna WJ, Thiene G, Nava A, et al. Diagnosis of arrhythmogenic right ventricular dysplasia/cardiomyopathy. Task Force of the Working Group Myocardial and Pericardial Disease of the European Society of Cardiology and of the Scientific Council on Cardiomyopathies of the International Society and Federation of Cardiology. Br Heart J 1994;71(3):215–8.
[52] Tandri H, Castillo E, Ferrari V, et al. Magnetic resonance imaging of arrhythmogenic right ventricular dysplasia. J Am Coll Cardiol 2006;48:2277–84.
[53] Bomma C, Rutberg J, Tandri H, et al. Misdiagnosis of arrhythmogenic right ventricular dysplasia/cardiomyopathy. J Cardiovasc Electrophysiol 2004; 15(3):300–6.
[54] Tandri H, Calkins H, Nasir K, et al. Magnetic resonance imaging findings in patients meeting task force criteria for arrhythmogenic right ventricular dysplasia. J Cardiovasc Electrophysiol 2003;14(5): 476–82.
[55] Auffermann W, Wichter T, Breithardt G, et al. Arrhythmogenic right ventricular disease: MR imaging vs angiography. AJR Am J Roentgenol 1993; 161(3):549–55.
[56] Sen-Chowdhry S, Prasad SK, Syrris P, et al. Cardiovascular magnetic resonance in arrhythmogenic right ventricular cardiomyopathy revisited: comparison with task force criteria and genotype. J Am Coll Cardiol 2006;48(10):2132–40.
[57] Tandri H, Saranathan M, Rodriguez ER, et al. Noninvasive detection of myocardial fibrosis in arrhythmogenic right ventricular cardiomyopathy using delayed-enhancement magnetic resonance imaging. J Am Coll Cardiol 2005;45(1):98–103.
[58] Giorgi B, Mollet NR, Dymarkowski S, et al. Clinically suspected constrictive pericarditis: MR imaging assessment of ventricular septal motion and configuration in patients and healthy subjects. Radiology 2003;228(2):417–24.
[59] Francone M, Dymarkowski S, Kalantzi M, et al. Assessment of ventricular coupling with real-time cine MRI and its value to differentiate constrictive pericarditis from restrictive cardiomyopathy. Eur Radiol 2006;16(4):944–51.
[60] Masui T, Finck S, Higgins CB. Constrictive pericarditis and restrictive cardiomyopathy: evaluation with MR imaging. Radiology 1992;182(2):369–73.
[61] Newman LS, Rose CS, Maier LA. Sarcoidosis. N Engl J Med 1997;336(17):1224–34.
[62] Sharma OP, Maheshwari A, Thaker K. Myocardial sarcoidosis. Chest 1993;103(1):253–8.
[63] Shammas RL, Movahed A. Sarcoidosis of the heart. Clin Cardiol 1993;16(6):462–72.
[64] Johns CJ, Michele TM. The clinical management of sarcoidosis. A 50-year experience at the Johns Hopkins Hospital. Medicine (Baltimore) 1999;78(2): 65–111.
[65] Silverman KJ, Hutchins GM, Bulkley BH. Cardiac sarcoid: a clinicopathologic study of 84 unselected patients with systemic sarcoidosis. Circulation 1978;58(6):1204–11.
[66] Roberts WC, McAllister HA Jr, Ferrans VJ. Sarcoidosis of the heart. A clinicopathologic study of 35 necropsy patients (group I) and review of 78 previously described necropsy patients (group II). Am J Med 1977;63(1):86–108.
[67] Iwai K, Sekiguti M, Hosoda Y, et al. Racial difference in cardiac sarcoidosis incidence observed at autopsy. Sarcoidosis 1994;11(1):26–31.
[68] Virmani R, Bures JC, Roberts WC. Cardiac sarcoidosis: a major cause of sudden death in young individuals. Chest 1980;77(3):423–8.
[69] Smedema JP, Snoep G, van Kroonenburgh MP, et al. Evaluation of the accuracy of gadolinium-enhanced cardiovascular magnetic resonance in the diagnosis of cardiac sarcoidosis. J Am Coll Cardiol 2005;45(10):1683–90.
[70] Tadamura E, Yamamuro M, Kubo S, et al. Effectiveness of delayed enhanced MRI for identification of cardiac sarcoidosis: comparison with radionuclide imaging. AJR Am J Roentgenol 2005;185(1):110–5.
[71] Patel M, Cawley P, Heitner JF, et al. Detection and prognostic significance of myocardial damage in patients with sarcoidosis using delayed-enhancement cardiac magnetic resonance. Circulation 2006; 114(Suppl II):408 [abstract].
[72] Falk RH, Comenzo RL, Skinner M. The systemic amyloidoses. N Engl J Med 1997;337(13):898–909.
[73] Falk RH. Diagnosis and management of the cardiac amyloidoses. Circulation 2005;112(13): 2047–60.
[74] Kholova I, Niessen H. Amyloid in the cardiovascular system: a review. J Clin Pathol 2005;58:125–33.
[75] Pellikka PA, Holmes DR Jr, Edwards WD, et al. Endomyocardial biopsy in 30 patients with primary amyloidosis and suspected cardiac involvement. Arch Intern Med 1988;148(3):662–6.
[76] Maceira AM, Joshi J, Prasad SK, et al. Cardiovascular magnetic resonance in cardiac amyloidosis. Circulation 2005;111(2):186–93.
[77] Perugini E, Rapezzi C, Piva T, et al. Non-invasive evaluation of the myocardial substrate of cardiac amyloidosis by gadolinium cardiac magnetic resonance. Heart 2006;92(3):343–9.
[78] White J, Patel M, Shah DJ, et al. Prognostic utility of delayed enhancement magnetic resonance imaging in patients with systemic amyloidosis and suspected cardiac involvement. Circulation 2006;114: 679 [abstract].

[79] Eng CM, Germain DP, Banikazemi M, et al. Fabry disease: guidelines for the evaluation and management of multi-organ system involvement. Genet Med 2006;8(9):539–48.
[80] Moon JC, Sachdev B, Elkington AG, et al. Gadolinium enhanced cardiovascular magnetic resonance in Anderson-Fabry disease. Evidence for a disease specific abnormality of the myocardial interstitium. Eur Heart J 2003;24(23):2151–5.
[81] Sachdev B, Takenaka T, Teraguchi H, et al. Prevalence of Anderson-Fabry disease in male patients with late onset hypertrophic cardiomyopathy. Circulation 2002;105(12):1407–11.
[82] Moon JC, Sheppard M, Reed E, et al. The histological basis of late gadolinium enhancement cardiovascular magnetic resonance in a patient with Anderson-Fabry disease. J Cardiovasc Magn Reson 2006;8(3):479–82.
[83] Ries M, Clarke JT, Whybra C, et al. Enzyme-replacement therapy with agalsidase alfa in children with Fabry disease. Pediatrics 2006;118(3):924–32.
[84] Beer M, Weidemann F, Breunig F, et al. Impact of enzyme replacement therapy on cardiac morphology and function and late enhancement in Fabry's cardiomyopathy. Am J Cardiol 2006;97(10): 1515–8.
[85] Borgna-Pignatti C, Rugolotto S, De Stefano P, et al. Survival and disease complications in thalassemia major. Ann N Y Acad Sci 1998;850:227–31.
[86] Olson LJ, Edwards WD, McCall JT, et al. Cardiac iron deposition in idiopathic hemochromatosis: histologic and analytic assessment of 14 hearts from autopsy. J Am Coll Cardiol 1987;10(6): 1239–43.
[87] Aldouri MA, Wonke B, Hoffbrand AV, et al. High incidence of cardiomyopathy in beta-thalassaemia patients receiving regular transfusion and iron chelation: reversal by intensified chelation. Acta Haematol 1990;84(3):113–7.
[88] Easley RM Jr, Schreiner BF Jr, Yu PN. Reversible cardiomyopathy associated with hemochromatosis. N Engl J Med 1972;287(17):866–7.
[89] Rahko PS, Salerni R, Uretsky BF. Successful reversal by chelation therapy of congestive cardiomyopathy due to iron overload. J Am Coll Cardiol 1986; 8(2):436–40.
[90] Anderson LJ, Holden S, Davis B, et al. Cardiovascular T2-star (T2*) magnetic resonance for the early diagnosis of myocardial iron overload. Eur Heart J 2001;22(23):2171–9.
[91] Westwood M, Anderson LJ, Firmin DN, et al. A single breath-hold multiecho T2* cardiovascular magnetic resonance technique for diagnosis of myocardial iron overload. J Magn Reson Imaging 2003;18(1):33–9.
[92] Tanner MA, Galanello R, Dessi C, et al. Myocardial iron loading in patients with thalassemia major on deferoxamine chelation. J Cardiovasc Magn Reson 2006;8(3):543–7.
[93] Anderson LJ, Westwood MA, Holden S, et al. Myocardial iron clearance during reversal of siderotic cardiomyopathy with intravenous desferrioxamine: a prospective study using T2* cardiovascular magnetic resonance. Br J Haematol 2004; 127(3):348–55.
[94] Jensen PD, Jensen FT, Christensen T, et al. Evaluation of myocardial iron by magnetic resonance imaging during iron chelation therapy with deferrioxamine: indication of close relation between myocardial iron content and chelatable iron pool. Blood 2003;101(11):4632–9.
[95] Ino T, Benson LN, Freedom RM, et al. Natural history and prognostic risk factors in endocardial fibroelastosis. Am J Cardiol 1988;62(7):431–4.
[96] De Letter EA, Piette MH. Endocardial fibroelastosis as a cause of sudden unexpected death. Am J Forensic Med Pathol 1999;20(4):357–63.
[97] Raman SV, Mehta R, Walker J, et al. Cardiovascular magnetic resonance in endocardial fibroelastosis. J Cardiovasc Magn Reson 2005;7(2):391–3.
[98] Alter P, Maisch B. Endomyocardial fibrosis in Churg-Strauss syndrome assessed by cardiac magnetic resonance imaging. Int J Cardiol 2006;108(1): 112–3.
[99] Petersen SE, Selvanayagam JB, Wiesmann F, et al. Left ventricular non-compaction: insights from cardiovascular magnetic resonance imaging. J Am Coll Cardiol 2005;46(1):101–5.
[100] Ritter M, Oechslin E, Sutsch G, et al. Isolated noncompaction of the myocardium in adults. Mayo Clin Proc 1997;72(1):26–31.
[101] Oechslin EN, Attenhofer Jost CH, Rojas JR, et al. Long-term follow-up of 34 adults with isolated left ventricular noncompaction: a distinct cardiomyopathy with poor prognosis. J Am Coll Cardiol 2000; 36(2):493–500.
[102] Rochitte CE, Oliveira PF, Andrade JM, et al. Myocardial delayed enhancement by magnetic resonance imaging in patients with Chagas' disease: a marker of disease severity. J Am Coll Cardiol 2005;46(8):1553–8.
[103] Bocchi EA, Kalil R, Bacal F, et al. Magnetic resonance imaging in chronic Chagas' disease: correlation with endomyocardial biopsy findings and gallium-67 cardiac uptake. Echocardiography 1998;15(3): 279–88.
[104] Baigent C, Burbury K, Wheeler D. Premature cardiovascular disease in chronic renal failure. Lancet 2000;356(9224):147–52.
[105] Mall G, Huther W, Schneider J, et al. Diffuse intermyocardiocytic fibrosis in uraemic patients. Nephrol Dial Transplant 1990;5(1):39–44.
[106] Aoki J, Ikari Y, Nakajima H, et al. Clinical and pathologic characteristics of dilated cardiomyopathy in hemodialysis patients. Kidney Int 2005; 67(1):333–40.
[107] Mark PB, Johnston N, Groenning BA, et al. Redefinition of uremic cardiomyopathy by contrast-

enhanced cardiac magnetic resonance imaging. Kidney Int 2006;69(10):1839–45.

[108] Bello D, Fieno DS, Kim RJ, et al. Infarct morphology identifies patients with substrate for sustained ventricular tachycardia. J Am Coll Cardiol 2005; 45(7):1104–8.

[109] Yan AT, Shayne AJ, Brown KA, et al. Characterization of the peri-infarct zone by contrast-enhanced cardiac magnetic resonance imaging is a powerful predictor of post-myocardial infarction mortality. Circulation 2006;114(1):32–9.

[110] Packer M, Antonopoulos GV, Berlin JA, et al. Comparative effects of carvedilol and metoprolol on left ventricular ejection fraction in heart failure: results of a meta-analysis. Am Heart J 2001;141(6): 899–907.

[111] Kim RJ, Wu E, Rafael A, et al. The use of contrast-enhanced magnetic resonance imaging to identify reversible myocardial dysfunction. N Engl J Med 2000;343(20):1445–53.

[112] Schvartzman PR, Srichai MB, Grimm RA, et al. Nonstress delayed-enhancement magnetic resonance imaging of the myocardium predicts improvement of function after revascularization for chronic ischemic heart disease with left ventricular dysfunction. Am Heart J 2003;146(3):535–41.

[113] Baks T, van Geuns RJ, Biagini E, et al. Effects of primary angioplasty for acute myocardial infarction on early and late infarct size and left ventricular wall characteristics. J Am Coll Cardiol 2006;47(1):40–4.

[114] McAlister FA, Ezekowitz JA, Wiebe N, et al. Systematic review: cardiac resynchronization in patients with symptomatic heart failure. Ann Intern Med 2004;141(5):381–90.

[115] Bleeker GB, Kaandorp TA, Lamb HJ, et al. Effect of posterolateral scar tissue on clinical and echocardiographic improvement after cardiac resynchronization therapy. Circulation 2006;113(7):969–76.

[116] White J, Yee R, Yuan X, et al. Delayed enhancement magnetic resonance imaging predicts response to cardiac resynchronization therapy in patients with intraventricular dysynchrony. J Am Coll Cardiol 2006;48(10):1953–60.

[117] Mollet NR, Dymarkowski S, Volders W, et al. Visualization of ventricular thrombi with contrast-enhanced magnetic resonance imaging in patients with ischemic heart disease. Circulation 2002; 106(23):2873–6.

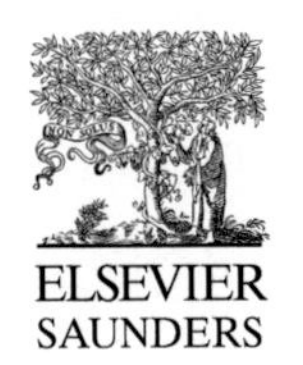

ELSEVIER
SAUNDERS

Cardiol Clin 25 (2007) 97–110

CARDIOLOGY
CLINICS

Clinical Applications of Cardiovascular Magnetic Resonance in Congenital Heart Disease

Anne Marie Valente, MD[a,b,*], Andrew J. Powell, MD[b]

[a]*Boston Adult Congenital Heart Service, Department of Cardiology, Children's Hospital Boston, Brigham and Women's Hospital, 300 Longwood Avenue, Boston, MA 02115, USA*
[b]*Department of Cardiology, Children's Hospital Boston, 300 Longwood Avenue, Boston, MA 02115, USA*

Cardiovascular malformations are the most common potentially lethal congenital defects and occur in approximately 1% of live births. Due to the successes of improved diagnostic techniques and therapeutic interventions, the early mortality of children who have these defects has been reduced substantially, and the long-term survival has improved [1]. Management issues in this population are challenging, and the application of cardiovascular magnetic resonance (CMR) to this group provides a wealth of diagnostic information to guide decision making. As the technical capabilities of CMR have advanced over the years since its initial application, the indications for CMR in patients who have congenital heart disease have grown [2,3]. This article provides an approach to the CMR evaluation of several common congenital heart lesions, including standard imaging protocols. The reader is cautioned, however, that one of the hallmarks of congenital heart disease is anatomic variation, and thus individualization of the protocol may be required to maximize diagnostic yield.

Shunt lesions

Atrial septal defects

Atrial septal defects (ASDs) are among the most common congenital heart defects, occurring in approximately 1 in 1500 live births [4]. The most common type of ASD, known as a secundum ASD, involves deficiency of a portion of the septum primum, (Fig. 1). These defects are associated with a left-to-right shunt leading to right heart volume overload. Defects that are large may present in childhood; however, many secundum ASDs first are diagnosed in adult life [5]. Transthoracic echocardiography is the primary imaging modality for ASDs in children; however, CMR increasingly is being used in the adolescent and adult populations, which often have limited transthoracic acoustic windows. The goal of the CMR examination is to delineate the number, location, and size of the defects, and identify the pulmonary venous drainage, as partial anomalous pulmonary venous connections may accompany this defect. CMR evaluation of ASDs involves high-resolution images of the atrial septum and adjacent structures, including the vena cavae, pulmonary veins, and atrioventricular (AV) valves.

Detailed anatomical information obtained from CMR has been used to determine the suitability for percutaneous device closure versus surgical repair. Durongpisitkul and colleagues [6] evaluated 66 adults and children older than 8 years who had secundum ASDs by echocardiography and CMR. CMR measurements of the major axis ASD diameter and measurement of the posterior–inferior rim were correlated closely with cardiac catheterization findings and useful in identifying patients suitable for device closure.

CMR is also useful in identifying rarer types of atrial-level shunt lesions, such as sinus venosus septal defect (Fig. 2), partial anomalous

* Corresponding author. Department of Cardiology, Children's Hospital Boston, 300 Longwood Avenue, Boston, MA 02115.
E-mail address: anne.valente@cardio.chboston.org (A.M. Valente).

0733-8651/07/$ - see front matter
doi:10.1016/j.ccl.2007.02.007

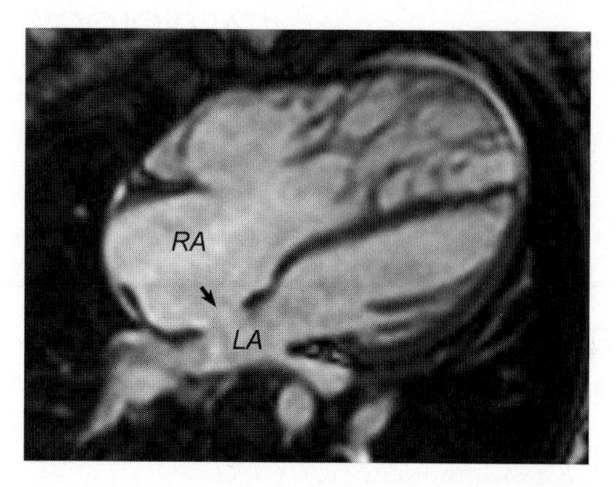

Fig. 1. Secundum atrial septal defect (*arrow*). Steady-state free precession cine MRI in the four-chamber plane. Note the dilated right atrium (RA) and right ventricle. LA, left atrium.

pulmonary venous return, and coronary sinus septal defects. These defects not uncommonly go undetected on transthoracic echocardiograms.

It is important to investigate the hemodynamic burden placed on the heart by shunt lesions. The right ventricular (RV) systolic pressure may be estimated by examination of the interventricular septal position in the short-axis plane in systole. As the RV pressure exceeds half systemic pressure, the ventricular septum flattens and then bows into the left ventricle. Care must be taken in interpretation of this finding, however, as it may be present with conduction delay (bundle branch block), or ventricular dyssynchrony.

The pulmonary-to-systemic flow ratio (Qp/Qs) ideally should be determined both by velocity-encoded cine (VEC) MRI and ventricular stroke volume comparison. The Qp/Qs ratio is determined by measuring flow in the ascending aorta and main pulmonary artery with VEC MRI (Fig. 3). The ventricular stoke volumes should approximate the stroke volumes in the great arteries providing that there is no significant valvular regurgitation or additional shunt. Pulmonary-to-systemic flow ratios measured by VEC MRI have been correlated closely with calculations obtained by oximetry during hemodynamic catheterization [7–9].

The authors' standard ASD protocol includes [10]:

- Three-plane localizing images
- ECG-gated, breath-held cine steady state free precession (SSFP) sequences in the following planes:
  - Two and four chamber
  - axial or oblique sagittal
  - short-axis plane from base-to-apex of the ventricles for quantitative assessment of ventricular size and function
- Gadolinium (Gd)-enhanced 3D cardiac magnetic angiography (MRA) to visualize pulmonary venous anatomy [11]

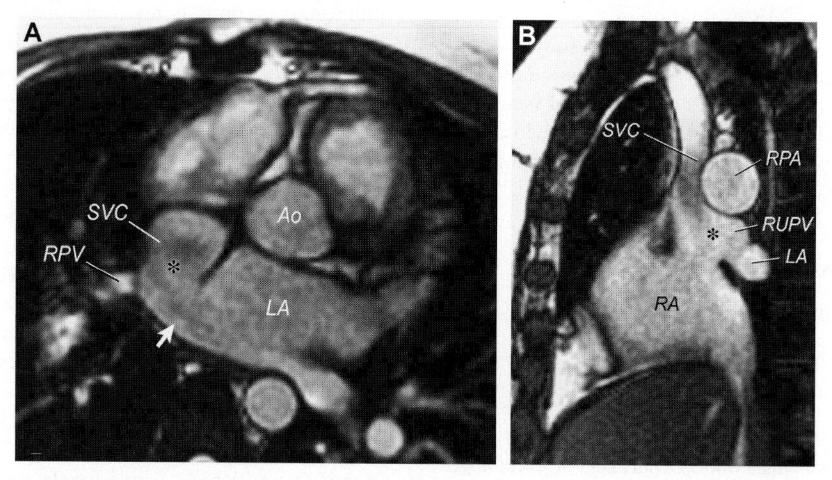

Fig. 2. Sinus venosus septal defect (superior vena cava type). Steady-state free precession cine MRI. (*A*) Axial plane image demonstrating the defect (*) in the wall that separates the superior vena cava (SVC) and the right upper pulmonary vein (RPV). The arrow indicates the orifice of the RPV through which blood can flow between the left atrium (LA) and the SVC. Ao, aorta. (*B*) Sagittal plane image demonstrating the defect (*) between the right upper pulmonary vein (RUPV) and the SVC. RA, right atrium; RPA, right pulmonary artery.

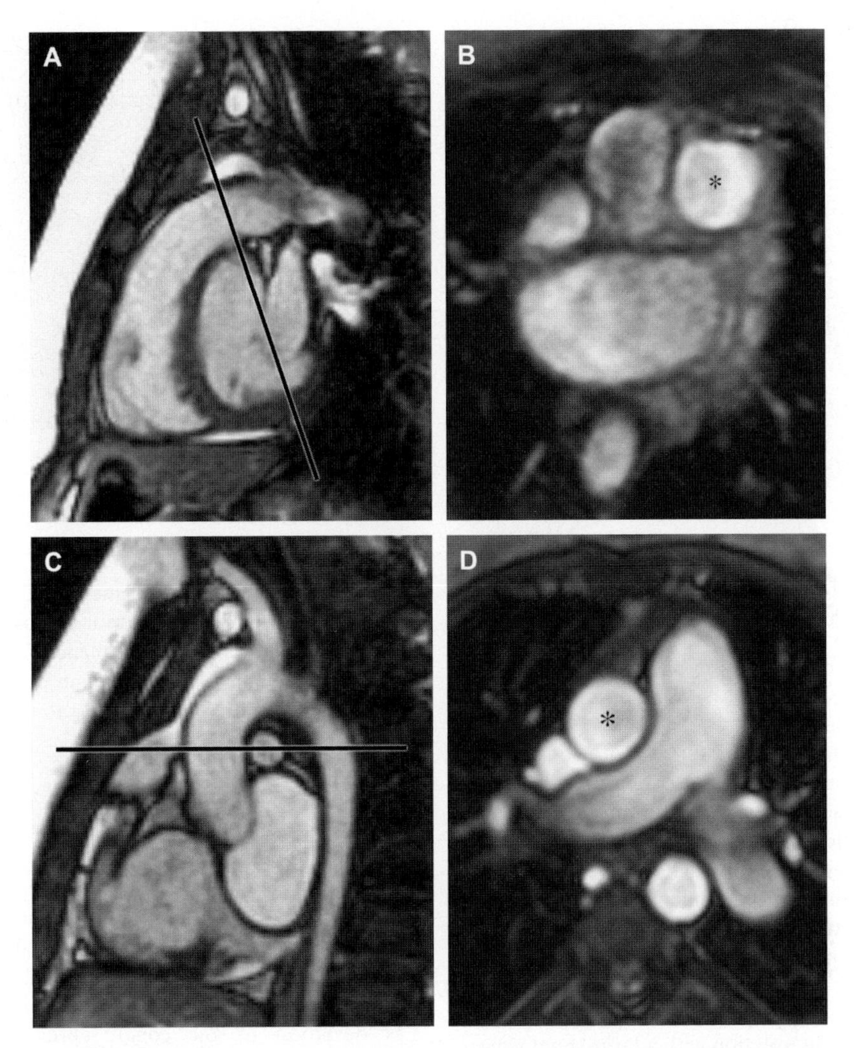

Fig. 3. Prescription for the velocity-encoded cine (VEC) MRI flow measurements. To measure flow in the main pulmonary artery, the VEC MRI sequence is planned from a right ventricular outflow tract view perpendicular to the direction of blood flow (*A, line*) so that the vessel (*) is imaged in cross section (*B, magnitude image*). To measure flow in ascending aorta, the VEC MRI sequence is planned from a sagittal view of the aorta perpendicular to the direction of blood flow (*C, line*) so that the vessel (*) is imaged in cross section (*D, magnitude image*).

ECG-gated VEC MRI sequences:

- in the plane of the septum to create an en face view, as well as in the corresponding orthogonal plane
- perpendicular to the main pulmonary artery and ascending aorta to measure flow

Ventricular septal defects

Ventricular septal defects (VSDs) also are encountered commonly in clinical practice, both as an isolated finding, and in association with complex congenital heart disease. VSDs may be classified as conoventricular (including perimembranous), muscular, conal septal, or atrioventricular canal type (Fig. 4) [12]. The clinical significance of VSDs depends on the defect location and size, and magnitude of the shunt; thus, these issues are the major imaging focal points of the CMR examination. The ventricular septum should be assessed by stacks of cine gradient echo or spin-echo sequences in at least two planes. Similar to the CMR analysis of ASDs, ventricular volumes, and function, and Qp/Qs should be quantified.

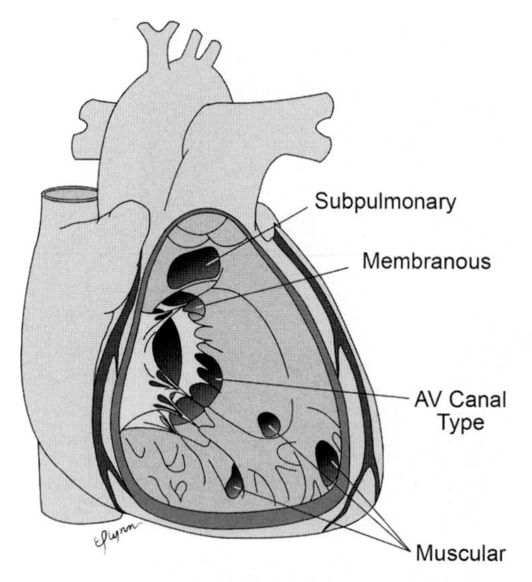

Fig. 4. Anatomical classification of ventricular septal defects.

The CMR examination of a patient who has a VSD must include assessment for associated defects. Perimembranous VSDs may be accompanied by tricuspid regurgitation [13]. Conal septal and perimembranous VSDs often are associated with prolapse of the right aortic valve cusp and resultant aortic insufficiency [14]. Rarely, VSDs may be associated with obstruction of the proximal portion of the os infundibulum, a condition called double-chamber right ventricle (Fig. 5) [15].

Long-term outcomes of adults who have small, restrictive VSDs are excellent [16]. Ventricular septal defects associated with other cardiac anomalies or those in isolation with a large shunt generally are repaired in childhood. Large VSDs that are not corrected surgically are associated with a large left-to-right shunt with progressive pulmonary artery and left heart dilation. The elevated pulmonary artery flow at high-pressure leads to irreversible pulmonary vascular changes and elevated pulmonary arterial resistance. The end result of this process is reversal in the ventricular level shunt to right-to-left shunting, arterial desaturation, cyanosis, and secondary erythrocytosis, known as Eisenmeger syndrome [17].

The authors' standard VSD protocol includes [10]:

Three-plane localizing images

ECG-gated, breath-held cine SSFP sequences in the following planes:

- In the four chamber plane to assess the base-to-apical location
- In the short-axis plane to define the VSD location in the anterior-to-posterior axis

ECG-gated VEC MRI sequences:

- perpendicular to the main pulmonary artery and ascending aorta to measure flow

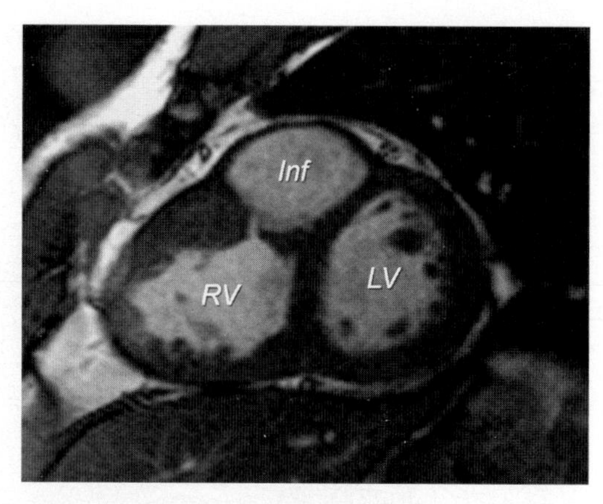

Fig. 5. Double chamber right ventricle (RV). SSFP cine MRI in the short-axis plane. There is muscular narrowing at the proximal os infundibulum between the RV sinus and the infundibulum (Inf). LV, left ventricle.

Conotruncal defects

Tetralogy of Fallot

Tetralogy of Fallot (TOF), the most frequent form of cyanotic congenital heart disease, has a prevalence of 0.26 to 0.8 per 1000 live births. The primary anatomical abnormality in this lesion is deviation of the conal septum anteriorly, superiorly, and leftward. As a result, it is characterized by varying degrees of obstruction of the RV outflow tract, a conoventricular septal defect, an aorta that overrides the ventricular septum, and right ventricular hypertrophy. Since the introduction of open-heart surgery for this condition, the 20-year survival rate has improved to nearly 90% [18–20]. Surgical repair typically involves patch closure of the conoventricular septal defect and an infundibular or transannular RV outflow tract patch to relieve the obstruction. Although surgical techniques for relieving the right outflow tract obstruction have been modified in recent years in attempts to preserve the integrity of the pulmonary valve, many adults who underwent tetralogy of Fallot surgery in childhood are now left with severe pulmonary valve regurgitation. Over time, this leads to RV dilation and dysfunction and predisposes these patients to exercise

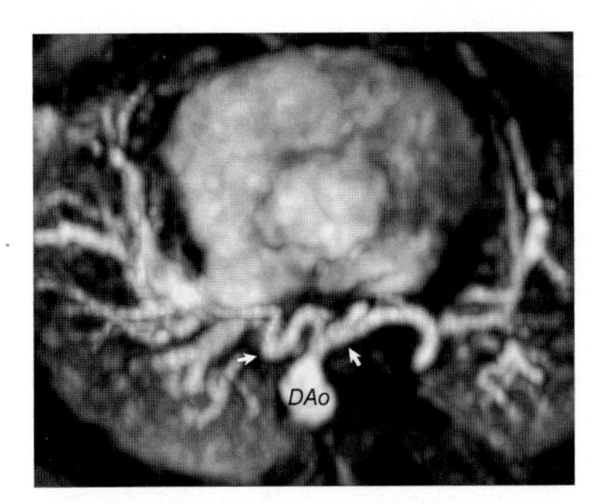

Fig. 6. Tetralogy of Fallot with pulmonary atresia. Axial subvolume maximum intensity projection (MIP) of a gadolinium-enhanced three-dimensional magnetic resonance angiogram showing a large aortopulmonary collateral arising from the descending aorta (DAo) and splitting into two branches (*arrows*), one to the left lung and one to the right lung.

intolerance, atrial and ventricular arrhythmias, and sudden cardiac death [18,20–22].

CMR is used most often in the preoperative assessment of TOF patients to delineate the sources of pulmonary blood flow, including pulmonary arteries, ductus arteriosus, and aorto–pulmonary collaterals (Fig. 6). Gd-enhanced three-dimensional MRA provides excellent visualization of these vessels [11]. Additionally, it is important to identify the origins and proximal course of the coronary arteries before surgical intervention, as in 5% to 6% of TOF patients a major coronary artery crosses the RV outflow tract [23]. Coronary artery imaging using a navigator and ECG-gated, three-dimensional SSFP with T2 preparation and fat saturation may be useful in obtaining this information [24].

The imaging focus in the repaired TOF patient focuses on identification and quantification of residual hemodynamic abnormalities, particularly RV dilation, pulmonary artery stenosis (Fig. 7), pulmonary regurgitation (Fig. 8), residual RV outflow tract obstruction, ventricular septal defects [25], RV and left ventricular (LV) systolic dysfunction [18], tricuspid valve regurgitation [26] and aortic root dilation [27], and aorto–pulmonary collaterals [28].

One of the most challenging management decisions in patients who have repaired TOF is the optimal timing for subsequent pulmonary valve replacement. This remains controversial, partly because of the limited ability of traditional assessment techniques to quantify relevant parameters in the right heart. CMR has become the gold standard for evaluating RV volumes, systolic function, and the degree of pulmonary valve regurgitation [21]. Pulmonary valve regurgitation should be quantified by VEC MRI and confirmed by RV and LV stoke volume comparison,

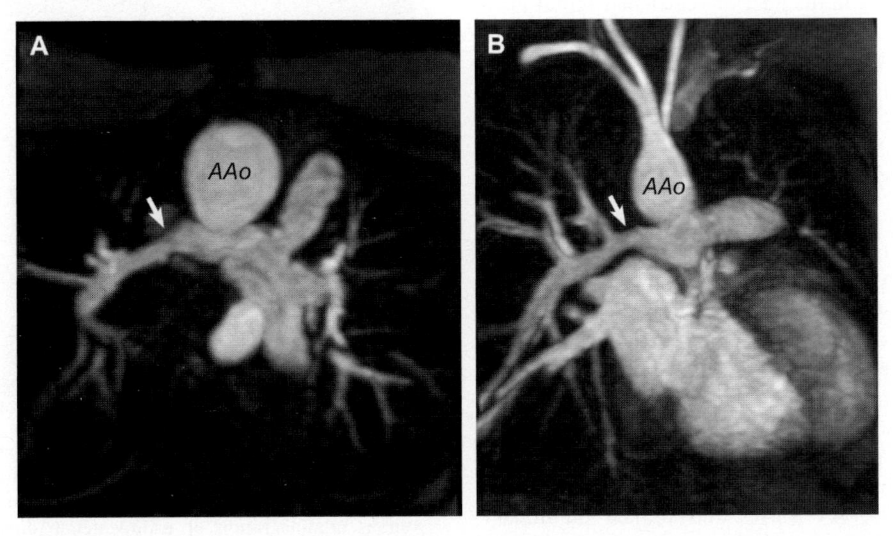

Fig. 7. Gadolinium-enhanced three-dimensional magnetic resonance angiogram in a patient with palliated tetralogy of Fallot. Axial (*A*) and coronal (*B*) MIP showing a hypoplastic right pulmonary artery with focal narrowing (*arrow*) at the site of previous Waterston shunt. AAo, ascending aorta.

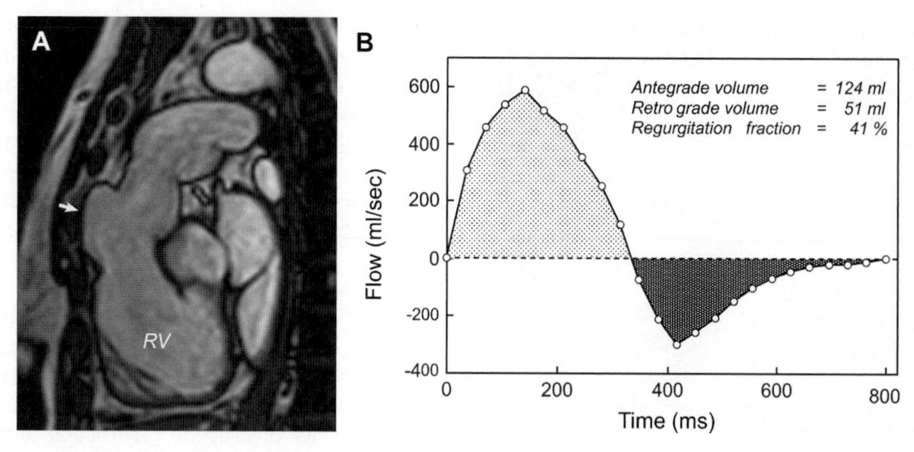

Fig. 8. Repaired tetralogy of Fallot. (*A*) Steady-state free precession cine MRI of the right ventricular outflow tract showing an aneurysm (*arrow*) of the transannular patch. RV, right ventricle. (*B*) Main pulmonary artery flow curve measured by velocity-encoded cine MRI. The area above the baseline is the antegrade volume, and the area below the baseline is the regurgitation volume.

provided there are no other regurgitant valves or shunts. CMR is being used in determining the hemodynamic effects of pulmonary valve replacement in patients who have previously repaired tetralogy of Fallot [21,29,30].

The CMR technique of myocardial-delayed enhancement (MDE) increasingly is being used in the population. MDE is found commonly at the site of the RV outflow patch (Fig. 9) [31,32]. Additionally, myocardial scarring remote from sites of direct surgical intervention is seen commonly, particularly in the inferior ventricular septal junction; however, the clinical significance of this finding is unknown [33].

The authors' standard TOF protocol includes [34]:

- Three-plane localizing images
- ECG-gated cine SSFP sequences in the following planes:
  - two and four chamber
  - short-axis plane from base-to-apex of the ventricles for quantitative assessment of ventricular size and function
  - parallel to the right ventricular outflow tract
- Gd-enhanced 3D MRA
- ECG-gated VEC MRI sequences perpendicular to the main pulmonary artery, ascending aorta, AV valves and branch pulmonary arteries.
- Post-gadolinium delayed myocardial enhancement to assess for myocardial fibrosis

Transposition of the great arteries

Transposition of the great arteries (TGA) is present when the aorta arises from the RV, and the pulmonary artery arises from the LV, and thus ventricular-to-great artery discordance is present. The most common type of TGA involves atrial–ventricular concordance, in which the

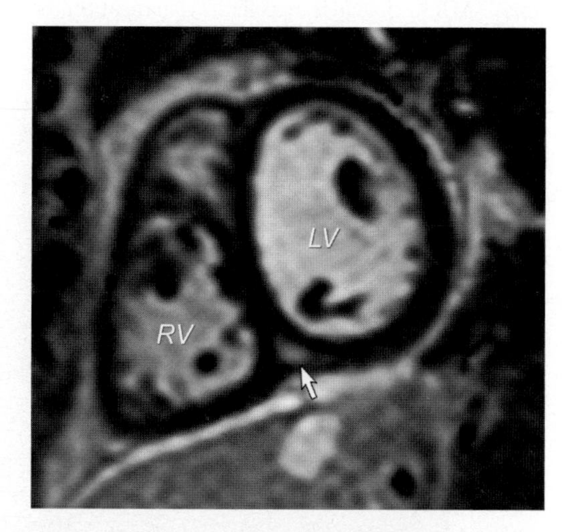

Fig. 9. Myocardial delayed enhancement imaging in repaired tetralogy of Fallot. Images were acquired in the short axis plane approximately 15 minutes after intravenous administration of gadopentetate dimeglumine (0.2 mmol/kg). Hyperenhancement (bright area in the myocardium indicated by arrow) indicates fibrosis at the inferior ventricular septal insertion.

systemic venous blood returns to the aorta, and the oxygenated pulmonary venous blood returns to the pulmonary artery. This physiology is not compatible with postnatal survival without a source of shunting present to allow mixing of saturated and desaturated blood. Shunting may be present at the atrial (ASD or patent foramen ovale), ventricular (VSD), or great artery level (patent ductus arteriosus). Surgical intervention usually is performed early in life, and CMR rarely is indicated in the preoperative TGA patient. One surgical treatment involves creation of atrial baffles to redirect blood flow so that systemic venous blood returns to the left ventricle and pulmonary artery. Oxygenated blood then returns to the right ventricle and out the aorta to the systemic circulation. These procedures, known as the Senning and Mustard operations, were performed several decades ago, and leave the RV in the systemic position. Long-term outcomes are generally favorable, yet over time many patients develop systemic RV dysfunction and atrial arrhythmias, and there is an increased incidence of sudden cardiac death [35–37].

The imaging goals in patients with TGA who have undergone an atrial switch procedure include assessment of RV (systemic ventricle) for size and function [38], the atrial baffle pathways for obstruction or leaks (Fig. 10) [39], the LV and RV outflow tracts for obstruction, the tricuspid valve for regurgitation, and the descending aorta for collateral vessels to the lungs.

Interestingly, one recent study of 36 patients with a previous atrial switch procedure for TGA concluded that the extent of late Gd enhancement correlated with age, ventricular dysfunction, electrophysiological parameters, and clinical events [40]. This small cross-sectional study illustrates the importance of further investigations into the area of abnormal myocardium in the setting of congenital heart disease.

The authors' standard TGA following atrial switch surgery protocol includes [34]:

Three-plane localizing images
ECG-gated cine SSFP sequences
- Axial plane with multiple contiguous slices from the level of the diaphragm to the level of the transverse arch to provide dynamic imaging of venous pathways, qualitative assessment of ventricular function, AV valve regurgitation, and great artery relationships
- Based on the previous sequence, multiple oblique coronal planes parallel to the superior and inferior vena cava pathways are obtained to image these pathways in long axis
- Short-axis plane from base-to-apex of the ventricles for quantitative assessment of ventricular size and function

Gd-enhanced 3D MRA
ECG-gated VEC MRI sequences perpendicular to the main pulmonary artery, ascending

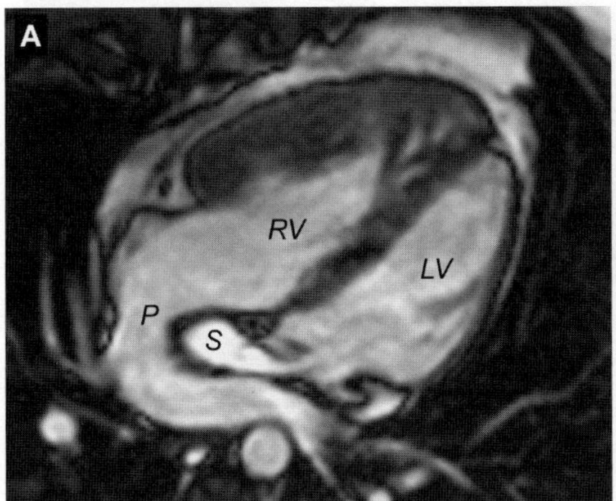

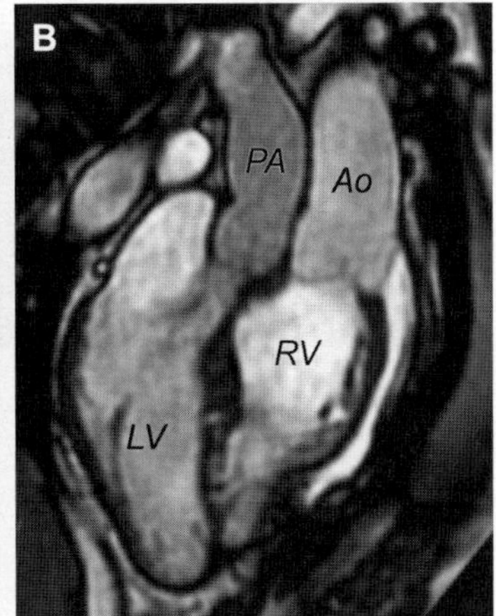

Fig. 10. Transposition of the great arteries status-post Mustard procedure. Steady-state free precession cine MRI in four-chamber (*A*) and outflow tract (*B*) planes. Note the pulmonary venous pathway (P) draining to the right ventricle (RV) and the systemic venous pathway (S) draining to the left ventricle (LV). The aorta (Ao) arises from the RV, and the pulmonary artery (PA) arises from the LV.

aorta, AV valves, and any further areas suspicious for obstruction
Post-gadolinium delayed myocardial enhancement to assess for myocardial fibrosis

As common with many congenital heart lesions, the surgical management of D-loop TGA has changed over time. Beginning in the late 1970s, the arterial switch procedure was introduced for surgical correction of TGA [41], and it now is performed routinely [42,43]. The arterial switch procedure involves transection of the aorta and pulmonary artery above the valve sinuses and reconnecting them to the other valve, translocation of the coronary arteries to the neo–aorta, and often moving the right pulmonary artery anterior to the aorta (Fig. 11). Compared with the atrial switch approach, the arterial switch operation has the advantage of avoidance of extensive atrial suture lines and establishing the LV as the systemic ventricle.

The CMR imaging focus in patients following the arterial switch procedure includes evaluation of the ventricles for size and systolic for function, the ventricular outflow tracts for obstruction [44], the pulmonary arteries for stenosis [45], the aortic valve for regurgitation [46,47], the aortic root for dilation, and the descending aorta for collateral vessels to the lungs.

The authors' standard TGA following arterial switch surgery protocol includes [34]:

Three-plane localizing images
ECG-gated cine SSFP sequences
- in the two and four chamber planes followed by a short-axis stack across the ventricles for quantitative assessment of ventricular dimensions and function
- in planes parallel to the left and right ventricular outflow tracts to rule out obstruction

Gd-enhanced 3D MRA
ECG-gated VEC MRI sequences perpendicular to the main and branch pulmonary arteries, ascending aorta
Post-gadolinium delayed myocardial enhancement to assess for myocardial fibrosis

In addition to the standard protocol, two other sequences may be employed:

Coronary artery imaging using a navigator and ECG-gated, 3D SSFP sequence with T2 preparation and fat saturation to evaluate the coronary artery origins, as they have

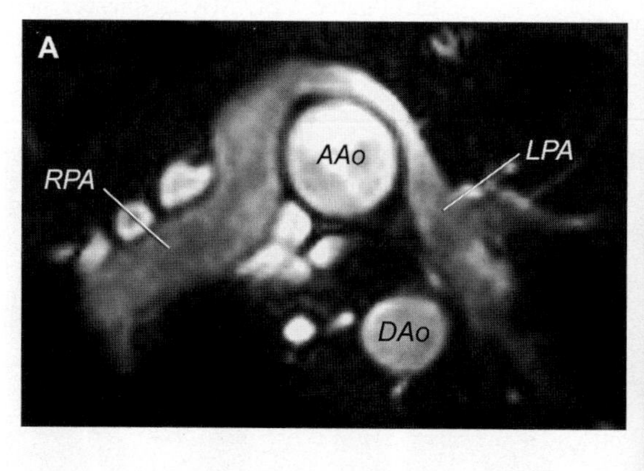

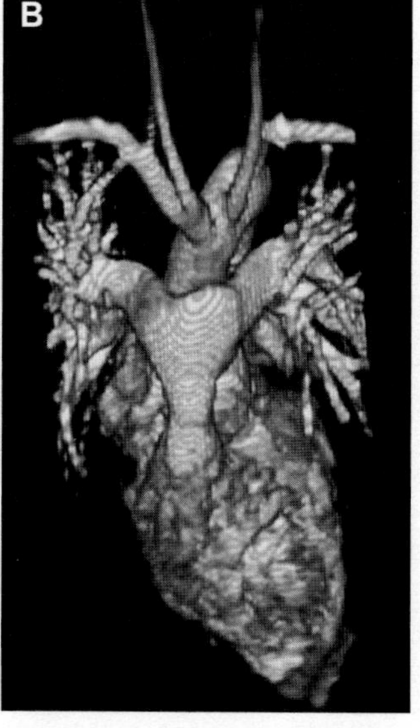

Fig. 11. Transposition of the great arteries status-post an arterial switch operation with the LeCompte maneuver. The proximal branch pulmonary arteries are positioned anterior to the ascending aorta as shown in (*A*) axial plane steady-state free precession cine MRI and (*B*) volume rendering of gadolinium-enhanced magnetic resonance angiogram. AAo, ascending aorta; LPA, left pulmonary artery; RPA, right pulmonary artery; DAo, descending aorta.

been transplanted to the neo-aortic root and may be compressed or stenotic.

Adenosine-stress perfusion or dobutamine stress MRI may also be performed to evaluate for myocardial ischemia. Inducible ischemia and perfusion abnormalities have been reported in this patient group using echocardiography and nuclear imaging [48,49].

CMR also is being performed increasingly in patients who have rarer conotruncal abnormalities including physiologically corrected TGA [50], double-outlet right ventricle [51], and truncus arteriosus [34].

Single ventricle physiology

Patients born with functionally single ventricles often undergo staged surgical palliation culminating in a Fontan operation. Since its initial application for tricuspid valve atresia in 1971, there have been many modifications to the Fontan procedure [52] . By convention, an operation that directs all systemic venous blood to the pulmonary arteries without passing through a functional ventricle is described as a Fontan procedure. The classic Fontan operation for tricuspid atresia involved an anastomosis between the superior vena cava and right pulmonary artery and placement of a valved conduit between the right atrium and left pulmonary artery, insertion of a valve into the inferior vena cava with closure of the ASD [52]. Other Fontan variations include right-atrial to pulmonary artery anastomosis, and total caval–pulmonary anastomosis with either an intracardiac lateral tunnel (Fig. 12) and extracardiac conduit.

CMR increasingly is being used in this patient population, because echocardiographic assessment often is limited by poor acoustic windows given their multiple surgeries and by difficulty visualizing the thoracic vasculature. The imaging focus includes assessment of the atrial septum, systemic ventricular outflow, Fontan pathway for obstruction, thrombus and baffle leaks, aortopulmonary collaterals, valve regurgitation, and ventricular function. Percutaneously implanted metallic devices such as endovascular coils or occlusion devices are relatively common in this patient group and may cause magnetic susceptibility artifact and limit image interpretation [53].

The authors' standard Fontan protocol includes:

Three-plane localizing images

ECG-gated cine SSFP sequences in the following planes:

- Axial to cover the thorax
- Two and four chamber, and short-axis
- Plane parallel to the Fontan connection

Gd-enhanced 3D MRA [54]

ECG-gated VEC MRI measurement perpendicular to the main and/or branch pulmonary arteries, ascending aorta, AV valves, and any other locations suspicious for obstruction

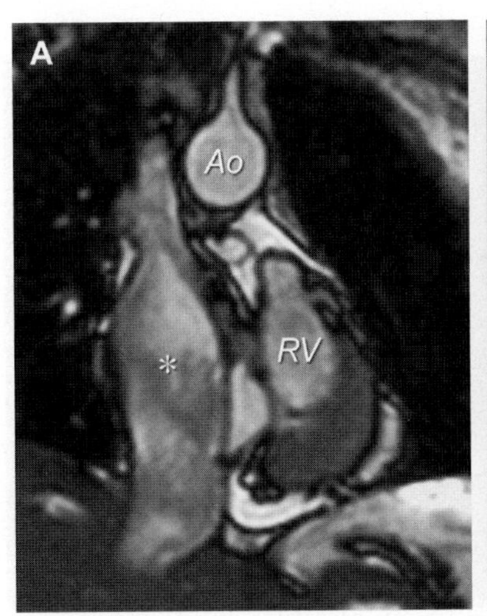

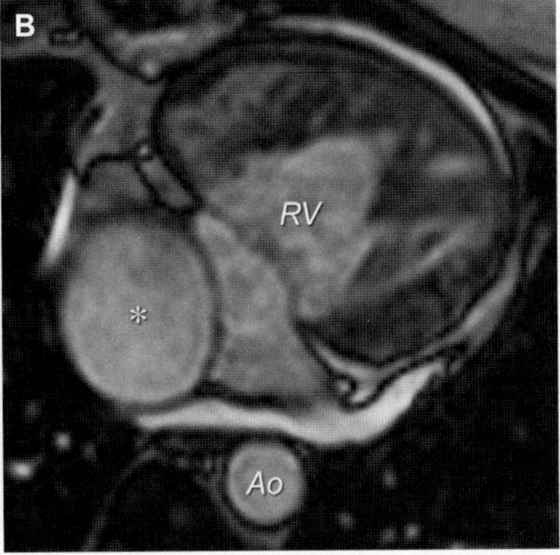

Fig. 12. Status-post lateral tunnel Fontan operation. Steady-state free precession cine MRI in the coronal (*A*) and axial (*B*) planes demonstrating the Fontan pathway (*). RV, right ventricle; Ao, aorta.

Obstructive lesions

Coarctation of the aorta

Coarctation of the aorta (CoA) is a discrete narrowing of the thoracic aorta, most commonly located at the aortic isthmus, just distal to the left subclavian artery (Fig. 13). It commonly is associated with a hypoplastic, elongated transverse aortic arch. There is also a high prevalence of bicomissural aortic valves (Fig. 14), mitral and aortic valve stenosis, ASD, VSD, patent ductus arteriosus, and conotruncal anomalies. The clinical presentation of the patient with CoA depends on several factors including patient age, associated lesions, and extent of collateral vessel formation. Infants may develop shock from inadequate perfusion to the descending aorta, whereas adults often may come to diagnosis after detection of asymptomatic hypertension.

The imaging goals of the CMR examination in the patient who has CoA include assessment of LV function and mass, the morphology of the aortic valve, the aortic arch caliber, the arch vessels, the collateral circulation, and any other left-sided obstructive lesions. Aortic wall complications are frequent in adults who have repaired CoA and include aneurysms (Fig. 15), dissection, fistulas, and aortic rupture [55]. In evaluating arch vessels, it is important to be aware of previous surgical interventions, as subclavian flap procedures will result in absence of the left subclavian artery origin from the aortic arch [56].

One component in evaluating the severity of aortic obstruction is to examine the descending aortic flow pattern distal to the obstruction. Characteristics that suggest a hemodynamically significant coarctation include decreased peak flow, decreased time average flow, delayed onset of descending aortic flow compared with ascending aortic flow, decreased acceleration rate, and

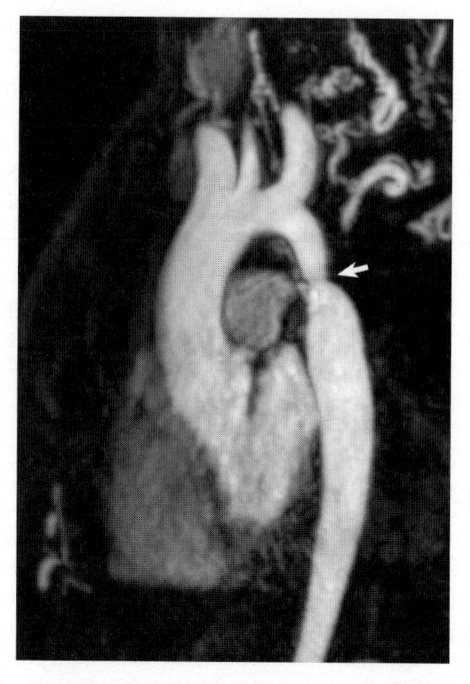

Fig. 13. Discrete coarctation (*arrow*) at the aortic isthmus. Oblique sagittal subvolume MIP from a gadolinium-enhanced three-dimensional magnetic resonance angiogram.

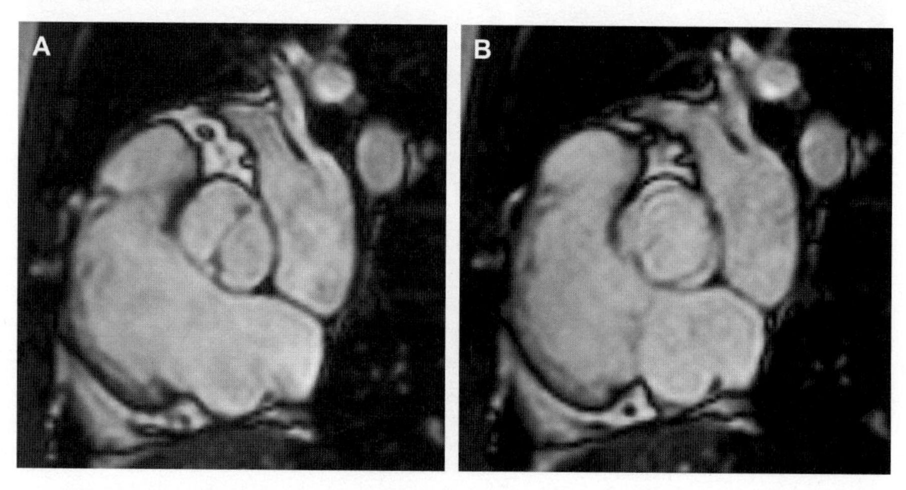

Fig. 14. Bicomissural aortic valve in with fusion of the intercoronary commissure. Steady-state free precession cine MRI in diastole (*A*) and systole (*B*).

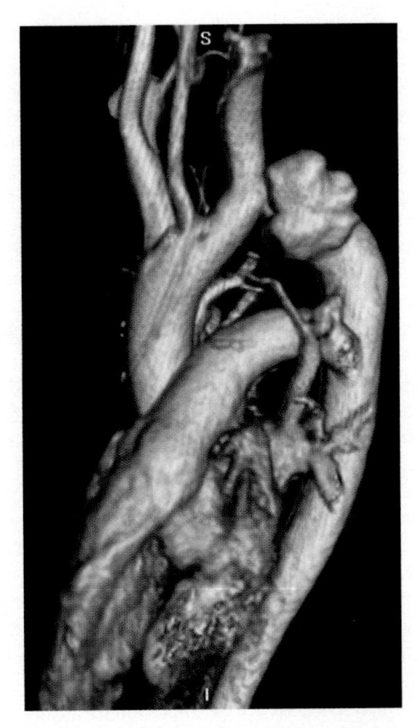

Fig. 15. Aneurysm at the aortic isthmus following balloon angioplasty for coarctation. Volume rendering of a gadolinium-enhanced three-dimensional magnetic resonance angiogram.

prolonged deceleration with increased antegrade diastolic flow (Fig. 16) [57–59]. VEC MRI also has been used to estimate the amount of collateral blood flow in patients who have CoA [60].

In addition to this standard imaging protocol, the authors advocate obtaining upper and lower blood pressure measurements at the time of the CMR to evaluate the pressure difference across the obstruction. In patients who have prominent collateral flow that bypasses the area of obstruction, little blood pressure differential may be present [61].

The authors' standard CoA protocol includes:

Three plane-localizing images

ECG-gated cine SSFP sequences in the following planes:

- Two and four chamber
- short-axis for quantitative assessment of left ventricular dimensions, systolic function, mass and mass-to-volume ratio
- parallel to the left ventricular outflow tract and cross-section to aortic valve and root
- long-axis view of the aortic arch (if high-velocity turbulent jets produce systolic signal voids on SSFP imaging, then cine gradient echo may be used; if there is artifact from previous endovascular stents then turbo spin echo is employed)

Gd-enhanced 3D MRA [54]

ECG-gated VEC MRI measurement in the ascending aorta and the descending aorta distal to the CoA

The authors' protocol additionally includes Gd-enhanced three-dimensional MRA [54] and ECG-gated VEC MRI measurement in the ascending aorta and the descending aorta distal to the CoA.

Summary

As the previous examples demonstrate, CMR is capable of providing important anatomical and physiological information in the pre- or post-operative patient who has congenital heart

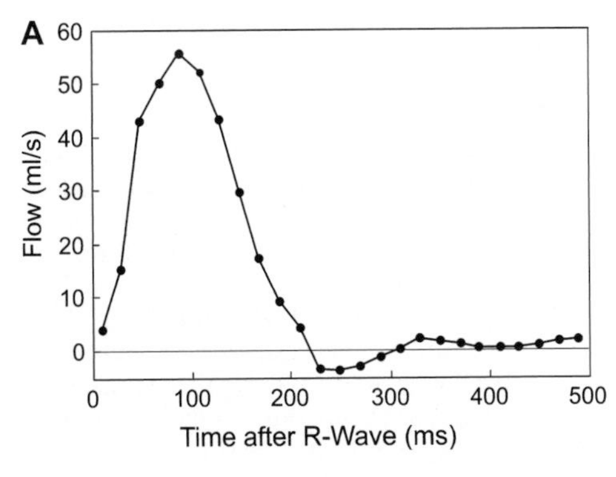

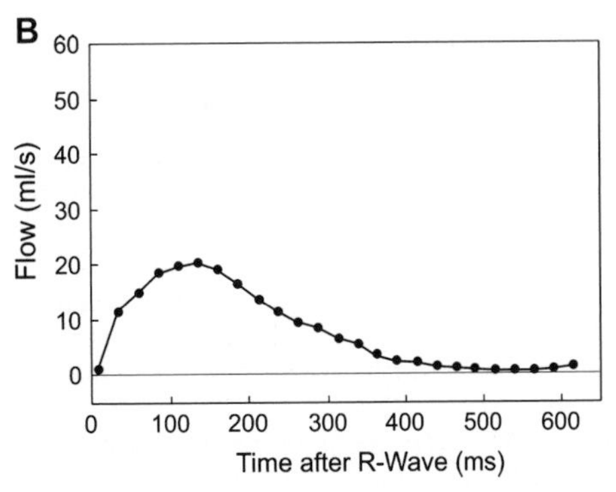

Fig. 16. Velocity-encoded cine MRI flow curves in the descending aorta in patients with no significant residual coarctation (*A*) and severe aortic coarctation (*B*).

disease. In many cases, it can serve as a noninvasive alternative to cardiac catheterization or transesophageal echocardiography. To maximize its diagnostic yield, however, a thorough understanding of the patient's underlying disease and medical history is necessary. The role of CMR in the management of these patients continues to evolve. Recently, the use of MRI-guided cardiac catheterization in children and adults who have congenital heart disease [62,63] and imaging of fetal cardiac anomalies [63] have been reported. There remains a need, however, for additional use studies to critically assess the clinical role of CMR in patients who have congenital heart disease. In addition, specialized training in congenital heart disease CMR must be made more widely available to afford more patients the benefits of this technology and to advance the field.

References

[1] Eskedal L, Hagemo PS, Eskild A, et al. Survival after surgery for congenital heart defects: does reduced early mortality predict improved long-term survival? Acta Paediatr 2005;94(4):438–43.

[2] Coats L, Khambadkone S, Derrick G, et al. Physiological and clinical consequences of relief of right ventricular outflow tract obstruction late after repair of congenital heart defects. Circulation 2006; 113(17):2037–44.

[3] Fenchel M, Greil GF, Martirosian P, et al. Three-dimensional morphological magnetic resonance imaging in infants and children with congenital heart disease. Pediatr Radiol 2006;36(12):1265–72.

[4] Samanek M. Children with congenital heart disease: probability of natural survival. Pediatr Cardiol 1992;13(3):152–8.

[5] Campbell M. Natural history of atrial septal defect. Br Heart J 1970;32(6):820–6.

[6] Durongpisitkul K, Tang NL, Soongswang J, et al. Predictors of successful transcatheter closure of atrial septal defect by cardiac magnetic resonance imaging. Pediatr Cardiol 2004;25(2):124–30.

[7] Powell AJ, Tsai-Goodman B, Prakash A, et al. Comparison between phase–velocity cine magnetic resonance imaging and invasive oximetry for quantification of atrial shunts. Am J Cardiol 2003;91(12): 1523–5, A9.

[8] Beerbaum P, Korperich H, Barth P, et al. Noninvasive quantification of left-to-right shunt in pediatric patients: phase contrast cine magnetic resonance imaging compared with invasive oximetry. Circulation 2001;103(20):2476–82.

[9] Hundley WG, Li HF, Lange RA, et al. Assessment of left-to-right intracardiac shunting by velocity-encoded, phase-difference magnetic resonance imaging. A comparison with oximetric and indicator dilution techniques. Circulation 1995;91(12): 2955–60.

[10] Wald RM, Powell AJ. Simple congenital heart lesions. J Cardiovasc Magn Reson 2006;8(4):619–31.

[11] Geva T, Greil GF, Marshall AC, et al. Gadolinium-enhanced 3-dimensional magnetic resonance angiography of pulmonary blood supply in patients with complex pulmonary stenosis or atresia: comparison with x-ray angiography. Circulation 2002; 106(4):473–8.

[12] Van Praagh R, Geva T, Kreutzer J. Ventricular septal defects: how shall we describe, name and classify them? J Am Coll Cardiol 1989;14(5):1298–9.

[13] Hagler DJ, Squarcia U, Cabalka AK, et al. Mechanism of tricuspid regurgitation in paramembranous ventricular septal defect. J Am Soc Echocardiogr 2002;15(4):364–8.

[14] Ishikawa S, Morishita Y, Sato Y, et al. Frequency and operative correction of aortic insufficiency associated with ventricular septal defect. Ann Thorac Surg 1994;57(4):996–8.

[15] Ibrahim T, Dennig K, Schwaiger M, et al. Images in cardiovascular medicine. Assessment of double chamber right ventricle by magnetic resonance imaging. Circulation 2002;105(22):2692–3.

[16] Gabriel HM, Heger M, Innerhofer P, et al. Long-term outcome of patients with ventricular septal defect considered not to require surgical closure during childhood. J Am Coll Cardiol 2002;39(6):1066–71.

[17] Hopkins WE, Waggoner AD. Severe pulmonary hypertension without right ventricular failure: the unique hearts of patients with Eisenmenger syndrome. Am J Cardiol 2002;89(1):34–8.

[18] Geva T, Sandweiss BM, Gauvreau K, et al. Factors associated with impaired clinical status in long-term survivors of tetralogy of Fallot repair evaluated by magnetic resonance imaging. J Am Coll Cardiol 2004;43(6):1068–74.

[19] Murphy JG, Gersh BJ, Mair DD, et al. Long-term outcome in patients undergoing surgical repair of tetralogy of Fallot. N Engl J Med 1993;329(9): 593–9.

[20] Nollert G, Fischlein T, Bouterwek S, et al. Long-term survival in patients with repair of tetralogy of Fallot: 36-year follow-up of 490 survivors of the first year after surgical repair. J Am Coll Cardiol 1997; 30(5):1374–83.

[21] Vliegen HW, van Straten A, de Roos A, et al. Magnetic resonance imaging to assess the hemodynamic effects of pulmonary valve replacement in adults late after repair of tetralogy of Fallot. Circulation 2002; 106(13):1703–7.

[22] Li W, Davlouros PA, Kilner PJ, et al. Doppler–echocardiographic assessment of pulmonary regurgitation in adults with repaired tetralogy of Fallot: comparison with cardiovascular magnetic resonance imaging. Am Heart J 2004;147(1):165–72.

[23] Need LR, Powell AJ, del Nido P, et al. Coronary echocardiography in tetralogy of Fallot: diagnostic

accuracy, resource utilization and surgical implications over 13 years. J Am Coll Cardiol 2000;36(4): 1371–7.
[24] Botnar RM, Stuber M, Kissinger KV, et al. Free-breathing 3D coronary MRA: the impact of isotropic image resolution. J Magn Reson Imaging 2000; 11(4):389–93.
[25] Walsh EP, Rockenmacher S, Keane JF, et al. Late results in patients with tetralogy of Fallot repaired during infancy. Circulation 1988;77(5):1062–7.
[26] Mahle WT, Parks WJ, Fyfe DA, et al. Tricuspid regurgitation in patients with repaired tetralogy of Fallot and its relation to right ventricular dilatation. Am J Cardiol 2003;92(5):643–5.
[27] Niwa K, Siu SC, Webb GD, et al. Progressive aortic root dilatation in adults late after repair of tetralogy of Fallot. Circulation 2002;106(11):1374–8.
[28] Knauth AL, Marshall AC, Geva T, et al. Respiratory symptoms secondary to aortopulmonary collateral vessels in tetralogy of Fallot absent pulmonary valve syndrome. Am J Cardiol 2004;93(4):503–5.
[29] Kleinveld G, Joyner RW, Sallee D III, et al. Hemodynamic and electrocardiographic effects of early pulmonary valve replacement in pediatric patients after transannular complete repair of tetralogy of Fallot. Pediatr Cardiol 2006;27(3):329–35.
[30] Therrien J, Provost Y, Merchant N, et al. Optimal timing for pulmonary valve replacement in adults after tetralogy of Fallot repair. Am J Cardiol 2005; 95(6):779–82.
[31] Prakash A, Powell AJ, Krishnamurthy R, et al. Magnetic resonance imaging evaluation of myocardial perfusion and viability in congenital and acquired pediatric heart disease. Am J Cardiol 2004; 93(5):657–61.
[32] Babu-Narayan SV, Kilner PJ, Li W, et al. Ventricular fibrosis suggested by cardiovascular magnetic resonance in adults with repaired tetralogy of fallot and its relationship to adverse markers of clinical outcome. Circulation 2006;113(3):405–13.
[33] Valente AM, Idriss SF, Cawley P, et al. Myocardial fibrosis patterns correlate with adverse right ventricular morphology and function in patients with repaired conotruncal heart defects. J Am Coll Cardiol 2004;43(5):390A.
[34] Dorfman AL, Geva T. Magnetic resonance imaging evaluation of congenital heart disease: conotruncal anomalies. J Cardiovasc Magn Reson 2006;8(4): 645–59.
[35] Kammeraad JA, van Deurzen CH, Sreeram N, et al. Predictors of sudden cardiac death after Mustard or Senning repair for transposition of the great arteries. J Am Coll Cardiol 2004;44(5):1095–102.
[36] Ebenroth ES, Hurwitz RA. Functional outcome of patients operated for d-transposition of the great arteries with the Mustard procedure. Am J Cardiol 2002;89(3):353–6.
[37] Dos L, Teruel L, Ferreira IJ, et al. Late outcome of Senning and Mustard procedures for correction of transposition of the great arteries. Heart 2005; 91(5):652–6.
[38] Lorenz CH, Walker Es, Graham TP Jr, et al. Right ventricular performance and mass by use of cine MRI late after atrial repair of transposition of the great arteries. Circulation 1995;92(9 Suppl): II233–9.
[39] Campbell RM, Moreau GA, Johns JA, et al. Detection of caval obstruction by magnetic resonance imaging after intra-atrial repair of transposition of the great arteries. Am J Cardiol 1987;60(8): 688–91.
[40] Babu-Narayan SV, Goktekin O, Moon JC, et al. Late gadolinium enhancement cardiovascular magnetic resonance of the systemic right ventricle in adults with previous atrial redirection surgery for transposition of the great arteries. Circulation 2005; 111(16):2091–8.
[41] Jatene AD, Fintes VF, Paulista PP, et al. Anatomic correction of transposition of the great vessels. J Thorac Cardiovasc Surg 1976;72(3):364–70.
[42] Wernovsky G, Jonas RA, Colan SD, et al. Results of the arterial switch operation in patients with transposition of the great arteries and abnormalities of the mitral valve or left ventricular outflow tract. J Am Coll Cardiol 1990;16(6):1446–54.
[43] Wernovsky G, Mayer JE Jr, Jonas RA, et al. Factors influencing early and late outcome of the arterial switch operation for transposition of the great arteries. J Thorac Cardiovasc Surg 1995;109(2): 289–301 [discussion: 301–2].
[44] Blakenberg F, Rhee J, Hardy C, et al. MRI vs echocardiography in the evaluation of the Jatene procedure. J Comput Assist Tomogr 1994;18(5):749–54.
[45] Beek FJ, Beekman RP, Dillon EH, et al. MRI of the pulmonary artery after arterial switch operation for transposition of the great arteries. Pediatr Radiol 1993;23(5):335–40.
[46] Schwartz ML, Gauvreau K, del Nido P, et al. Long-term predictors of aortic root dilation and aortic regurgitation after arterial switch operation. Circulation 2004;110(11 Suppl 1):II128–32.
[47] Marino BS, Wernovsky G, McElhinney DB, et al. Neo-aortic valvar function after the arterial switch. Cardiol Young 2006;16(5):481–9.
[48] Colan SD, Trowitzsch E, Wernovsky G, et al. Myocardial performance after arterial switch operation for transposition of the great arteries with intact ventricular septum. Circulation 1988;78(1):132–41.
[49] Weindling SN, Wernovsky G, Colan SD, et al. Myocardial perfusion, function and exercise tolerance after the arterial switch operation. J Am Coll Cardiol 1994;23(2):424–33.
[50] Sunger B, Sechtem U, Schicha H. [Magnetic resonance tomography findings in adult patients with congenital corrected transposition of great arteries]. Z Kardiol 1995;84(4):316–22 [in German].
[51] Beekmana RP, Roest AA, Helbing WA, et al. Spin echo MRI in the evaluation of hearts with a double

outlet right ventricle: usefulness and limitations. Magn Reson Imaging 2000;18(3):245–53.
[52] Fontan F, Baudet E. Surgical repair of tricuspid atresia. Thorax 1971;26(3):240–8.
[53] Garg R, Powell AJ, Sena L, et al. Effects of metallic implants on magnetic resonance imaging evaluation of Fontan palliation. Am J Cardiol 2005;95(5): 688–91.
[54] Bogaert J, Kuzo R, Dymarkowski S, et al. Follow-up of patients with previous treatment for coarctation of the thoracic aorta: comparison between contrast-enhanced MR angiography and fast spin echo MR imaging. Eur Radiol 2000;10(12): 1847–54.
[55] Oliver JM, Gallego P, Gonzalez A, et al. Risk factors for aortic complications in adults with coarctation of the aorta. J Am Coll Cardiol 2004; 44(8):1641–7.
[56] Scholz TD, Sato Y, Bolinger L. Aortic aneurysm following subclavian flap repair: diagnosis by magnetic resonance imaging. Pediatr Cardiol 2001;22(2): 153–5.
[57] Muhler EG, Neuerburg JM, Ruben A, et al. Evaluation of aortic coarctation after surgical repair: role of magnetic resonance imaging and Doppler ultrasound. Br Heart J 1993;70(3):285–90.
[58] Mohiaddin RH, Kilner PJ, Rees S, et al. Magnetic resonance volume flow and jet velocity mapping in aortic coarctation. J Am Coll Cardiol 1993;22(5): 1515–21.
[59] Nielsen JC, Powell AJ, Gauvreau K, et al. Magnetic resonance imaging predictors of coarctation severity. Circulation 2005;111(5):622–8.
[60] Steffens JC, Bourne MW, Sakuma H, et al. Quantification of collateral blood flow in coarctation of the aorta by velocity- encoded cine magnetic resonance imaging. Circulation 1994;90(2):937–43.
[61] Araoz PA, Reddy GP, Tarnoff H, et al. MR findings of collateral circulation are more accurate measures of hemodynamic significance than arm–leg blood pressure gradient after repair of coarctation of the aorta. J Magn Reson Imaging 2003;17(2): 177–83.
[62] Razavi R, Hill DL, Keevil SF, et al. Cardiac catheterisation guided by MRI in children and adults with congenital heart disease. Lancet 2003;362(9399): 1877–82.
[63] Fogel MA, Wilson RD, Flake A, et al. Preliminary investigations into a new method of functional assessment of the fetal heart using a novel application of real-time cardiac magnetic resonance imaging. Fetal Diagn Ther 2005;20(5):475–80.

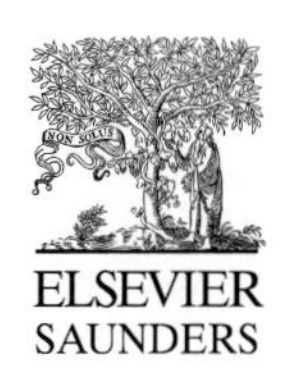

ELSEVIER
SAUNDERS

Cardiol Clin 25 (2007) 111–140

CARDIOLOGY CLINICS

Magnetic Resonance Imaging of Pericardial Disease and Cardiac Masses

John D. Grizzard, MD[a,*], Gregory B. Ang, MD[b]

[a]*Department of Radiology, Noninvasive Cardiovascular Imaging, Virginia Commonwealth University Medical Center, 1250 East Marshall Street, Post Office Box 980615, Richmond, VA 23298, USA*
[b]*Duke Cardiovascular Magnetic Resonance Center, Division of Cardiology, Duke University Medical Center, Box 31074, Durham, NC 27710, USA*

Multiple imaging modalities are now available for the comprehensive evaluation of pericardial disease and cardiac masses. Plain film radiography long has been superseded by CT for evaluating pericardial calcification, and echocardiography is currently the mainstay of cardiac imaging diagnosis. MRI, however, has several advantages over echocardiography and the competing modality of CT (Table 1).

Echocardiography is inexpensive, rapidly performed, and portable. In addition, it is ubiquitous, being readily available in virtually all hospital settings. It is often the first modality used in the evaluation of suspected pericardial disease or cardiac masses. It has limitations, however. Specifically, in many patients, the acoustic windows are limited, allowing only partial visualization of the global cardiac structure, as well as of the adjacent mediastinal contents. Many patients have a large body habitus that also significantly degrades image quality. In addition, pericardial thickening can be very difficult to detect with echocardiography, as can calcification. Finally, echocardiography is limited in its ability to provide tissue characterization [1].

CT has emerged as a vigorous competitor to MRI and echocardiographic imaging. Like MRI, CT is capable of high-resolution thin section imaging, and can be gated to the cardiac cycle, allowing cinematic displays of cardiac motion, although with a lower temporal resolution than MRI. It is more sensitive than MRI for detecting calcification, and this represents an often-cited advantage relative to MR imaging. Current multislice CT scanners allow multiplanar reconstructions using isotropic voxels, resulting in high-resolution imaging in virtually any plane. The resultant improvement in multiplanar imaging with current-generation CT scanner technology has lessened to some extent the prior advantage of multiplanar MR imaging. CT, however, requires the use of ionizing radiation, and gated CT examinations can result in a radiation dose that exceeds that of cardiac catheterization [2,3]. Also, it usually requires the administration of iodinated contrast, with the attendant risks of nephrotoxicity and potential allergic reactions. Its efficacy in tissue characterization is inferior to that of MRI.

For various reasons, MRI remains the gold standard for the comprehensive imaging of pericardial disease and cardiac masses. MRI provides direct multiplanar imaging without the need for reconstructions, and in any freely selectable imaging plane. There are no limitations regarding acoustic windows. No radiation is required, and no nephrotoxic contrast media are administered. Gadolinium is frequently administered, but it is widely regarded as significantly safer than iodinated contrast material.

Most importantly, MRI provides superior tissue characterization relative to both CT and echocardiography. Various imaging sequences, including fast spin echo (T1 weighted and T2 weighted), cine, and delayed-enhancement techniques provide a broad palette that the examiner can choose from to localize and characterize

* Corresponding author.
E-mail address: jdgrizzard@vcu.edu (J.D. Grizzard).

doi:10.1016/j.ccl.2007.02.004

Table 1
Comparison of cross-sectional imaging modalities

Modality	Multiplanar capability	Soft tissue contrast	Temporal resolution	Windows
Echocardiography	+++	+	++++	Limited
CT	++	++	+	Unlimited
MRI	++++	++++	+++	Unlimited

various pericardial and cardiac disorders [4,5]. Fat suppression can be added as needed to characterize suspected fatty tumors. Perfusion imaging can be performed for evaluating tumor vascularity. Finally, MRI using real-time sequences can provide depiction of dynamic processes, thereby furnishing hemodynamic and structural information. Therefore, the multisequence, multiplanar capability of MRI makes it the ideal method for evaluating pericardial diseases, and pericardial and cardiac masses.

Although pericardial disease and cardiac masses are clearly separate and discrete entities, there are significant similarities in the utility of MRI for their diagnosis, and overlap in the MR techniques used. Thus, these disorders will be considered together in this article.

MRI techniques

In early implementations, cardiac MRI for evaluating masses and pericardial disease was performed with gated spin-echo examinations without breath holding. Typically, two signal acquisitions were averaged to diminish breathing-induced motion artifacts, and a study yielding five dual-echo slices required 45 minutes to obtain.

Subsequently, fast spin-echo sequences were developed that allowed image acquisition in a single breath hold. A single image using this technique requires between 10 and 15 heartbeats, however, and a comprehensive examination of the entire chest requires 5 to 10 minutes for one sequence type. Pre- and postcontrast T1 weighted imaging, and comprehensive T2 weighted imaging of the entire chest using this type of sequence are therefore time-consuming exercises. In addition, this sequence often results in suboptimal T1weighting because of the long repetition time used, and breathing artifact often diminishes image quality.

In the last several years, significant technical improvements have been made to MRI scanner hardware such as powerful gradients capable of more rapid imaging and coils that facilitate parallel imaging. Additionally, software improvements in the form of new and robust sequences have been developed that provide unique information not previously available with the older imaging sequences [6,7]. These changes have resulted in a significant improvement in image quality, and decreases in scan time. For example, dark-blood morphologic survey imaging of the entire chest now is performed with HASTE (half-Fourier acquisition single-shot turbo spin echo) imaging in approximately one minute. Similarly, cine imaging now is performed with the steady-state free-precession (SSFP) sequence, resulting in improved image quality and diminished scan time. Certain compromises have been made, as will be described, and in selected instances conventional fast spin echo T1 or T2 weighted sequences may be appropriate. Nonetheless, the more modern techniques usually demonstrate superior image quality with less respiratory artifact and better spatial resolution [8].

Standard cardiac MRI examination

A cardiac examination designed for evaluation of cardiac masses or pericardial disease should begin with the standard sequences used in essentially all cardiac MRI: initial static morphologic images and high-resolution cine images of the heart. These sequences then are supplemented by delayed-enhancement and perfusion imaging for tissue characterization. The examination also should be tailored to the specific clinical circumstance, and various other sequences can be added as necessary (Table 2).

Previously, dark blood morphologic sequences were most often performed with fast spin-echo imaging, which as described previously, could be quite time-consuming. Recently, the HASTE sequence largely has replaced the older fast spin-echo technique as it allows dark blood imaging with a greatly reduced acquisition time, with one entire image acquisition occurring at every other heartbeat. This represents a tremendous acceleration relative to the former technique. There is slightly increased blurring with this technique relative to standard gated spin-echo techniques, however. The resistance of the single-shot

Table 2
Suggested imaging protocol

Sequence	Planes	Coverage
Core examination		
Localizer	Axial, coronal, sagittal	Entire chest
HASTE	Axial, sagittal, or coronal	Entire chest
Steady-state free precession (SSFP) cines	Short- and long-axis views	Heart from base to apex
Single-shot SSFP delayed-enhancement images with inversion time set to null normal myocardium	Short- and long-axis views	Copy the cines
Single-shot SSFP delayed-enhancement images with inversion time of 600 ms (for thrombus detection)	Short- and long-axis views	Copy the cines
Optional for masses		
Perfusion images	Tailored to mass	Copy cine image that best shows the mass
T1 and T2 gated fast spin echo imaging	Tailored to mass	As needed for evaluation
As with fat-suppression	Tailored to mass	Can be added to HASTE or standard fast spin echo to characterize fatty lesions
Volumetric interpolated breath-hold examination (VIBE)	Axial	Entire chest
Optional for pericardium		
Real-time steady-state free precession cine images	Short-axis and four chamber views during deep inspiration	To evaluate septal motion

sequence to respiratory motion artifact, which frequently degrades spin-echo image quality, usually offsets this minimal disadvantage.

Cine imaging through the entire myocardium in the short and long axis planes as routinely performed for cardiac evaluation is appropriate for the imaging of suspected pericardial disease and masses. SSFP imaging is now the standard used for cine imaging, as it demonstrates improved image quality in comparison with segmented gradient echo imaging techniques [6]. The signal intensity in the SSFP technique depends upon the T2/T1 ratio. Therefore, structures with a high T2/T1 ratio such as fat, fluid, and intracavitary blood demonstrate similar high signal despite their significantly different T1 and T2 properties. The myocardium is relatively low in signal intensity on precontrast images, providing excellent contrast between the blood pool and the endocardium. This is often quite helpful in the delineation of intracavitary lesions. In addition, the impact of masses upon the myocardium and the valvular structures of the heart can be assessed readily.

In addition, newer scanners also are often able to perform real-time cine image acquisitions, which allow images to be performed without breath holding, and without segmentation. These nongated SSFP images are acquired in the cine mode in real-time, and can be used for evaluating dynamic processes [9].

Uncommonly, sequences using tagging to evaluate for pericardial/myocardial adhesions also can be performed. In this sequence, a grid of saturation bands is placed over the heart, and their deformation can provide information about regional wall motion. This sequence also has been used to depict abnormal adherence of the visceral pericardium to the parietal pericardium or of the pericardium to the chest wall [10]. (The grid lines remain unbroken as opposed to demonstrating the normal disruption caused by cardiac motion). Given the high-resolution imaging possible with SSFP, however, tagging sequences usually are not required on a routine basis.

Perfusion sequences are used to evaluate the vascularity of a lesion and can be obtained in multiple imaging planes with one injection. These are heavily T1 weighted imaging sequences that can provide information regarding vascularity (or the absence thereof), and they are helpful in evaluating masses and thrombi.

The same delayed-enhancement sequences that are used for detecting myocardial infarction (MI) also are used for evaluating masses. The standard delayed-enhancement sequence is a segmented T1 weighted inversion recovery gradient echo sequence with an inversion time chosen that provides nulling of the signal of normal myocardium, accentuating the contrast differences between normal myocardium and areas of infarction [7]. The same sequence can be used for the characterization of masses, which typically demonstrate hyperenhancement. Moreover, single-shot delayed-enhancement images using an inversion recovery single-shot SSFP sequence can provide similar information in a fraction of the imaging time. The same sequences also can be performed with a long inversion time (>600 milliseconds), which is often very helpful in detecting thrombus, as will be described.

In certain circumstances, fat saturation can be added to conventional fast spin-echo or single-shot fast spin-echo sequences for additional tissue characterization.

In the evaluation of masses, a breath-hold fat-saturated volumetric three-dimensional image acquisition with T1 weighting (VIBE) can be performed in less than 20 seconds before and following the administration of contrast material. These often provide additional helpful information regarding tissue characterization, and three-dimensional volumetric assessment of masses.

Pericardial disease

The pericardium is a mesothelial-lined serous sac, into which the heart has been invaginated, much as placing one's hand into a balloon and then deflating it. The visceral pericardium is composed of a thin layer of mesothelial cells overlying the epicardial surface of the heart. The parietal pericardium is a somewhat thicker and more collagenous layer. The normal thickness of the pericardium is less than 2 mm on MRI, and even this measurement actually represents a summation of both pericardial layers, as well as a small amount of intervening fluid usually present, along with chemical shift artifact [11]. The actual pericardial thickness is probably less than 1.5 mm. Normally, between 25 and 50 mL of clear serous fluid is present in the pericardial sac, providing lubrication. The normal pericardium is depicted readily on MRI as a thin low-signal intensity line on static morphologic or cine images [11]. It usually is seen most easily overlying the right ventricular (RV) free wall and at the left ventricular (LV) apex (Fig. 1).

The pericardium normally provides a barrier to the spread of infection, and limits the degree to which the myocardium can be distended acutely. In addition, a certain amount of physiologic ventricular coupling is facilitated by the presence of the intact pericardium. It is infrequently the subject of consideration, except in instances of a significant alteration of sensation or function. These disorders usually fall into one of a few clinical syndromes: acute pericarditis, pericardial effusion (with or without tamponade), and constrictive pericarditis.

Acute pericarditis

Acute pericarditis is usually a clinical diagnosis, and it infrequently requires imaging. It is likely that 90% or more of isolated cases of acute pericarditis are either idiopathic or viral in origin, but various causes, including uremia, acute MI, and neoplasm can result in the clinical pattern of acute pericarditis. Specifically, causes of acute pericarditis/pericardial effusion include:

- Idiopathic
- Infection—viral, bacterial, fungal/TB
- Injury—radiation, surgery, trauma, MI
- After injury—post-MI, postpericardiotomy
- Connective tissue disease—rheumatoid arthritis, systemic lupus
- Malignancies—breast, lung, lymphoma
- Metabolic—uremia

On imaging, one may observe a small amount of pericardial effusion, and minimal pericardial thickening may be seen. Significant pericardial thickening usually implies chronicity, however, and this would be uncommon in acute pericarditis [12]. Occasionally, pericardial enhancement may be seen [13]. Most cases respond readily to conservative therapy and treatment with nonsteroidal anti-inflammatory agents.

Pericardial effusion

Any of the disorders that can cause acute pericarditis also may result in pericardial effusion. Although echocardiography is the usual initial imaging modality chosen to detect and characterize pericardial effusions, MRI is nonetheless helpful in various circumstances. It is more sensitive than echocardiography for detecting small effusions, and it is superior to echocardiography in detecting loculated effusions, or those effusions complicated by pericardial thickening [14–16].

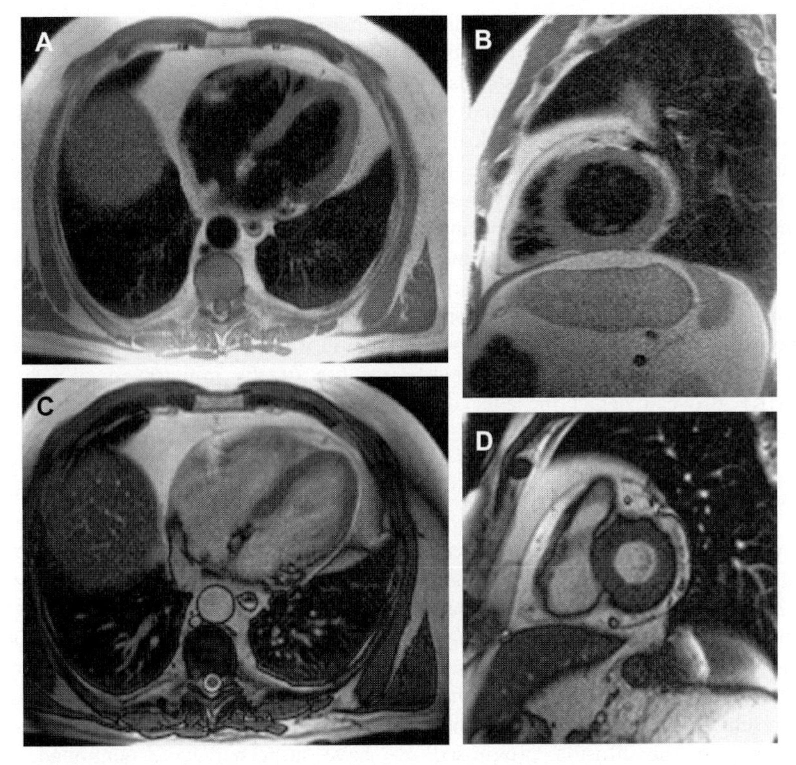

Fig. 1. Four-chamber (*A*) and short-axis (*B*) dark-blood half-fourier acquisition single-shot turbo spin echo images and four-chamber (*C*) and short-axis (*D*) bright-blood steady-state free-precession (SSFP) images showing normal pericardium.

MRI findings

Uncomplicated effusions are usually low in signal intensity on T1 weighted images, and high in signal intensity on T2 weighted images. In addition, cine gradient echo images performed with SSFP often will demonstrate pericardial effusions as having uniformly high signal intensity. This high signal intensity on cine and T2 weighted images allows clear differentiation from the fibrous pericardium, which is low in signal on these sequences (Fig. 2).

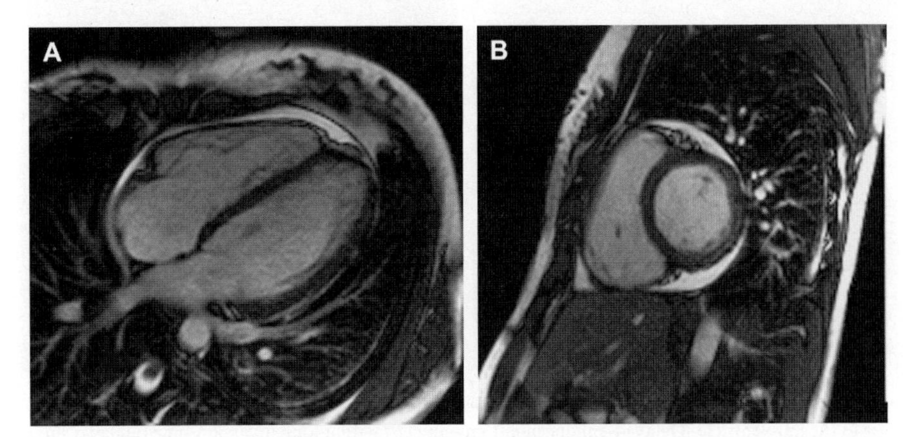

Fig. 2. Small, simple effusion on four-chamber (*A*) and short-axis (*B*) cine SSFP images. Note the uniform high signal.

Complicating hemorrhage can be suspected when high signal intensity is seen within the pericardial sac on T1 weighted images. Also, hemorrhage or infection should be suspected on cine imaging when the effusion fluid is clearly complex and inhomogeneous, containing regions of different signal intensity [17–20]. Delayed-enhancement imaging can demonstrate abnormal pericardial enhancement, indicative of inflammation or infection. Imaging with a delayed-enhancement sequence using a long inversion time also can demonstrate intrapericardial thrombus as a region of low signal intensity (Fig. 3). Most importantly, MRI also can depict the effect of the effusion upon the myocardium.

Cardiac tamponade

The pericardium normally demonstrates a very steep pressure/volume curve, such that even small increases in volume beyond a certain point result in a significant rise in intrapericardial pressure [21–23]. This is particularly true in the acute setting, where the rapid development of a pericardial effusion may result in cardiac tamponade that would not develop if the effusion progressed more slowly. Specifically, the slow, progressive development of pericardial effusion (or progressive cardiomegaly) results in a shift of the pressure/volume relationship to the right, and also produces flattening of the slope of the curve such that greater volumes of intrapericardial fluid are tolerated before a significant rise in pressure occurs. Also, the rate at which a small volume increase results in a pressure increase is also diminished. Hence, as little as 200 to 250 mL of pericardial fluid can result in tamponade if it develops rapidly, whereas a significantly larger effusion may be tolerated if it develops slowly.

Clinically, patients with large pericardial effusions producing hemodynamic compromise often will demonstrate venous distention and peripheral edema. The lungs may be relatively clear, although the patient frequently will complain of dyspnea [24]. In patients who have cardiac tamponade, the stroke volume cannot be increased because of the impairment of ventricular filling, and tachycardia often is seen as a physiologic response to maintain cardiac output. The diagnosis of cardiac tamponade often can be suspected clinically, with noninvasive imaging used to confirm the presence of a significant pericardial effusion. Transthoracic echocardiography is the imaging modality of choice because of its portability and rapid availability in the acute setting. MRI can be used to confirm findings on echocardiography. The need for rapid diagnosis and management in patients with hemodynamic instability, however, makes it impractical to perform in patients who have suspected acute tamponade. It sometimes may be helpful in nonemergent situations, however, in which echocardiography findings are equivocal, such as the evaluation of a chronic effusion that is of uncertain hemodynamic significance.

A large circumferential pericardial effusion is usually evident, although a focal loculated effusion that significantly impairs RV filling may

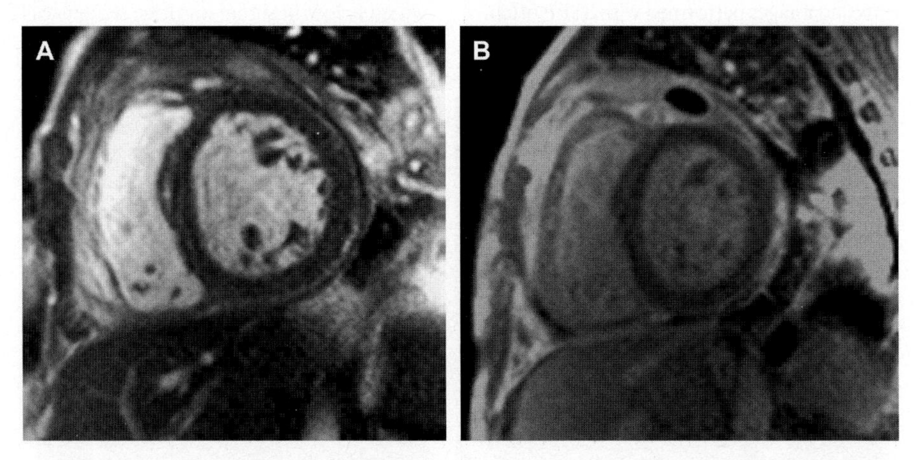

Fig. 3. Postcontrast cine image (*A*) showing a complex effusion in a patient with uremic pericarditis. Note the small oval mass superior to the left ventricle. Delayed-enhancement imaging (*B*) with a long inversion time (600 ms) shows the mass has low signal intensity consistent with thrombus.

produce significant hemodynamic impairment. The character of the effusion may be inferred as described previously. Large effusions may be present without producing tamponade, however. A finding indicative of the likely presence of significant hemodynamic compromise is the observation of right atrial and ventricular collapse in diastole [25–27]. This finding is best observed on cine imaging (Fig. 4A). Real-time cine imaging has some theoretical advantages over breath-hold cine imaging given that the degree of atrial or ventricular collapse may be variable in certain phases of the respiratory cycle, being more prominent after the first two or three heartbeats following the initiation of breath holding (Fig. 4B) [28].

Real-time imaging demonstrating abnormal septal movement indicative of abnormal ventricular interdependence is also helpful in confirming the hemodynamic significance of a large pericardial effusion [29]. Specifically, images acquired in the short-axis plane while the patient takes a deep inspiration can be observed for septal flattening or inversion. This usually is observed on the first two heartbeats after a deep inspiration, after which the septal flattening reverses. This sequence allows visual representation of the hemodynamic significance of the pathologic anatomy. Septal flattening or inversion in this circumstance indicates that the distensibility of the pericardial sac has reached its limit, such that any augmentation of RV filling as results from a deep inspiration will result in diminished LV filling and displacement of the septum to the left (Fig. 4C). Conversely, a lack of septal flattening or inversion despite the presence of significant effusion would imply that residual distensibility

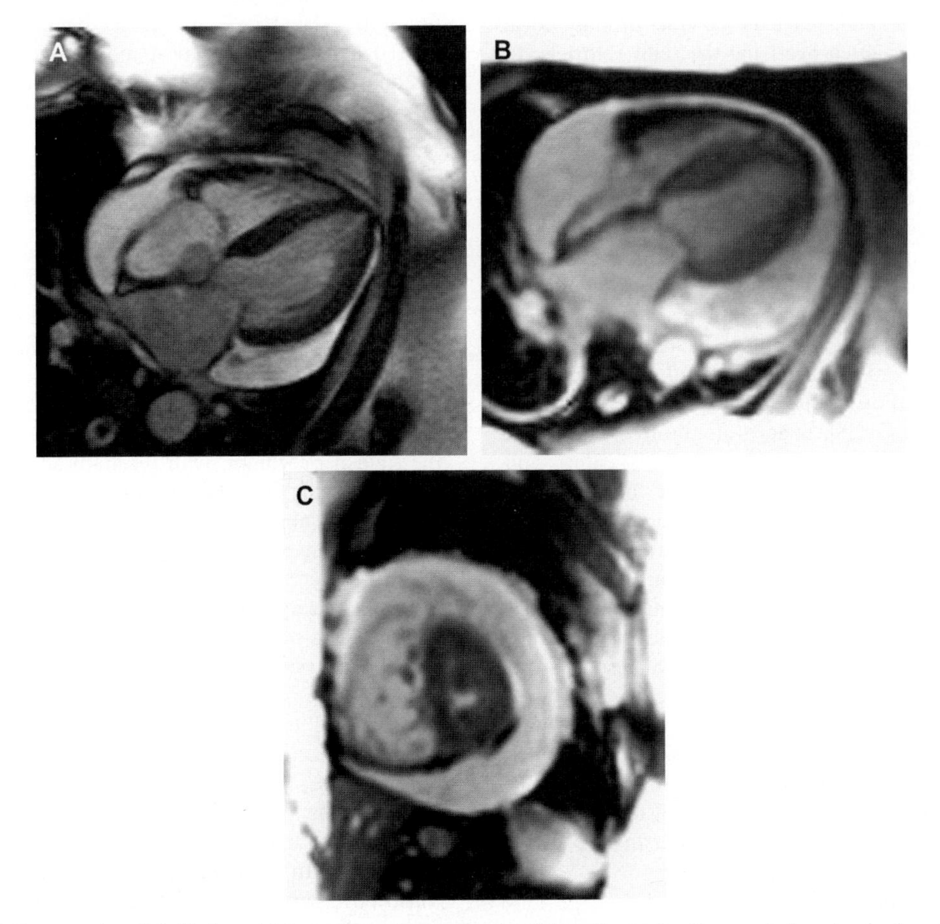

Fig. 4. Large pericardial effusion with hemodynamic compromise. Diastolic atrial collapse noted on standard segmented cine image (*A*) is seen better on real-time cine image (*B*). Real-time cine imaging during a deep inspiration (*C*) demonstrates marked septal flattening.

of the pericardium persists despite the volume of pericardial fluid present.

Constrictive pericarditis

Constrictive pericarditis usually results from abnormal thickening of the pericardium, which subsequently limits distention of the heart, resulting in impairment of diastolic ventricular filling. It was formerly most often caused by tuberculosis, but this is presently an uncommon cause. At present, the most common identifiable causes include prior surgery and prior irradiation, but many cases are idiopathic in origin [30–35]. Many of the previously listed causes of acute pericarditis also can result in chronic constrictive pericarditis.

Histologically, constrictive pericarditis results from fibrosis of the pericardium, resulting in encasement of the heart in a noncompliant rigid structure. In the recent literature, global pericardial thickening still predominates, but a significant percentage of cases may be due to only focal thickening, often overlying the right ventricle. In less than 5% of cases, gross pericardial thickening is not evident, although usually areas of adhesion between the visceral and parietal pericardium are seen on microscopic examination [35,36].

The clinical differentiation between constrictive pericarditis and restrictive cardiomyopathy can be quite difficult. The distinction is of critical importance, however, as pericardiectomy can be curative for the appropriate patient. Although various imaging techniques including echocardiography and CT can be helpful in making this determination, MR imaging is the preferred technique [37,38]. Echocardiography is limited in its ability to detect pericardial thickening, and given that the thickening may be focal and not global, this is an important limitation. CT is superior to MRI in detecting calcification, but given that constriction can occur without calcification, and calcification can occur without constriction, this advantage is of limited clinical importance [32]. Although the excellent spatial resolution of CT provides superb definition of static processes, the significantly lower temporal resolution limits its use for the detection of hemodynamic processes that can be depicted readily with MRI. In addition, MR is superior to CT in differentiating pericardial thickening from small effusions [18].

MRI findings

MRI imaging provides excellent differentiation between high signal epicardial fat and pericardial fluid and the low signal of fibrous pericardium. Thus it allows clear detection of pericardial thickening. Thickening of the pericardium is diagnosed when its width exceeds 4 mm (Fig. 5A, B) [12]. Small focal areas of thickening should be sought in the appropriate clinical circumstance, as constriction may result from focal thickening as described previously.

Ancillary findings such as atrial dilatation, distention of the inferior vena cava, hepatomegaly, and ascites may be seen with restrictive cardiomyopathy and constrictive pericarditis (Fig. 5C). Morphologic images showing pericardial thickening and a normal appearing myocardium, however, are highly predictive of the presence of constriction in the appropriate clinical setting. These findings of abnormal pathologic anatomy are helpful in making the diagnosis; nonetheless, given that ultimately the diagnosis of constriction is one of altered physiology, direct or indirect demonstration of the abnormal hemodynamics is desirable. Therefore, cine images demonstrating altered hemodynamics are a more direct means of confirming the diagnosis of constriction.

Dynamic imaging

Cine imaging in constrictive pericarditis can demonstrate abnormal interventricular dependence caused by the lack of pericardial distensibility. An abnormal configuration of the ventricular septum frequently is observed in early diastole on cine imaging. This septal bounce, or shivering septum is a manifestation of the abnormal ventricular filling dynamics. Specifically, this reflects the limitation of RV filling secondary to the rigid pericardium, with resultant shift of the septum to the left during early diastole. This results in an abnormal septal curvature, which is normally convex to the right; in patients with constrictive pericarditis, reports indicate that loss of this convexity is frequently seen [39]. This sign has excellent sensitivity and specificity for diagnosing constrictive pericarditis, being present in over 85% of patients, and none of the normal controls (Fig. 6A, B).

Real-time cine imaging during a deep inspiration also has been reported to be helpful in distinguishing patients who have restrictive cardiomyopathy from those who have constrictive pericarditis. In a small series of patients with constrictive pericarditis, all constrictive pericarditis patients were differentiated clearly from those who had restrictive cardiomyopathy on real-time cine imaging performed with the patient taking

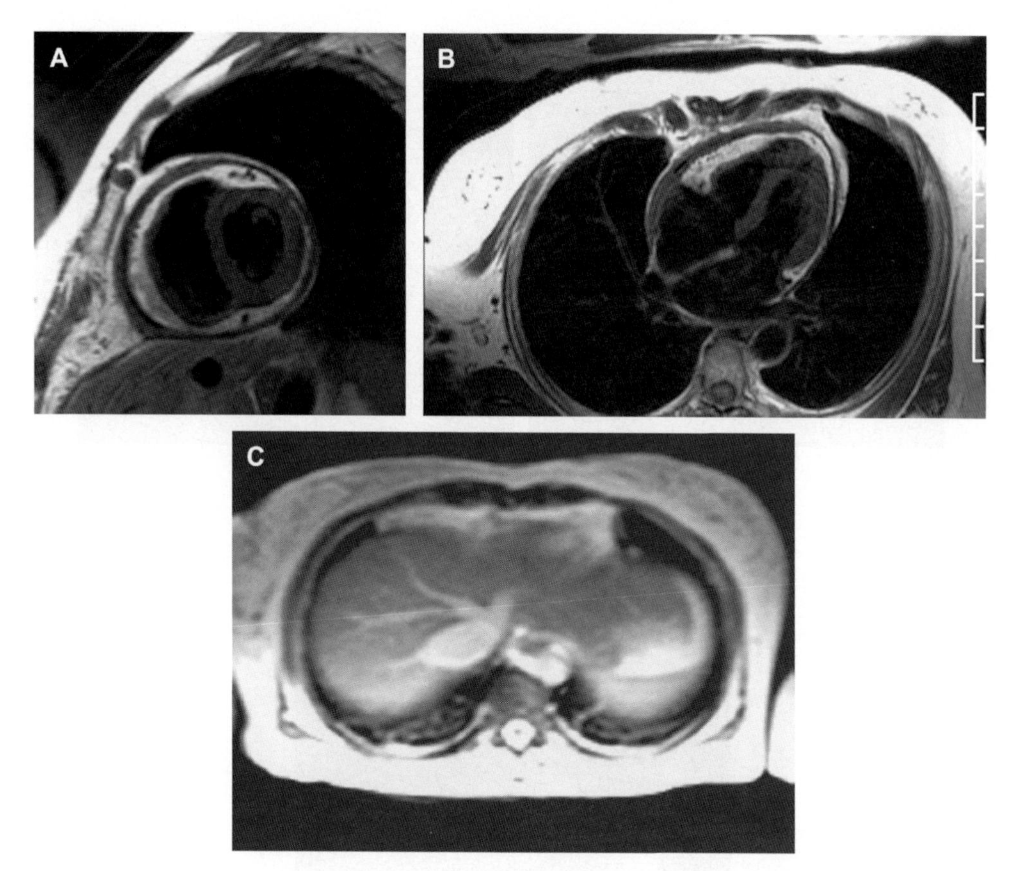

Fig. 5. Short-axis (*A*) and four-chamber views (*B*) demonstrating global pericardial thickening in a patient with constrictive pericarditis. Note the atrial dilatation seen in image (*B*). Atrial and caval dilatation (*C*) may be seen in both constrictive pericarditis and restrictive cardiomyopathy.

a deep inspiration. In the patients who had constrictive pericarditis, septal flattening or inversion was observed, while this finding was absent in those with restrictive cardiomyopathy [29]. The septal inversion noted in these cases is indicative of the diminished compliance of the pericardium, such that any increase in RV filling (such as that caused by a deep inspiration) results in shift of the septum to the left (Fig. 6C). Patients who had restrictive cardiomyopathy did not show such septal abnormalities.

Effusive/constrictive pericarditis

This disorder represents a combination of a significant pericardial effusion producing increased intrapericardial pressure along with pericardial thickening. The diagnosis is based on the persistence of abnormal pericardial dynamics even after the raised intrapericardial pressure secondary to the effusion has been relieved [40,41]. It is seen most often following radiation therapy. It is diagnosed at cardiac catheterization where pressure measurements before and after pericardiocentesis confirm the hemodynamic alterations. Some authors feel that this may represent an intermediate phase in the transition from acute effusive pericarditis to the development of chronic fibrous pericarditis.

Other pericardial disorders

Congenital absence of the pericardium

This is a rare developmental abnormality in which the pericardium may be partially or completely absent. The overwhelming majority of cases are comprised of partial agenesis of the pericardium, usually involving the left side. It may be associated with underlying congenital heart disease, including atrial septal defects, patent ductus arteriosus. and other disorders.

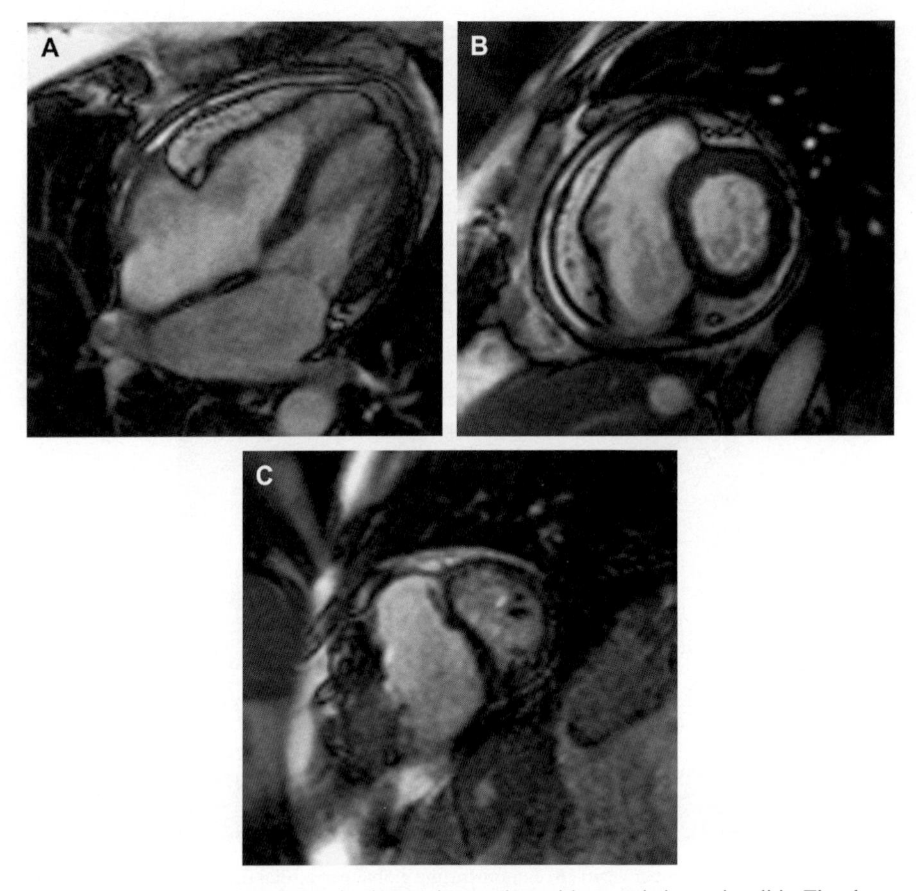

Fig. 6. Four-chamber (*A*) and short-axis (*B*) cine images in a patient with constrictive pericarditis. The abnormal septal curvature seen on standard cine images obtained in diastole (*A*, *B*) is indicative of impaired right ventricular diastolic filling. Real-time cine imaging (*C*) shows septal inversion apparent during a deep inspiration, consistent with abnormal ventricular interdependence.

It is recognized most often on chest radiography, which demonstrates the characteristic abnormal rotation of the heart into the left side of the chest in the usual case of left-sided partial agenesis. The left atrial appendage is often abnormally prominent, and rare cases of herniation of the left atrial appendage through the defect with resultant strangulation have been reported [18,42,43].

It is recognized on MRI when lung tissue is seen interposed between the aorta and pulmonary artery, an appearance not possible with intact pericardium. Also, occasionally lung tissue can be observed inferior to the heart and interposed between the heart and diaphragm.

Pericardial masses

Primary pericardial masses most commonly are caused by pericardial cysts. These benign lesions are felt to originate from portions of the pericardium being pinched off from the remainder of the pericardium during embryologic development. They most commonly occur along the right cardiophrenic angle, and are less commonly left-sided. They can occur anywhere along the margin of the pericardium, however.

MRI findings. Pericardial cysts are low in signal intensity on T1 images, and high in signal intensity on T2 images, consistent with their fluid character. They do not enhance, and they usually are unilocular (Fig. 7A–D) [44,45].

Other pericardial tumors

Other benign pericardial tumors are quite rare and include teratomas, solitary benign fibrous tumors of the pericardium, and hemangiomas [46].

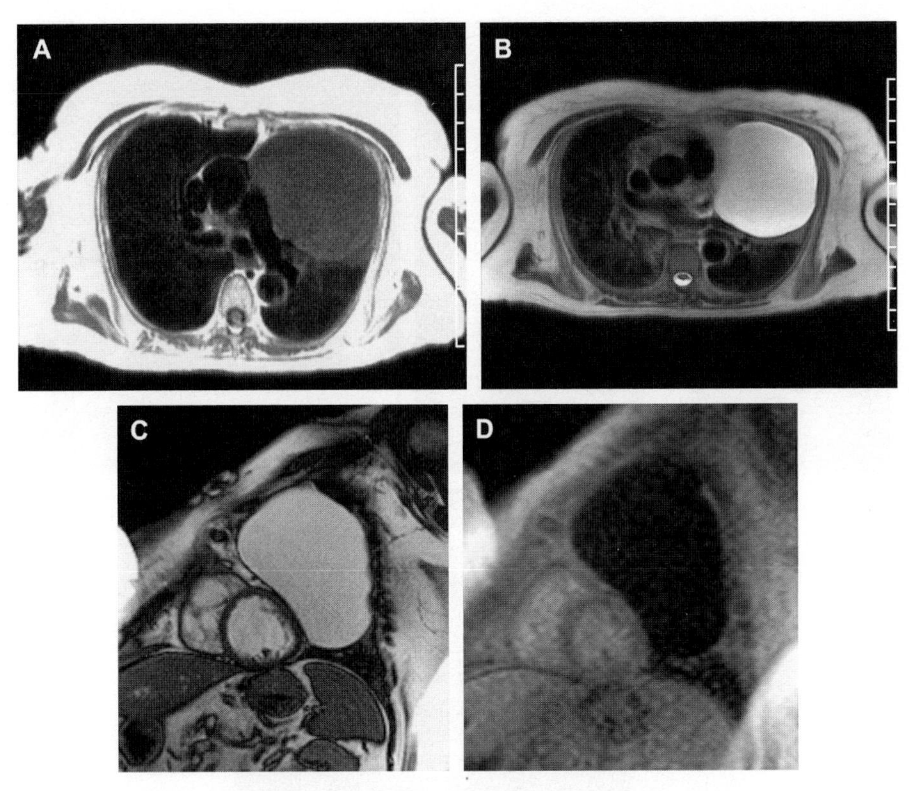

Fig. 7. Multisequence comprehensive MRI study of a pericardial cyst. Note the low signal intensity on the T1 weighted image (*A*), the high signal on the T2 weighted and cine images (*B, C*), and the lack of enhancement on the perfusion image (*D*). Note how the comprehensive nature of the MRI examination allows one to visualize the relationship of the lesion to the myocardium and to characterize this lesion as a simple, nonenhancing cyst lacking solid elements.

Primary malignant tumors of the pericardium are also quite rare, and metastatic disease is significantly more common. Mesothelioma is the most common primary malignant tumor, although sarcomas occasionally may be seen also. Mesothelioma may present with multiple confluent soft-tissue masses that engulf the heart. MRI findings include the presence of pericardial effusion along with a nodular appearance of the pericardium [46].

Secondary or metastatic tumors of the pericardium will be considered with metastatic cardiac masses in the following sections.

Cardiac and pericardial masses

Evaluation of a suspected or known cardiac mass is a frequent source of referrals for cardiac MRI. In addition, cardiac MRI often is requested for further evaluation of a mass suspected but incompletely imaged on echocardiography [47]. Another frequent source of referrals is for evaluation of a possible pseudomass, with clarification desired as to the significance of the finding in question. In all of these instances, the superior tissue characterization, as well as high-resolution imaging capable with MRI, usually provides a definitive evaluation.

Pseudomasses

Any discussion of cardiac masses should begin with a discussion of lesions that can mimic a significant cardiac or paracardiac mass. The most common of these entities is the right atrial pseudotumor produced by a prominent crista terminalis (Fig. 8A), which can be mistaken for a right atrial mass on echocardiography. A prominent Chiari network also can be mistaken for a right atrial mass, as can a prominent Eustachian valve. All of these normal structures can be well-visualized on MRI, and a true mass can be excluded [48].

Extrinsic mass lesions that can simulate cardiac pathology include large hiatal hernias. These can produce significant displacement of the atria.

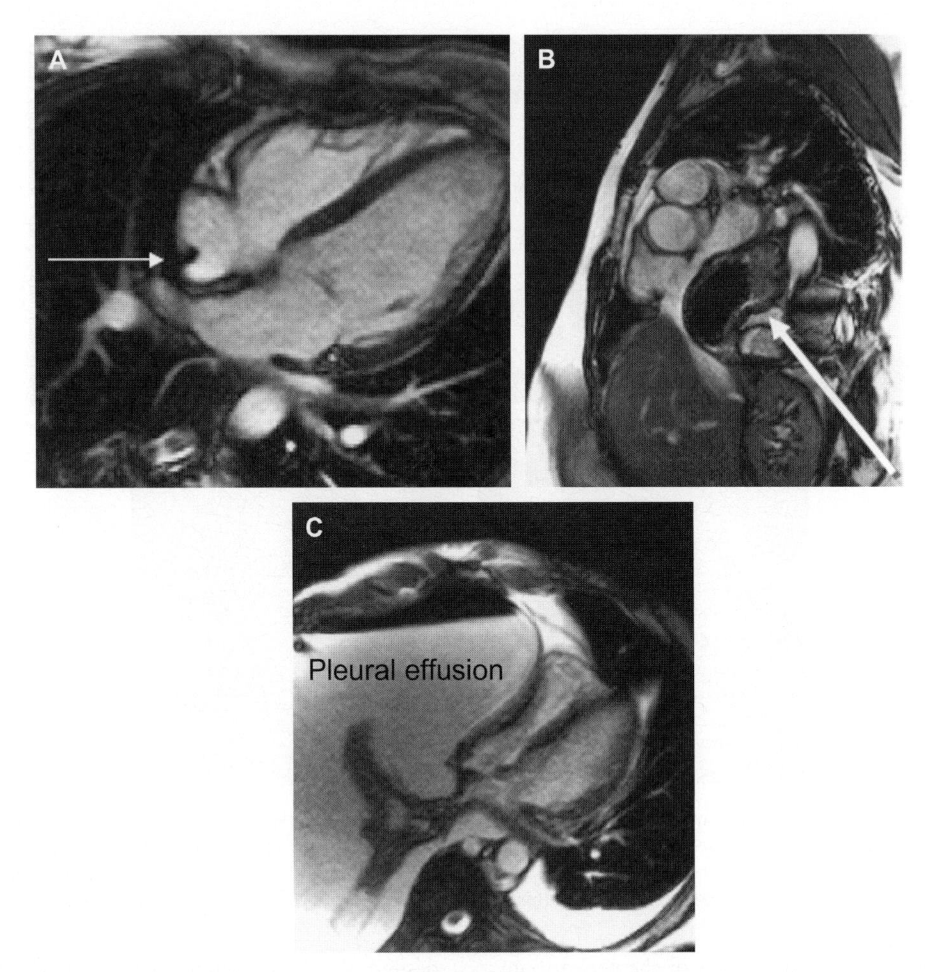

Fig. 8. (*A*) Cine image demonstrating a prominent crista terminalis (*arrow*) producing a right atrial pseudomass. (*B*) Cine image showing a large hiatal hernia (*arrow*) indenting the atria. (*C*) A large right pleural effusion is noted to compress the right atrium and ventricle. Note the air-fluid level along the anterior margin of the effusion from prior thoracentesis.

In addition, their heterogenous internal architecture can lead to significant confusion on echocardiography [47]. They are depicted clearly with MRI, and their true nature can be discerned easily (Fig. 8B). Pleural effusions likewise can produce mass-effect upon the heart occasionally, and can result in a confusing echocardiographic appearance. Their relationship to the pleural space and their internal architecture can be clarified readily with MRI (Fig. 8C).

True cardiac masses

Although not a neoplasm, thrombus is actually the most common cardiac mass. Thrombi occur predominantly in the left atrial appendage and within the ventricular chambers. Left atrial appendage thrombus most often arises in the setting of atrial fibrillation.

Ventricular thrombi most commonly occur in the setting of cardiomyopathy, most often ischemic in nature. The diminished ejection fraction and regional wall motion abnormalities likely contribute to the formation of these thrombi. In addition, denudation of the endothelium by prior infarction also likely contributes, as ventricular thrombi most often are found adherent to sites of prior infarction. In particular, thrombi often are noted along the endocavitary aspect of ventricular aneurysms (Fig. 9A).

Right atrial thrombi often will develop adjacent to long-standing central venous catheters (Fig. 9B) [49].

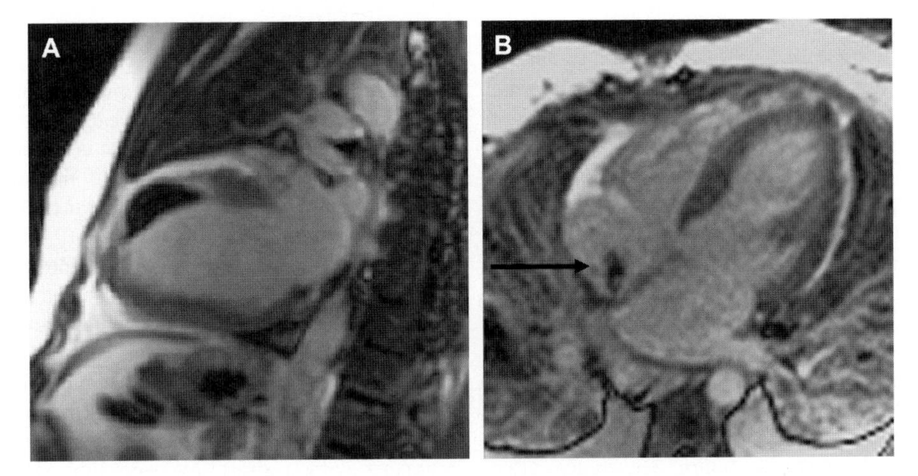

Fig. 9. Delayed-enhancement images with a long inversion time (600 ms) showing mural thrombus lining an anterior wall aneurysm (*A*) and a large peri-catheter thrombus (*arrow*) in the right atrium (*B*).

Cardiac MRI is significantly more sensitive than echocardiography for detecting ventricular thrombi. Studies have demonstrated an approximately twofold increase in sensitivity for the detection of ventricular thrombi when comparison is made with echocardiography [50–52]. The sensitivity of MRI for detecting ventricular thrombi is significantly improved by the administration of intravenous contrast material. Precontrast cine imaging often will fail to detect ventricular thrombi that clearly are seen as low signal intensity foci following the administration of contrast. In addition, postcontrast delayed-enhancement inversion recovery images with a long inversion time are exquisitely sensitive for the detection of even small thrombi [53]. In this instance, the long inversion time allows recovery of signal by virtually all tissues except thrombus, which remains low in signal intensity and therefore dark on imaging (see Fig. 9A, B).

Primary and secondary cardiac neoplasms

True neoplasms of the heart, whether primary or secondary, are relatively uncommon in clinical practice. Autopsy figures from the presurgical era demonstrated an incidence rate of approximately 0.05% for primary cardiac tumors. Significantly higher figures often are seen in autopsy rates from referral centers. Of the primary cardiac tumors, 75% are benign, and 25% are malignant. Of the malignant primary tumors, the overwhelming majority represents some form of sarcoma, as will be described in following sections [54].

Metastatic disease is significantly more common, with incidence rates 20 to 40 times that of primary cardiac tumors. Although it is estimated that between 10% and 12% of patients dying from cancer will demonstrate metastatic involvement of the heart and pericardium at autopsy, a far smaller percentage comes to clinical attention [55–58].

A thorough knowledge of the clinical presentations and imaging characteristics of the primary cardiac tumors often will allow one to make a reasonably intelligent differential diagnosis of the various diagnostic possibilities, and sometimes a specific diagnosis, based on MRI. A detailed evaluation of the imaging characteristics of the lesion often will allow the interpreting physician to have a sense of the likely aggressive or benign nature of the lesion in question. The following section first considers the histology of the primary cardiac tumors, as well as their different clinical presentations and imaging characteristics. Subsequently, the imaging characteristics and pattern of spread of metastatic disease will be considered. In addition, findings that favor metastatic disease will be addressed. It will become apparent to the reader that the MRI characteristics usually will mirror the histology of the lesion in question.

Primary benign cardiac tumors

Myxoma

Cardiac myxomas make up approximately 50% of all primary benign cardiac neoplasms. They demonstrate a female predominance that is as high as 3 to 1 in some series, and closer to 1.5 to 1 in others. The average patient age at presentation is approximately 50, with most cases occurring between the ages of 30 and 60. They are rarely diagnosed in childhood except for instances where they arise as part of a syndrome [59].

Myxomas may present with a bewildering variety of clinical manifestations. The classic clinical triad of constitutional symptoms (such as fever and malaise), valvular obstruction, and embolic phenomena, however, are seen to some degree in most cases.

They are usually solitary tumors, with less than 5% of cases demonstrating multiple lesions. Patients who have multiple lesions should be strongly suspected of having syndromic myxomas, the most common manifestation of which is the Carney syndrome. In this disorder, atrial myxomas are commonly seen and they may be multiple and may demonstrate tumor recurrence after surgery. In addition, these patients also demonstrate abnormal skin pigmentation, Sertoli cell tumor of the testes, cutaneous myxomas, myxoid fibroadenoma of the breast, melanotic schwannomas, adrenocortical hyperplasia, and pituitary hyperplasia. A gene deletion at the 17q22 locus has been reported in these patients [60–64].

Myxomas are located in the left atrium in approximately 75% to 80% of cases, and they usually are attached to the fossa ovalis. Approximately 15% to 20% arise in the right atrium, with a small percentage extending across the fossa ovalis to involve both atria. Approximately 2% arise in each respective ventricle. They are always intracavitary in location.

The exact cell of origin is uncertain. Histologically, the diagnosis is based on the finding of typical cardiac myxoma cells in a myxoid background. The myxoma cell is histologically different from that of the soft tissue myxomas. The tumors often have a gelatinous appearance, because of the abundance of myxoid matrix. They frequently are attached to the interatrial septum by either a broad base or a narrow stalk. Lesions arising on a stalk frequently will demonstrate significant mobility, and they may prolapse through the mitral or tricuspid valves.

Frequently, organized thrombi are noted on the surface, which can lead to a confusing appearance on imaging. In addition, superficial calcifications are noted frequently [65].

MRI findings. MRI closely parallels the previously described findings. Specifically, a myxoma frequently presents as a well-defined mass arising from the fossa ovalis and extending into the left atrium on dark blood morphologic imaging (Fig. 10A). Given their gelatinous nature, they often will demonstrate high signal on T2 weighted images. Their appearance on gradient echo imaging is often complex given the presence of coating thrombus and superficial calcifications along their outer margin, and older gradient echo cine imaging often resulted in low signal intensity [65]. SSFP cine images often will demonstrate higher signal intensity, owing to the high T2/T1 ratio of the myxoid matrix present. Also, cine imaging is useful in visualizing the possible hemodynamic effects of these mobile lesions, which can obstruct the atrioventricular valves (Fig. 10B) [5,66]. Perfusion imaging often demonstrates subtle increased vascularity. The lesions usually will demonstrate heterogenous enhancement on delayed-enhanced images with a short inversion time (Fig. 10C). Any associated thrombus overlying the lesion will be low in signal intensity on delayed-enhancement inversion recovery images with a long inversion time. The central portion of the lesion will demonstrate enhancement on these sequences, however.

Papillary fibroelastomas

These represent benign avascular papillomas of the endocardium, and they are similar in many respects to Lambl's excrescences. They are noted to be larger and more gelatinous, however, and they are frequently present on the valves away from the sites of closure, as opposed to Lambl's excrescences, which are by definition at the sites of valve closure [67].

The exact incidence is unknown, because the entity is seldom sought at autopsy and rarely causes symptoms. In several series, however, it was felt to represent the second most common primary cardiac tumor [58,68]. There is no sex predilection, and the average age at presentation is 60. They most often are discovered incidentally on an echocardiogram performed for another indication, but they have been reported to cause neurological symptoms, presumably on an embolic basis.

Their gross anatomic appearance has been likened to that of a sea anemone. They usually measure less than 1 cm in size. They may have a minimal short stalk. Over 90% of lesions occur on valve surfaces, making them the most common tumor originating along the valve surfaces. When they occur along the atrioventricular valve, they have a predilection for the atrial surface, but there is no specific predilection regarding the semilunar valves.

MRI findings. Because of their small size and their location on valvular surfaces, they are

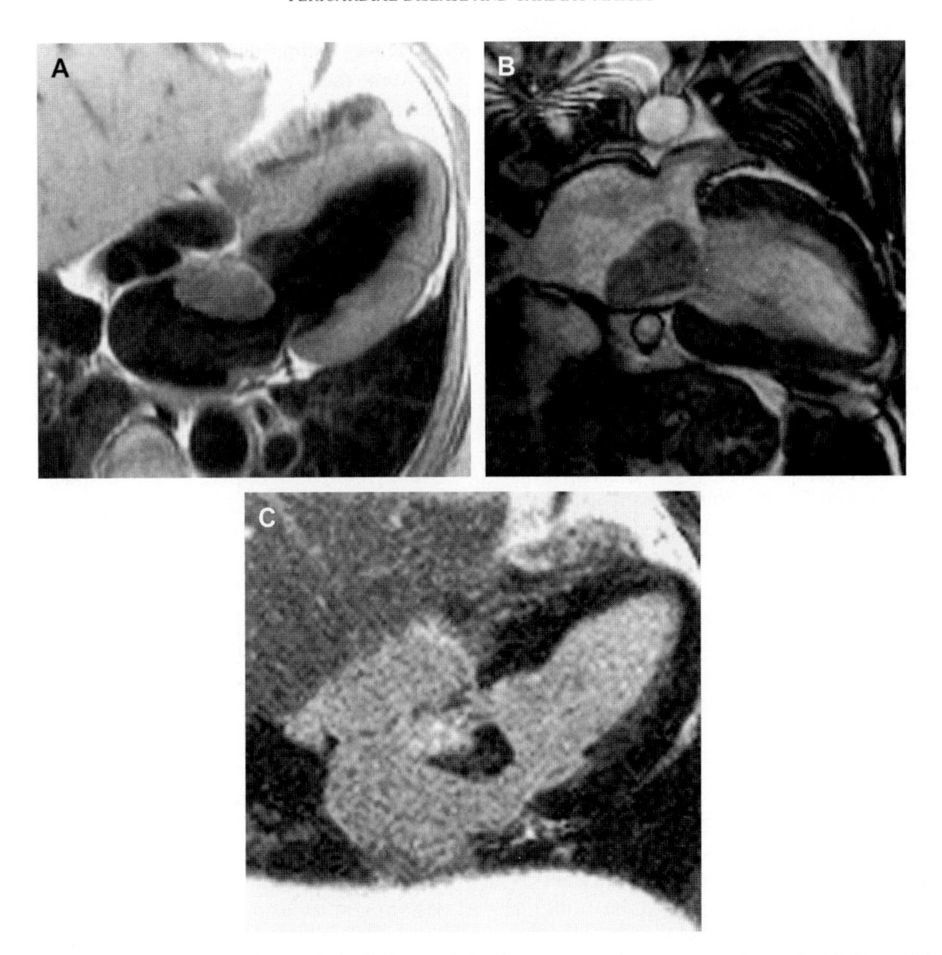

Fig. 10. Four-chamber dark-blood morphologic image (*A*) of a myxoma demonstrates the typical left atrial location with attachment to the fossa ovalis. Two-chamber steady-state free-precession cine image (*B*) demonstrates the effect of the lesion on transmitral flow. Four-chamber inversion recovery delayed enhancement image (*C*) shows the typical heterogeneous enhancement.

uncommonly visualized on MRI. When seen, they usually are visualized as small sessile lesions that demonstrate signal intensity similar to the endocardium [69,70].

Cardiac rhabdomyoma

Cardiac rhabdomyomas likely represent hamartomas rather than true neoplasms. Although uncommon, they represent the most common cardiac mass in childhood, accounting for 50% to 75% of pediatric cardiac tumors [71–74]. They frequently are associated with tuberous sclerosis, with a prevalence that depends on the age at which the patient is imaged. Specifically, most infants with tuberous sclerosis will demonstrate cardiac masses consistent with rhabdomyomas at echocardiography. Sixty percent of the older children and less than 25% of adults with tuberous sclerosis, however, will have detectable cardiac masses [54]. This apparent decrease in incidence likely is predominantly because of the tendency of these lesions to regress spontaneously [75,76]. There is no sex predilection.

Occasional cases are seen in the absence of tuberous sclerosis, and these are termed sporadic. In these instances, approximately 50% of the lesions are single. These rhabdomyomas often do not demonstrate spontaneous regression, and they may require surgery [77].

Histologically, the tumors are composed of atypical myocytes containing abundant glycogen. They have a predilection for the ventricles, and they often involve the interventricular septum. They vary widely in size, but they are usually 1 to 3 cm in size.

MRI findings. Given their histological makeup, it is not surprising that the MRI appearance of these lesions is most often that of mass-like regions of otherwise normal-appearing myocardium. They usually present as multiple intramural masses that produce distortion of the normal ventricular anatomy. Their signal intensity is similar to that of normal myocardium, but they can be recognized on cine imaging as mass-like regions of focal altered contraction [78,79].

Fibroma

Cardiac fibromas are uncommon tumors that nonetheless comprise the second most common cardiac mass seen in childhood. They represent benign congenital tumors that present usually as a discrete focal mass composed predominantly of fibroblasts and collagen. They are felt to be congenital in origin, and they may in fact represent a hamartoma rather than a neoplasm. The overwhelming majority occur in children, with one third of the lesions presenting before 1 year of age. The mean age of presentation is 13 years, and a small percentage may not present until adulthood [57,58,71].

Approximately one third of patients present with arrhythmias, one third with heart failure or cyanosis, and one third are detected incidentally [80]. They are usually solitary lesions, in contrast to rhabdomyomas, which tend to be multiple. Cardiac fibromas are associated with Gorlin syndrome, which is characterized by multisystem involvement including basal cell carcinomas of the skin, odontogenic keratocysts, rib and vertebral anomalies, and multiple skin lesions [81,82].

These lesions tend to involve the ventricular septum, the LV free wall, the right ventricle, and the atria in that order. Histologically, they represent a homogenous proliferation of fibroblasts. Abundant collagen is also frequently present. Calcification is a frequent finding, although it may not be apparent on MRI [80].

MRI findings. MRI often will allow a fairly specific diagnosis of cardiac fibroma. On standard dark blood imaging, cardiac fibroma is recognized as an intramural mass, often protruding into the ventricular cavity as well as distorting the epicardial surface of the heart. Cardiac fibromas are nearly isointense on T1 weighted images, but they are hypointense on T2 weighted images [60,66]. This is a helpful finding. The lesions are relatively hypovascular on perfusion imaging when comparison is made with normal myocardium. Delayed-enhancement imaging of fibromas also has been reported recently [83], and this has demonstrated intense uptake of contrast by the lesions, which became quite hyperintense on images where the inversion time was chosen to null the normal myocardium (Fig. 11).

Lipomatous hypertrophy of the interatrial septum and lipomas

These lesions are considered together because of their similar signal characteristics on MRI. The lesions are quite distinct both histologically and clinically, however.

Lipomatous hypertrophy of the interatrial septum is not a true neoplasm, and it is not truly hypertrophy of the adipocytes. Rather, it represents a nonencapsulated hyperplasia of otherwise

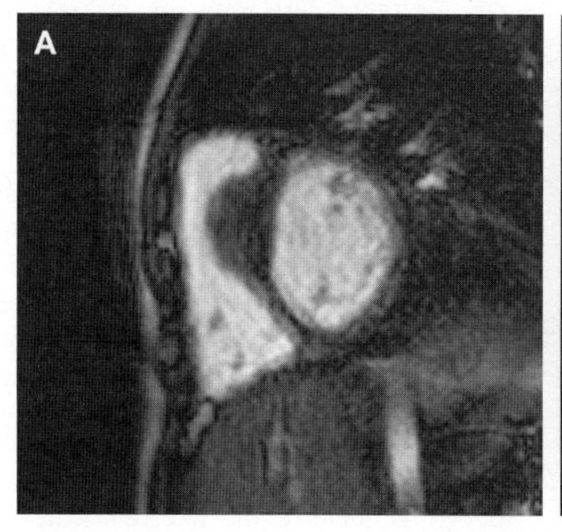

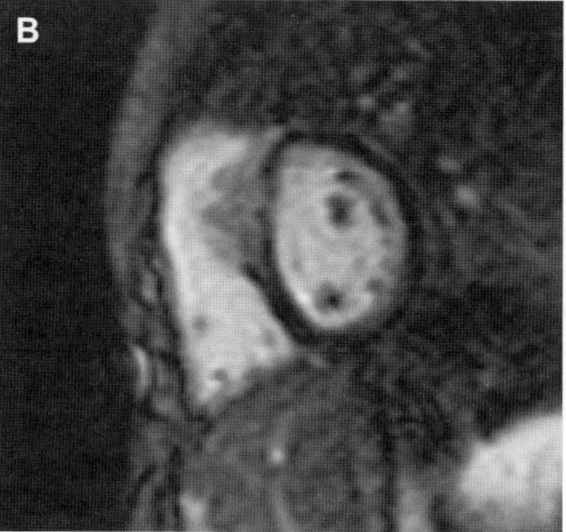

Fig. 11. Cardiac fibroma evident as a septal mass on cine imaging (*A*), which demonstrates hyperenhancement on delayed enhancement imaging (*B*).

normal fatty cells within the interatrial septum. This diagnosis is based on the finding of fatty deposits in the interatrial septum resulting in a diameter exceeding 2 cm in transverse dimension [78,84].

The exact etiology is unknown, but it appears to be associated with obesity and advanced age. The average age at diagnosis is approximately 69 years, and there appears to be a slight male predominance. It is said to be associated with tachyarrhythmias, predominantly atrial in origin.

The exact incidence of this disorder is difficult to discern, as some series do not separate this disorder from lipomas. It increasingly is recognized, however, based on echocardiographic imaging and MRI. The pathologic findings noted in this disorder include thickening of the atrial septum by mature fat cells and myocytes. Sparing of the fossa ovalis is usually apparent [58,85].

MRI findings. MRI is quite specific in this disorder. Thickening of the interatrial septum to a diameter greater than 2 cm is noted, and sparing of the fossa ovalis is apparent. This often results in a dumbbell- or barbell-like appearance (Fig. 12A). The fatty hyperplasia results in high signal on T1 weighted images through the interatrial septum. The addition of fat saturation to the imaging sequences results in signal dropout confirming the fatty nature of these lesions (Fig. 12B, C). In addition, cine imaging with SSFP sequences results in a characteristic chemical shift artifact at the interface between the fatty portions of the septum and the remainder of the myocardium (see Fig. 12A) [84].

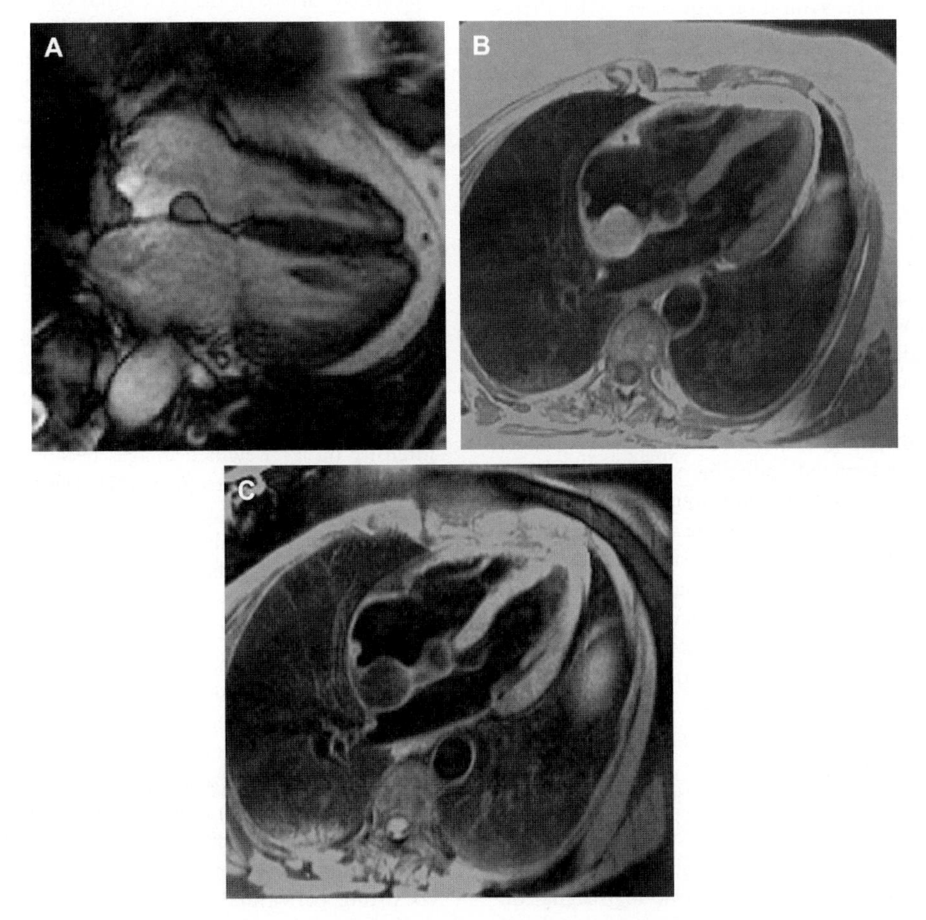

Fig. 12. Lipomatous hypertrophy of the interatrial septum. (*A*) Cine image demonstrating the characteristic barbell appearance. HASTE images without (*B*) and with fat-suppression (*C*) demonstrate signal drop-out of the lipomatous septum on the fat-suppressed image (*C*).

Lipoma

Cardiac lipomas are probably quite rare, although the exact incidence is difficult to define, given that some pathologic series combine these lesions with lipomatous hypertrophy of the interatrial septum. They are benign neoplasms composed of encapsulated mature adipose tissue, similar to extracardiac lipomas. There does not appear to be any sex predilection. They are usually discovered in adulthood.

Histologically, they represent well-encapsulated deposits of mature adipocytes [58,85]. Most occur along the epicardial surface of the heart, although approximately 25% to 30% rise in an intramural location, and they can protrude into the cardiac cavities.

MRI findings. Given their fatty nature, cardiac lipomas are high in signal intensity on T1 weighted sequences, and they show evidence of signal dropout on fat saturation sequences. MRI therefore provides a specific diagnosis of these lesions [60,84].

Paragangliomas

These are tumors originating from neuroendocrine cells, and formerly, they were termed pheochromocytomas. The preferred term at present, however, is functioning paraganglioma.

Most of these lesions present with symptoms of catecholamine excess. Specifically, many patients present with hypertension, tachyarrhythmias, and heart failure. Patients range in age from adolescence to middle age, but the lesions are most common in adults between 25 and 40 years of age. Although paragangliomas often arise as part of a more widespread endocrine syndrome, cardiac paragangliomas are usually sporadic [86–88].

Grossly, the lesions may be well-encapsulated, and they tend to originate at sites of the normal cardiac ganglia. Specifically, they tend to occur in the atria, along the atrioventricular sulcus, and at the roots of the great vessels. The interatrial septum is also a common location. They are typically quite hypervascular in nature. They average between 3 and 12 cm in dimension. Histologically, they are usually benign tumors of neuroendocrine cells, and resection is usually curative [57,86].

MRI findings. Like paragangliomas elsewhere, these lesions have a characteristic high signal on T2 weighted images, and they have been termed light-bulb bright [60]. They tend to be intramural masses that are isointense to normal myocardium on T1 images before the administration of contrast but demonstrate extensive heterogenous hyperenhancement following the administration of contrast (Fig. 13) [89,90].

Hemangiomas/lymphangiomas

These are benign neoplasms composed of endothelial lined thin-walled spaces that contain either blood (hemangioma) or lymph (lymphangioma). These are rare tumors, and the exact incidence is unknown. The age at presentation is quite variable, ranging from infancy to late adulthood [57,86].

Many hemangiomas are asymptomatic and are discovered incidentally at cardiac surgery. Lymphangiomas are probably less common, and they tend to occur in childhood or adolescence. Whereas hemangiomas can occur in any portion of the heart [91], lymphangiomas have a predilection for the epicardial surface or the pericardial sac.

On histologic examination, both entities are characterized by the presence of vascular channels. Lymphangiomas often will be filled with fluid, and the endothelial-lined spaces may become quite large and cystic in appearance. Hemangiomas tend to demonstrate minimally prominent endothelial channels, with a variable proportion of fat.

MRI findings. Both lymphangiomas and hemangiomas demonstrate high signal on T2 weighted images. Hemangiomas also demonstrate high signal on T1 weighted images, likely because of the frequent presence of areas of interspersed fat. Lymphangiomas, however, will be low in signal intensity on T1 weighted images because of their extensive cystic nature [60,92,93]. Hemangiomas usually will demonstrate heterogenous prolonged enhancement; the enhancement pattern of lymphangiomas has not been well-reported.

Malignant cardiac tumors

Malignant tumors make up approximately 25% of primary cardiac neoplasms. The great majority represents some form of sarcoma, with lymphoma making up most of the remainder. The imaging characteristics of these malignant tumors are fairly similar, with most lesions demonstrating invasion of surrounding structures and normal myocardium, poor border definition, and frequent coexisting pericardial effusions. Most cannot be distinguished based on imaging characteristics as discrete entities, but findings favoring malignancy usually can be detected.

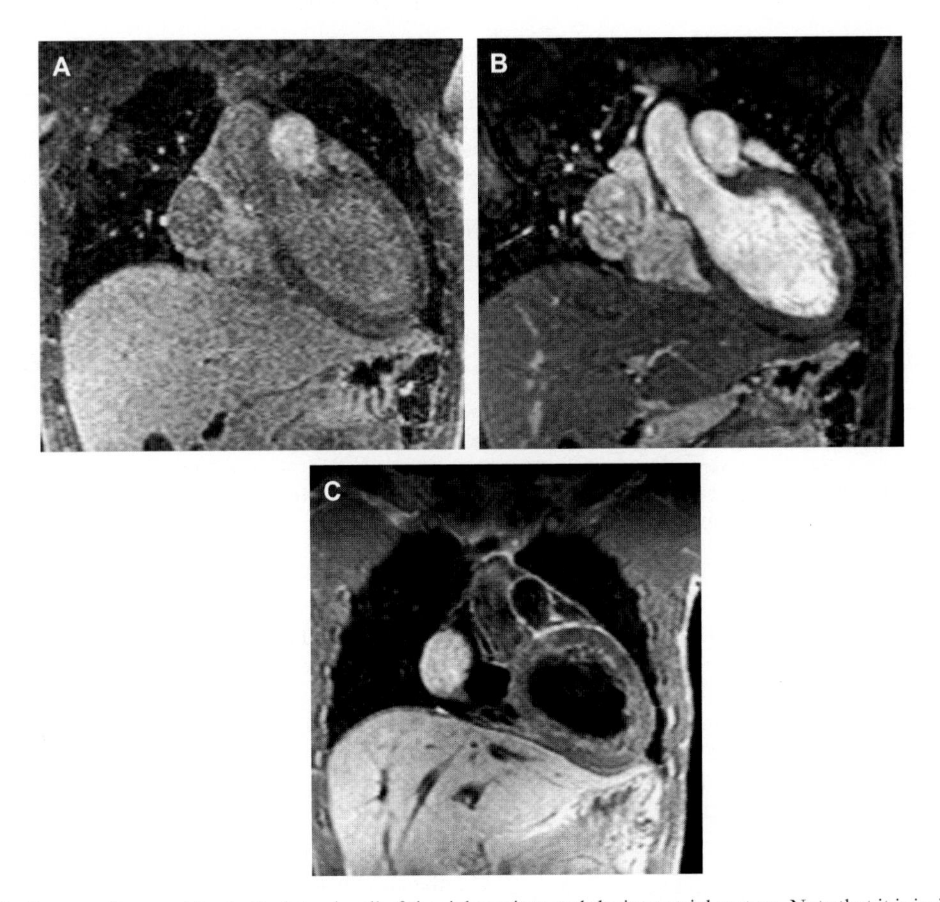

Fig. 13. Paraganglioma arising in the lateral wall of the right atrium and the interatrial septum. Note that it is isointense to myocardium on the precontrast coronal T1 weighted image (*A*) and shows heterogenous enhancement on the post-contrast T1 weighted image (*B*). Note the characteristic high signal on the T2 weighted image (*C*).

The various cardiac sarcomas have many features in common, although differentiating features that may favor one or the other histologic subtype often can be detected. Distinguishing characteristics are listed in Table 3. Because most of the sarcomas demonstrate imaging features that are similar, angiosarcoma will be discussed in detail, and the differentiation of the other histologic subtypes from this archetype then will be made.

Angiosarcoma

Angiosarcoma is the most common form of cardiac sarcoma, accounting for approximately 40% of cases, and most series demonstrate a slight male predominance. It is a tumor of endothelial origin, and it has a predilection for involvement of the right atrium [94]. This location represents a differentiating feature in that most of the other sarcomas have a left atrial predilection [95,96]. Because of its site of origin, patients often present with signs of right heart failure and/or cardiac tamponade. Pericardial invasion is frequent and often results in a bloody pericardial effusion.

On pathologic examination, these sarcomas are usually hemorrhagic, necrotic, and adherent to the pericardium. They frequently demonstrate infiltration of normal adjacent myocardium, and compression of cardiac chambers and direct extension to the pericardium. They often protrude into the atrial cavity, also [58].

MRI findings. Angiosarcomas are typically bulky, infiltrating masses that are isointense on T1 imaging, with areas of internal higher signal often noted because of the frequent presence of hemorrhage (Fig. 14). They usually demonstrate intense enhancement. Cases of extensive pericardial infiltration often result in contrast enhancement, giving rise to what some have described as

Table 3
Differentiating features of cardiac sarcomas

Tumor type	Imaging characteristics	Notes
Angiosarcoma	Bulky mass extending to pericardium. Frequent internal hemorrhage. Right atrial origin in 90%	Most common primary malignancy, approximately 40% of sarcomas
MFH	Posterior wall of left atrium in approximately 85%; results in pulmonary venous congestion	Must be distinguished from myxoma
Undifferentiated sarcoma	Left atrial origin in two thirds; also can present with pulmonary venous congestion	Improved diagnostic techniques results in fewer cases
Osteosarcoma	95+% originate in left atrium; often involve the mitral valve	Primary lesions in left atrium; mets in right
Leiomyosarcoma	Posterior wall of LA in approximately 80%	Must be distinguished from myxoma
Fibrosarcoma	Most common sarcoma to involve the ventricles	Frequently involve the pericardium
Rhabdomyosarcoma	Slight left atrial predominance; can arise anywhere; most common sarcoma to involve the valves	Most common cardiac sarcoma in children

a "sunray" appearance [95,97]. Postcontrast imaging results in a heterogenous pattern of enhancement. Areas of coexisting thrombus will result in typical low signal intensity on delayed-enhanced images with a long inversion time. Occasionally, pulmonary metastases will be evident from these predominantly right-sided tumors.

Other sarcomas

Most of the other sarcomas arising within the heart are also bulky, infiltrating masses. No significant male/female predominance is noted. The usual age range of affected patients is between 30 and 50 years, except for rhabdomyosarcoma, which has a mean age of 14. Most of these lesions have a tendency to involve the left atrium (Table 3), distinguishing them from the more common angiosarcoma that has a predilection for the right atrium [95].

Malignant fibrous histiocytoma. This is the second most common identified cardiac sarcoma in most series. It preferentially involves the left atrium, and can mimic a left atrial myxoma. Malignant fibrous histiocytoma, however, usually arise along the posterior border of the left atrium, rather than the fossa ovalis as seen with myxomas. Its clinical presentation relates to its left atrial location, with the predominant symptoms related to pulmonary venous congestion and left atrial obstruction.

Undifferentiated sarcoma. The relative proportion of undifferentiated sarcoma has diminished over time, in large measure because of improved diagnostic techniques using immuno-histochemistry. Nonetheless, this remains the second or third most common category. It also has left atrial predominance.

Osteosarcoma. Primary cardiac osteosarcomas almost always (>95%) originate within the left atrium. They are usually bulky masses measuring 4 to 10 cm in diameter, and they commonly invade the atrial wall and the mitral valve (Fig. 15). Calcification may be present although difficult to detect on MRI.

Leiomyosarcoma. These lesions originate in the left atrium in approximately 80% cases, usually from the posterior wall. Therefore, they must be distinguished from myxomas. They also tend to present with pulmonary vascular congestion.

Fibrosarcoma. These lesions not infrequently (22%) involve the pericardium. They also involve the ventricles in one third of cases. Approximately 50% of cases originate within the left atrium.

Rhabdomyosarcomas. These lesions are the most common sarcomas in the pediatric age group. They may arise in any cardiac chamber, and they are the most likely sarcoma to involve the valvular structures.

Other sarcomas including liposarcoma, synovial cell sarcoma, and malignant peripheral nerve sheath tumors also have been reported, but they are extraordinarily rare [46,58,68].

MRI findings. All of the previously mentioned tumors are bulky masses that usually are located within the left atrium, with the exception of

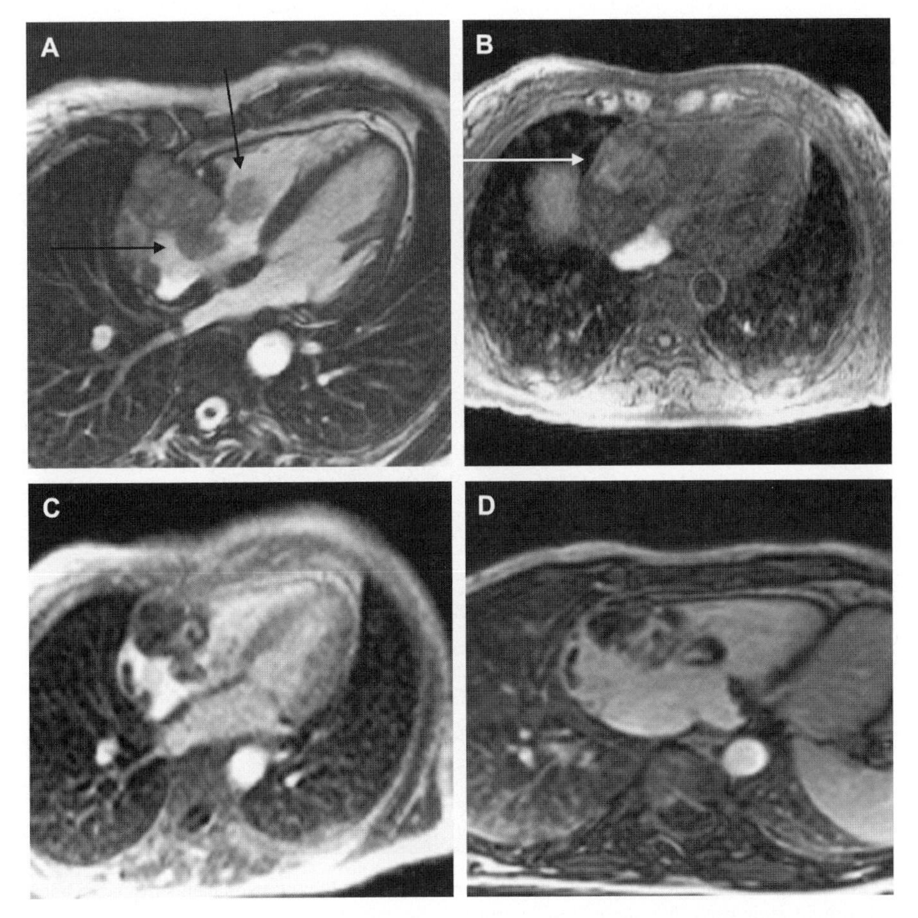

Fig. 14. Multisequence comprehensive imaging of a right atrial angiosarcoma demonstrates extensive infiltration of the atrial wall with extension to the pericardium on the still-frame cine image (*A*). Note also the attached, pedunculated masses (*arrows*) that were mobile on cine imaging. A fat-suppressed T1 weighted precontrast (*B*) image shows high signal in the mass (*arrow*) before contrast consistent with internal hemorrhage. A perfusion image (*C*) demonstrates heterogenous enhancement. Delayed- enhancement image (*D*) with an inversion time of 600 ms shows associated thrombus as low in signal intensity.

rhabdomyosarcoma and fibrosarcoma, which have a more generalized pattern. Importantly, these lesions need to be distinguished from the benign atrial myxoma. As opposed to myxomas that originate from the fossa ovalis, these lesions tend to have a broad-based origin from the posterior wall of the left atrium [95,98], and they often will demonstrate findings indicative of their aggressive nature (see Fig. 15). Specifically, pericardial effusion and infiltration of the myocardium are important findings suggestive of malignancy. A bizarre pattern of enhancement is suggestive, and a high index of suspicion should be maintained for any left atrial lesion that does not arise from the fossa ovalis.

Primary cardiac lymphoma

By definition, these malignancies are distinct from systemic lymphoma with cardiac involvement, particularly non-Hodgkin's lymphoma, which may aggressively involve the mediastinum. It is estimated that up to 24% of patients who have disseminated lymphoma will demonstrate cardiac involvement [55,95,99].

These neoplasms are almost always aggressive B-cell lymphomas. They have increased prevalence in immunocompromised patients, particularly those who have HIV infection, but they also can arise in previously immunocompetent patients. The incidence is unknown, but the disorder is felt to be rare. The average age at presentation is

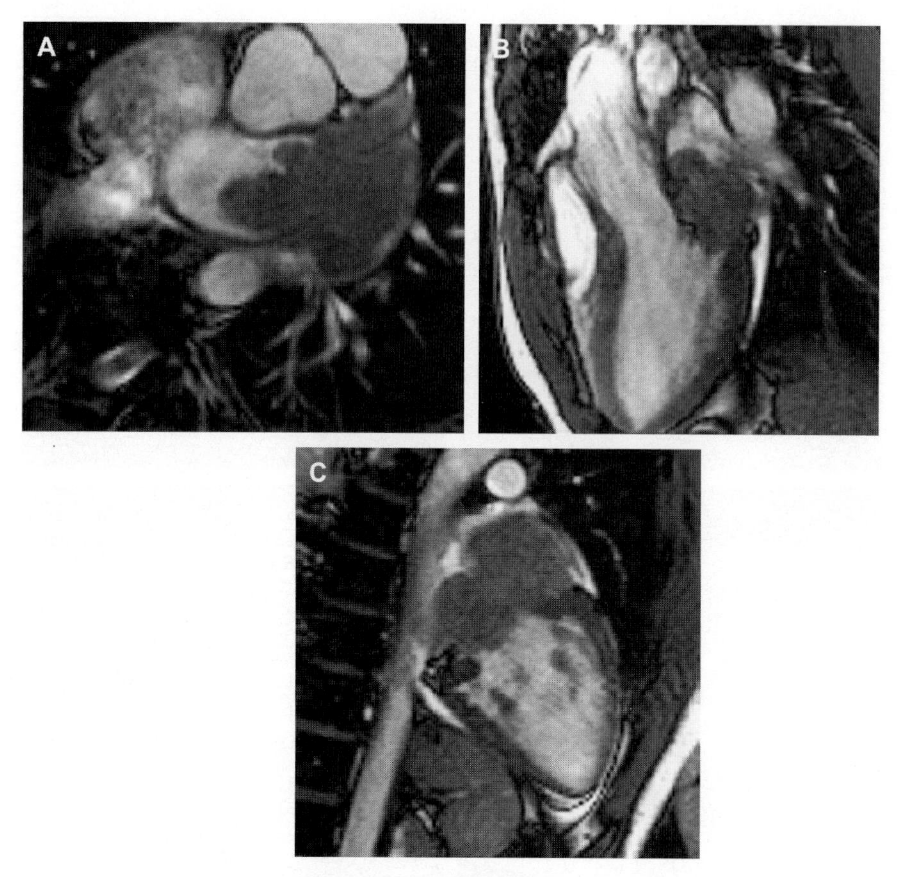

Fig. 15. Left atrial osteosarcoma–oblique short-axis (*A*), three-chamber (*B*), and two-chamber (*C*) cine images demonstrating a bulky, infiltrating mass that almost-totally obstructs the mitral valve.

approximately 58 years. Males appear to have a slight predominance.

Clinically, cardiac lymphomas frequently present with shortness of breath, arrhythmias, superior vena cava obstruction, or cardiac tamponade. This latter finding is related to the frequent involvement of the pericardium, and pericardial effusions are commonly present.

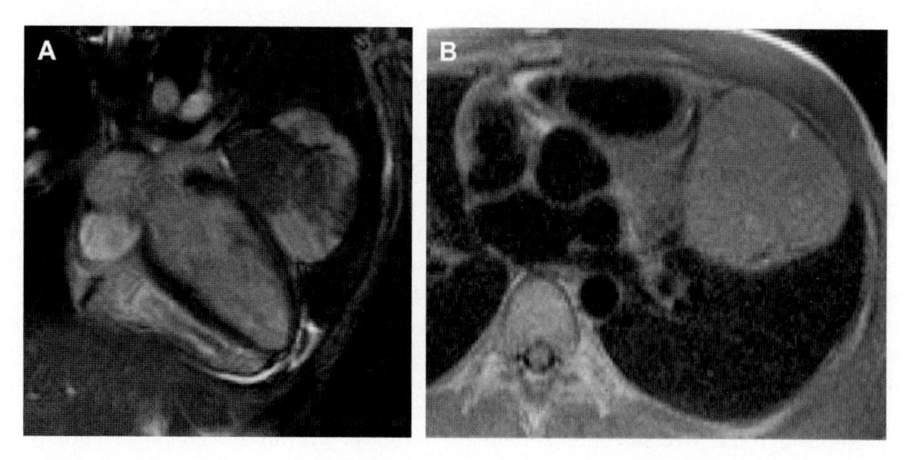

Fig. 16. (*A, B*) Four-chamber cine and axial HASTE images showing a malignant thymoma extending to involve the pericardium.

At pathologic examination, multiple nodules of varying sizes most often characterize primary cardiac lymphoma. They frequently involve the epicardium and extend to involve the pericardium. The right atrium is affected most commonly, followed by the right ventricle. More than one cardiac chamber is involved in over 75% in cases. They are less likely than sarcomas to demonstrate internal necrosis or to invade the cardiac chambers [95].

MRI findings. The imaging findings parallel those of the clinical pathology; that is, frequent involvement of the epicardial surface of the heart is apparent, along with extensive pericardial involvement. Pericardial effusion is present in the overwhelming majority of cases, and it is usually quite large [100,101].

The tumor nodules may be relatively hypointense on T1 weighted images and hyperintense on T2 weighted images, but the appearance is variable. Contrast enhancement is frequent and may be homogenous or heterogenous. Delayed-enhancement imaging using an inversion time chosen to null the normal myocardium has been

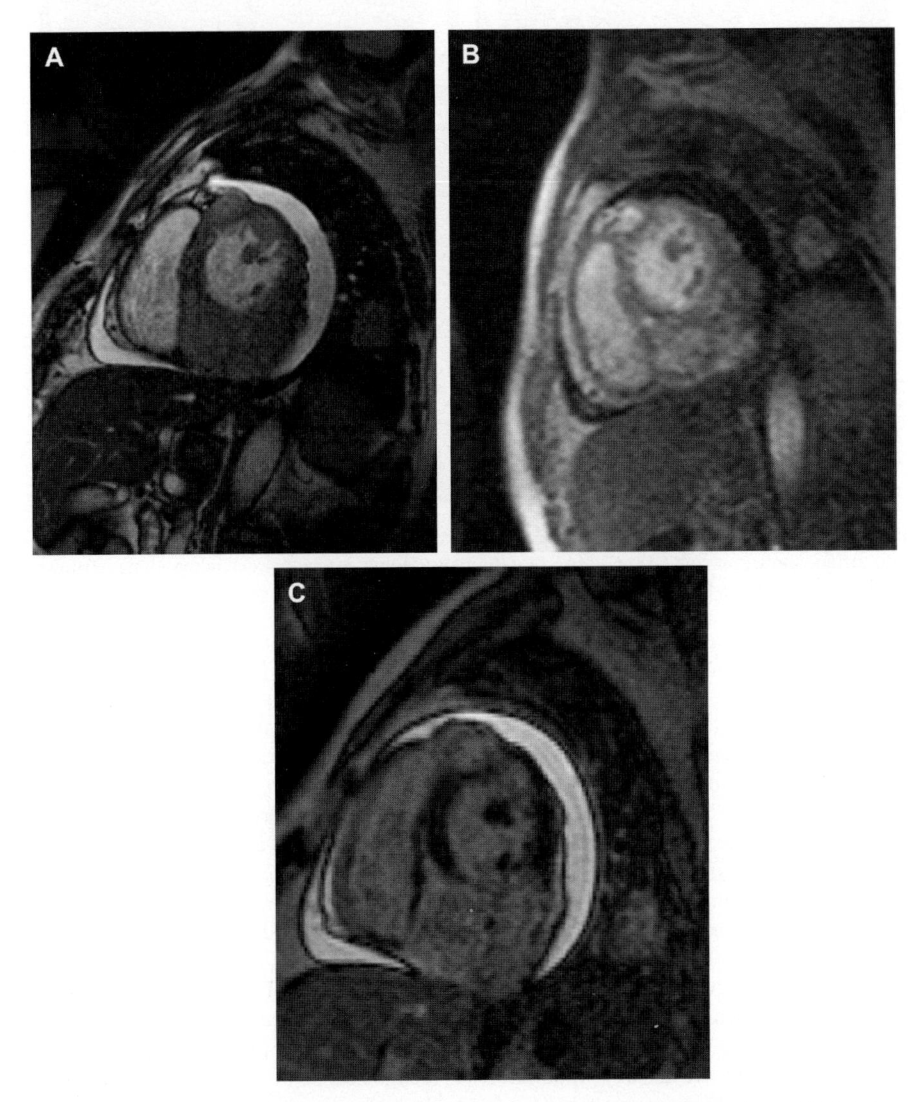

Fig. 17. Short-axis cine (*A*), perfusion (*B*), and delayed enhancement (*C*) images demonstrating multiple intramural nodules caused by renal cell carcinoma metastases. Note the extensive vascularity of the myocardial and pulmonary metastases shown by perfusion imaging. Also note the extensive hyperenhancement noted on delayed-enhancement imaging (*C*). A large pericardial effusion also noted.

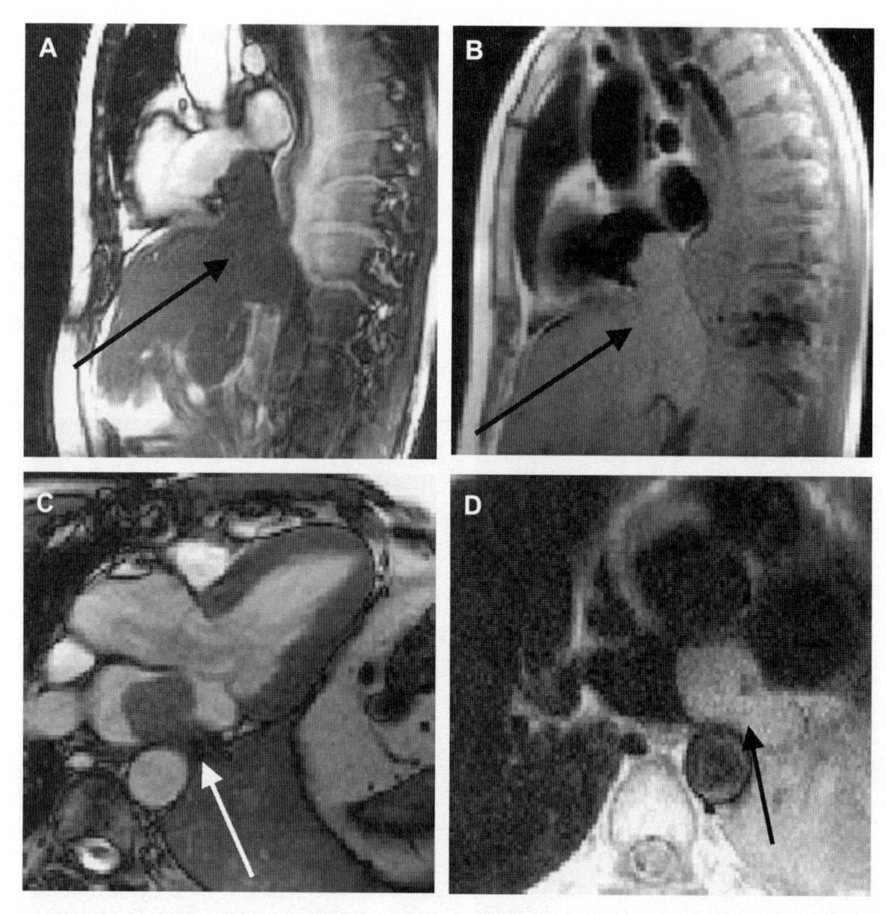

Fig. 18. Transvenous extension of tumor. Hepatocellular carcinoma extending up the inferior vena cava (*arrow*) and into the right atrium shown on cine (*A*) and HASTE (*B*) images. Lung carcinoma extending along left lower lobe pulmonary vein (*arrow*) into the left atrium shown on cine (*C*) and HASTE (*D*) images.

reported to aid in the localization of an infiltrating lymphoma [102].

Metastatic disease of the heart and pericardium

Tumors metastasizing to the heart often involve the pericardium also. As noted previously, metastatic disease is reported to be 20 to 40 times more common than primary cardiac neoplasia, but the true incidence may be even higher. Multiple series have demonstrated that approximately 10% to 12% of patients dying of cancer will demonstrate autopsy evidence of metastatic cardiac or pericardial disease. These lesions are rarely the presenting manifestation of the patient's malignancy, however, and are usually apparent only in the later phases of the patient's illness [55,56].

Although metastatic melanoma is the most likely malignancy to spread to the heart (46% to 64% of patients) [103,104], its low prevalence relative to other malignancies makes neoplasms such as lung carcinoma and breast carcinoma more common primary sites of disease. Hematologic malignancies such as leukemia and lymphoma are represented disproportionately because of their frequent cardiac involvement. A recent series reported that lung carcinoma was the primary site in 36% of patients who had cardiac metastases; nonsolid primary malignancies (leukemia, lymphoma) represented 20%, carcinoma of the breast 7%, and carcinoma of the esophagus 6% [56].

Many of these lesions are clinically silent, and even those that produce symptoms may go unrecognized or be mistaken for findings related to the patient's primary tumor. Findings suggestive of cardiac involvement include the frequent presence of pericardial effusions, unexplained shortness of breath, and the new development of an arrhythmia in a patient with a known malignancy. This latter finding in particular should raise the suspicion of myocardial involvement in a patient who has a known malignancy [55,57]. In approximately 10% to 25% of patients who have metastatic cardiac disease, the cause of death is related to this involvement. This often results from malignant pericardial effusion producing cardiac tamponade, congestive heart failure, coronary arterial involvement, or arrhythmia.

There are four pathways by which malignancy can reach the heart: direct extension from an adjacent primary tumor, retrograde extension by means of the lymphatics from adjacent mediastinal lymph node involvement, hematogenous spread, and transvenous extension [55]. Many lesions demonstrate a combination of one or more of these pathways:

Direct extension to involve the heart or pericardium is a finding often observed in lung carcinomas, as well as primary mediastinal tumors such as malignant thymoma (Fig. 16).

Retrograde extension by means of the lymphatics is a common pathway for those carcinomas that frequently spread to the pulmonary hilar or mediastinal lymph nodes (lung and esophageal carcinoma). The pericardium frequently is involved in cases of retrograde lymphatic extension, and large pericardial effusions may be associated.

Hematogenous spread is the usual route by which melanoma, sarcomas, leukemia, and renal cell carcinoma metastasize to the heart. This route of dissemination is manifested most often by multiple intramyocardial metastatic deposits (Fig. 17).

Transvenous extension to the right side of the heart is seen frequently with renal cell carcinoma, adrenal carcinoma, or hepatocellular carcinoma extending up the inferior vena cava. Transvenous extension to the left atrium is seen most often in primary lung carcinoma (Fig. 18).

MRI findings. Given the extensive variety of possible mechanisms of involvement, and the variable primary tumors, the MRI findings of secondary cardiac malignancies span a range of possibilities. Pericardial effusion is probably the most common imaging manifestation of metastatic disease, although it may be seen in other disorders also. The presence of nodular implants upon the pericardium should be viewed with a high degree of suspicion, however. Complex pericardial effusions or loculated pericardial effusions are also suggestive findings.

Intramural nodular deposits within the myocardium in an adult who has a known primary malignancy would be highly suspicious, and should prompt consideration of those disorders that tend to spread by means of hematogenous pathways. Metastases often produce extensive infiltration of normal structures, and cine imaging is very helpful for the depiction of altered myocardial and valvular function (see Fig. 17). Myocardial parenchymal lesions may demonstrate intense enhancement following administration of contrast material, and these may demonstrate evidence of hypervascularity on perfusion imaging. Delayed-enhanced imaging also will demonstrate intense enhancement often (see Fig. 17).

Melanomas may demonstrate characteristic nodular deposits with high signal on T1 weighted images, which is virtually pathognomonic of this diagnosis (Fig. 19).

Tumors or intracavitary lesions directly extending from a primary noncardiac malignancy usually present no diagnostic difficulty.

To summarize, metastatic malignancies will usually demonstrate infiltration of normal structures, abnormal enhancement, and associated pericardial effusions. Nodular pericardial deposits also may be seen. Any of these findings in a patient

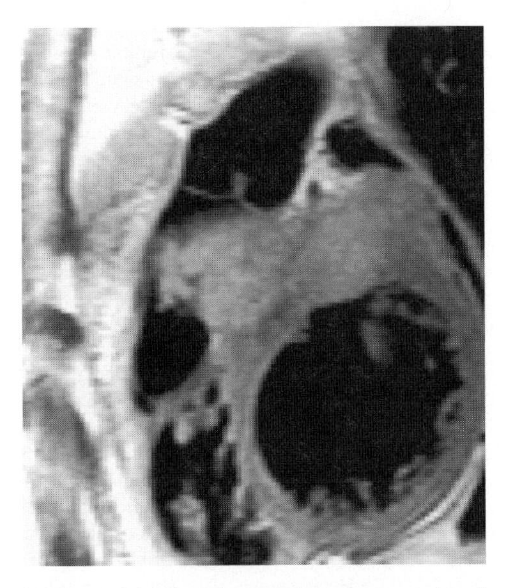

Fig. 19. Nodular deposits secondary to metastatic melanoma in the anterior septum and anterior wall that extend into the right ventricular outflow tract. Note the high signal of the lesions on this T1 weighted image.

who has a known primary malignancy should be viewed with a high degree of suspicion. In the absence of a known primary malignancy, there may be occasional diagnostic difficulty in distinguishing between a primary cardiac malignancy such as a sarcoma and a secondary cardiac malignancy. In these cases, a biopsy may be necessary to make the final determination.

Differential diagnosis

In the differential diagnosis of cardiac masses (as in restaurants), location is everything. The diagnostic considerations can be simplified significantly if one has localized the lesion accurately, as can be seen in Table 4. It should be noted that localizing the lesion also means assessing its boundaries, and whether it invades or simply displaces normal structures. Following localization, evaluation of the signal characteristics of the lesion is critically important, as many lesions have nearly pathognomonic features (eg, tumors composed of fat or fibrous tissue). Finally, the enhancement pattern can be quite helpful. For instance, myxomas and thrombi can be very similar in location (left atrium) and behavior (mobile), but myxomas usually demonstrate heterogenous enhancement, while thrombi are almost always very low in signal on delayed-enhancement images with a long inversion time.

Although exceptions to these guidelines can certainly occur, they represent a conceptual framework that hopefully will provide the reader with a starting point in evaluating patients with cardiac masses. The importance of accurate

Table 4
Differential diagnosis by location

Location	Lesion	Typical MRI features	Specific diagnostic features
Intracavitary	Myxoma	Oval, mobile left atrial lesion, heterogenous enhancement	Attachment to fossa ovalis
	Thrombus	Left atrium/appendage or ventricles at sites of stasis/infarction	Low-signal (dark) on delayed enhancement images with a long inversion time
	Vegetations	Irregular nodules or masses arising along valvular surfaces and peri-valvular tissues	Signal intensity similar to thrombus; may have associated septic pulmonary emboli
	Metastases	Transvenous extension of tumor	Lesions extend in continuity from primary lesion to heart
Intramural—children	Rhabdomyomas	Multiple masses with signal intensity similar to muscle	Infants and children with tuberous sclerosis
	Fibromas	Solitary mass distorting normal anatomy	Low in signal intensity on T2 weighted images
Intramural—adults	Metastases	Variable—pericardial effusions very common; typically known late-stage malignancy; lesions usually enhance	Melanoma metastases may show high signal on T1 weighted images
	Lipomatous hypertrophy of interatrial septum	Thickening of septum to >2cm; typically spares fossa ovalis; high signal on T1 weighted images	Signal drop-out on fat-saturation images
	Lipoma	Epicardial/intramural lesion with high signal on T1 weighted images	Signal drop-out on fat-saturation images
	Paraganglioma	Well-defined lesion arising in atrial walls or septum	Light-bulb bright on T2 weighted images
Epicardial/pericardial	Metastases	Variable, pericardial metastases more common than myocardial; large pericardial effusions common	Direct tumor extension; extensive adjacent adenopathy very suggestive
	Pericardial cyst	Well-defined nonenhancing lesion contiguous with pericardium	Signal follows fluid on all sequences
	Hemangioma	Multicystic enhancing lesions, may involve epicardium and pericardium	High in signal on T1 and T2
	Lymphangioma	Rare multicystic lesions may be intramural, epicardial, or pericardial	Low in signal on T1 weighted images, high on T2

diagnosis cannot be overemphasized, as appropriate management strategies can vary from watchful waiting and continued observation (as in the case of benign tumors or pseudomasses) to anticoagulation (as in the case of thrombi) to surgical resection (in the case of myxomas and malignant tumors). The superior ability of cardiac MRI to aid in this endeavor, as compared with other modalities, thus makes it the gold standard for evaluating cardiac and paracardiac masses.

Summary

MRI is superior to echocardiography and CT in the comprehensive evaluation of pericardial disease and cardiac masses.

In the modern MRI examination, the older spin-echo morphologic sequences have been replaced by HASTE imaging, and SSFP cine imaging has replaced gradient echo techniques. Improved tissue characterization is provided by the combination of perfusion and delayed enhancement imaging.

Pericardial effusions and thickening whether global or localized can be well-depicted with MRI.

In addition to imaging the anatomic abnormality present in constrictive pericarditis, MRI with real-time cine imaging can demonstrate the pathologic hemodynamics.

Thrombus is the most common cardiac mass, and MRI detects twice as many as echo.

Metastases are 20 to 40 times more common than primary cardiac tumors; of the primary tumors, 75% are benign, and at least half are myxomas.

Twenty-five percent of primary cardiac tumors are malignant, and almost all are some form of sarcoma.

Specific diagnoses of cardiac masses are often possible.

Acknowledgment

The authors wish to thank Ms. Fifi LeBlanc for her invaluable secretarial assistance, and Dr. Sarah Joyner for her helpful suggestions.

References

[1] Gulati G, Sharma S, Kothari SS, et al. Comparison of echo and MRI in the imaging evaluation of intracardiac masses. Cardiovasc Intervent Radiol 2004;27(5):459–69.

[2] Budoff MJ, Achenbach S, Blumenthal RS, et al. Assessment of coronary artery disease by cardiac computed tomography: a scientific statement from the American Heart Association Committee on Cardiovascular Imaging and Intervention, Council on Cardiovascular Radiology and Intervention, and Committee on Cardiac Imaging, Council on Clinical Cardiology. Circulation 2006; 114(16):1761–91.

[3] Coles DR, Smail MA, Negus IS, et al. Comparison of radiation doses from multislice computed tomography coronary angiography and conventional diagnostic angiography. J Am Coll Cardiol 2006; 47(9):1840–5.

[4] Semelka RC, Shoenut JP, Wilson ME, et al. Cardiac masses: signal intensity features on spin echo, gradient echo, gadolinium-enhanced spin echo, and TurboFLASH images. J Magn Reson Imaging 1992;2(4):415–20.

[5] Hoffmann U, Globits S, Schima W, et al. Usefulness of magnetic resonance imaging of cardiac and paracardiac masses. Am J Cardiol 2003;92(7): 890–5.

[6] Pereles FS, Kapoor V, Carr JC, et al. Usefulness of segmented trueFISP cardiac pulse sequence in evaluation of congenital and acquired adult cardiac abnormalities. AJR Am J Roentgenol 2001;177(5): 1155–60.

[7] Simonetti OP, Kim RJ, Fieno DS, et al. An improved MR imaging technique for the visualization of myocardial infarction. Radiology 2001; 218(1):215–23.

[8] Fuster V, Kim RJ. Frontiers in cardiovascular magnetic resonance. Circulation 2005;112(1): 135–44.

[9] Kuhl HP, Spuentrup E, Wall A, et al. Assessment of myocardial function with interactive nonbreath hold real-time MR imaging: comparison with echocardiography and breath-hold cine MR imaging. Radiology 2004;231(1):198–207.

[10] Reichek N. MRI myocardial tagging. J Magn Reson Imaging 1999;10(5):609–16.

[11] Sechtem U, Tscholakoff D, Higgins CB. MRI of the normal pericardium. AJR Am J Roentgenol 1986;147(2):239–44.

[12] Sechtem U, Tscholakoff D, Higgins CB. MRI of the abnormal pericardium. AJR Am J Roentgenol 1986;147(2):245–52.

[13] Teraoka K, Hirano M, Yannbe M, et al. Delayed-contrast enhancement in a patient with perimyocarditis on contrast-enhanced cardiac MRI: case report. Int J Cardiovasc Imaging 2005;21(2–3): 325–9.

[14] Rienmuller R, Groll R, Lipton MJ. CT and MR imaging of pericardial disease. Radiol Clin North Am 2004;42(3):587–601, vi.

[15] Breen JF. Imaging of the pericardium. J Thorac Imaging 2001;16(1):47–54.

[16] White CS. MR evaluation of the pericardium. Top Magn Reson Imaging 1995;7(4):258–66.
[17] Kastler B, Germain P, Dietemann JL, et al. Spin echo MRI in the evaluation of pericardial disease. Comput Med Imaging Graph 1990;14(4):241–7.
[18] Wang ZJ, Reddy GP, Gotway MB, et al. CT and MR imaging of pericardial disease. Radiographics 2003;23:S167–80.
[19] Glockner JF. Imaging of pericardial disease. Magn Reson Imaging Clin N Am 2003;11(1):149–62, vii.
[20] Frank H, Globits S. Magnetic resonance imaging evaluation of myocardial and pericardial disease. J Magn Reson Imaging 1999;10(5):617–26.
[21] Refsum H, Junemann M, Lipton MJ, et al. Ventricular diastolic pressure–volume relations and the pericardium. Effects of changes in blood volume and pericardial effusion in dogs. Circulation 1981; 64(5):997–1004.
[22] Freeman GL, LeWinter MM. Pericardial adaptations during chronic cardiac dilation in dogs. Circ Res 1984;54(3):294–300.
[23] Freeman GL, LeWinter MM. Determinants of intrapericardial pressure in dogs. J Appl Physiol 1986;60(3):758–64.
[24] Little WC, Freeman GL. Pericardial disease. Circulation 2006;113(12):1622–32.
[25] Tsang TS, Oh JK, Seward JB. Diagnosis and management of cardiac tamponade in the era of echocardiography. Clin Cardiol 1999;22(7):446–52.
[26] Tsang TS, Barnes ME, Hayes SN, et al. Clinical and echocardiographic characteristics of significant pericardial effusions following cardiothoracic surgery and outcomes of echo-guided pericardiocentesis for management: Mayo Clinic experience, 1979–1998. Chest 1999;116(2):322–31.
[27] Singh S, Wann LS, Schuchard GH, et al. Right ventricular and right atrial collapse in patients with cardiac tamponade—a combined echocardiographic and hemodynamic study. Circulation 1984; 70(6):966–71.
[28] Appleton CP, Hatle LK, Popp RL. Cardiac tamponade and pericardial effusion: respiratory variation in transvalvular flow velocities studied by Doppler echocardiography. J Am Coll Cardiol 1988;11(5): 1020–30.
[29] Francone M, Dymarkowski S, Kalantzi M, et al. Real-time cine MRI of ventricular septal motion: a novel approach to assess ventricular coupling. J Magn Reson Imaging 2005;21(3):305–9.
[30] Myers RB, Spodick DH. Constrictive pericarditis: clinical and pathophysiologic characteristics. Am Heart J 1999;138(2 Pt 1):219–32.
[31] Ling LH, Oh JK, Schaff HV, et al. Constrictive pericarditis in the modern era: evolving clinical spectrum and impact on outcome after pericardiectomy. Circulation 1999;100(13):1380–6.
[32] Ling LH, Oh JK, Breen JF, et al. Calcific constrictive pericarditis: is it still with us? Ann Intern Med 2000;132(6):444–50.
[33] Nishimura RA. Constrictive pericarditis in the modern era: a diagnostic dilemma. Heart 2001; 86(6):619–23.
[34] Nishimura RA, Connolly DC, Parkin TW, et al. Constrictive pericarditis: assessment of current diagnostic procedures. Mayo Clin Proc 1985;60(6): 397–401.
[35] Oh KY, Shimizu M, Edwards WD, et al. Surgical pathology of the parietal pericardium: a study of 344 cases (1993–1999). Cardiovasc Pathol 2001; 10(4):157–68.
[36] Talreja DR, Edwards WD, Danielson GK, et al. Constrictive pericarditis in 26 patients with histologically normal pericardial thickness. Circulation 2003;108(15):1852–7.
[37] Mertens LL, Denef B, De Geest H. The differentiation between restrictive cardiomyopathy and constrictive pericarditis: the impact of the imaging techniques. Echocardiography 1993;10(5): 497–508.
[38] Masui T, Finck S, Higgins CB. Constrictive pericarditis and restrictive cardiomyopathy: evaluation with MR imaging. Radiology 1992;182(2): 369–73.
[39] Giorgi B, Mollet NR, Dymarkowski S, et al. Clinically suspected constrictive pericarditis: MR imaging assessment of ventricular septal motion and configuration in patients and healthy subjects. Radiology 2003;228(2):417–24.
[40] Hancock EW. A clearer view of effusive-constrictive pericarditis. N Engl J Med 2004;350(5):435–7.
[41] Hancock EW. Subacute effusive-constrictive pericarditis. Circulation 1971;43(2):183–92.
[42] Yamano T, Sawada T, Sakamoto K, et al. Magnetic resonance imaging differentiated partial from complete absence of the left pericardium in a case of leftward displacement of the heart. Circ J 2004;68(4):385–8.
[43] Faridah Y, Julsrud PR. Congenital absence of pericardium revisited. Int J Cardiovasc Imaging 2002; 18(1):67–73.
[44] Oyama N, Oyama N, Komuro K, et al. Computed tomography and magnetic resonance imaging of the pericardium: anatomy and pathology. Magn Reson Med Sci 2004;3(3):145–52.
[45] Vander Salm TJ. Unusual primary tumors of the heart. Semin Thorac Cardiovasc Surg 2000;12(2): 89–100.
[46] Gilkeson RC, Chiles C. MR evaluation of cardiac and pericardial malignancy. Magn Reson Imaging Clin N Am 2003;11(1):173–86, viii.
[47] Link KM, Lesko NM. MR evaluation of cardiac/juxtacardiac masses. Top Magn Reson Imaging 1995;7(4):232–45.
[48] Meier RA, Hartnell GG. MRI of right atrial pseudomass: is it really a diagnostic problem? J Comput Assist Tomogr 1994;18(3):398–401.
[49] Negulescu O, Coco M, Croll J, et al. Large atrial thrombus formation associated with tunneled

cuffed hemodialysis catheters. Clin Nephrol 2003; 59(1):40–6.
[50] Mollet NR, Dymarkowski S, Volders W, et al. Visualization of ventricular thrombi with contrast-enhanced magnetic resonance imaging in patients with ischemic heart disease. Circulation 2002; 106(23):2873–6.
[51] Srichai MB, Junor C, Rodriguez LL, et al. Clinical imaging and pathological characteristics of left ventricular thrombus: a comparison of contrast-enhanced magnetic resonance imaging, transthoracic echocardiography, and transesophageal echocardiography with surgical or pathological validation. Am Heart J 2006;152(1):75–84.
[52] Barkhausen J, Hunold P, Eggebrecht H, et al. Detection and characterization of intracardiac thrombi on MR imaging. AJR Am J Roentgenol 2002;179(6):1539–44.
[53] Bruder O, Waltering KU, Hunold P, et al. Detection and characterization of left ventricular thrombi by MRI compared to transthoracic echocardiography [German]. Rofo 2005;177(3):344–9.
[54] Burke A, Virmani R, Armed Forces Institute of Pathology (U.S.) Tumors of the heart and great vessels. Washington, DC: Published by the Armed Forces Institute of Pathology: Available at: American Registry of Pathology; 1996.
[55] Chiles C, Woodard PK, Gutierrez FR, et al. Metastatic involvement of the heart and pericardium: CT and MR imaging. Radiographics 2001;21(2): 439–49.
[56] Klatt EC, Heitz DR. Cardiac metastases. Cancer 1990;65(6):1456–9.
[57] Lam KY, Dickens P, Chan AC. Tumors of the heart. A 20-year experience with a review of 12,485 consecutive autopsies. Arch Pathol Lab Med 1993;117(10):1027–31.
[58] Basso C, Valente M, Poletti A, et al. Surgical pathology of primary cardiac and pericardial tumors. Eur J Cardiothorac Surg 1997;12(5):730–7 [discussion: 737–38].
[59] Grebenc ML, Rosado-de-Christenson ML, Green CE, et al. Cardiac myxoma: imaging features in 83 patients. Radiographics 2002;22(3):673–89.
[60] Araoz PA, Mulvagh SL, Tazelaar HD, et al. CT and MR imaging of benign primary cardiac neoplasms with echocardiographic correlation. Radiographics 2000;20(5):1303–19.
[61] Bourdeau I, Matyakhina L, Stergiopoulos SG, et al. 17q22-24 chromosomal losses and alterations of protein kinase a subunit expression and activity in adrenocorticotropin-independent macronodular adrenal hyperplasia. J Clin Endocrinol Metab 2006;91(9):3626–32.
[62] Edwards A, Bermudez C, Piwonka G, et al. Carney's syndrome: complex myxomas. Report of four cases and review of the literature. Cardiovasc Surg 2002;10(3):264–75.
[63] Schmutz GR, Fisch-Ponsot C, Sylvestre J. Carney syndrome: radiologic features. Can Assoc Radiol J 1994;45(2):148–50.
[64] Carney JA. The complex of myxomas, spotty pigmentation, and endocrine overactivity. Arch Intern Med 1987;147(3):418–9.
[65] Masui T, Takahashi M, Miura K, et al. Cardiac myxoma: identification of intratumoral hemorrhage and calcification on MR images. AJR Am J Roentgenol 1995;164(4):850–2.
[66] Sparrow PJ, Kurian JB, Jones TR, et al. MR imaging of cardiac tumors. Radiographics 2005;25(5): 1255–76.
[67] Boone SA, Campagna M, Walley VM. Lambl's excrescences and papillary fibroelastomas: are they different? Can J Cardiol 1992;8(4):372–6.
[68] Tazelaar HD, Locke TJ, McGregor CG. Pathology of surgically excised primary cardiac tumors. Mayo Clin Proc 1992;67(10):957–65.
[69] Wintersperger BJ, Becker CR, Gulbins H, et al. Tumors of the cardiac valves: imaging findings in magnetic resonance imaging, electron beam computed tomography, and echocardiography. Eur Radiol 2000;10(3):443–9.
[70] Gowda RM, Khan IA, Nair CK, et al. Cardiac papillary fibroelastoma: a comprehensive analysis of 725 cases. Am Heart J 2003;146(3):404–10.
[71] Wang JN, Yao CT, Chen JS, et al. Cardiac tumors in infants and children. Acta Paediatr Taiwan 2003; 44(4):215–9.
[72] Becker AE. Primary heart tumors in the pediatric age group: a review of salient pathologic features relevant for clinicians. Pediatr Cardiol 2000;21(4): 317–23.
[73] Freedom RM, Lee KJ, MacDonald C, et al. Selected aspects of cardiac tumors in infancy and childhood. Pediatr Cardiol 2000;21(4):299–316.
[74] Abushaban L, Denham B, Duff D. 10-year review of cardiac tumours in childhood. Br Heart J 1993; 70(2):166–9.
[75] Stiller B, Hetzer R, Meyer R, et al. Primary cardiac tumours: when is surgery necessary? Eur J Cardiothorac Surg 2001;20(5):1002–6.
[76] Fesslova V, Villa L, Rizzuti T, et al. Natural history and long-term outcome of cardiac rhabdomyomas detected prenatally. Prenat Diagn 2004;24(4): 241–8.
[77] Bosi G, Lintermans JP, Pellegrino PA, et al. The natural history of cardiac rhabdomyoma with and without tuberous sclerosis. Acta Paediatr 1996; 85(8):928–31.
[78] Restrepo CS, Largoza A, Lemos DF, et al. CT and MR imaging findings of benign cardiac tumors. Curr Probl Diagn Radiol 2005;34(1):12–21.
[79] Kiaffas MG, Powell AJ, Geva T. Magnetic resonance imaging evaluation of cardiac tumor characteristics in infants and children. Am J Cardiol 2002; 89(10):1229–33.

[80] Burke AP, Rosado-de-Christenson M, Templeton PA, et al. Cardiac fibroma: clinicopathologic correlates and surgical treatment. J Thorac Cardiovasc Surg 1994;108(5):862–70.
[81] Vaughan CJ, Veugelers M, Basson CT. Tumors and the heart: molecular genetic advances. Curr Opin Cardiol 2001;16(3):195–200.
[82] Herman TE, Siegel MJ, McAlister WH. Cardiac tumor in Gorlin syndrome. Nevoid basal cell carcinoma syndrome. Pediatr Radiol 1991;21(3):234–5.
[83] Yan AT, Coffey DM, Li Y, et al. Images in cardiovascular medicine. Myocardial fibroma in Gorlin syndrome by cardiac magnetic resonance imaging. Circulation 2006;114(10):e376–9.
[84] Salanitri JC, Pereles FS. Cardiac lipoma and lipomatous hypertrophy of the interatrial septum: cardiac magnetic resonance imaging findings. J Comput Assist Tomogr 2004;28(6):852–6.
[85] O'Connor S, Recavarren R, Nichols LC, et al. Lipomatous hypertrophy of the interatrial septum: an overview. Arch Pathol Lab Med 2006;130(3):397–9.
[86] Grebenc ML, Rosado de Christenson ML, Burke AP, et al. Primary cardiac and pericardial neoplasms: radiologic–pathologic correlation. Radiographics 2000;20(4):1073–103.
[87] Jimenez JF, Warren ET, Shroff RK, et al. Primary cardiac paraganglioma. J Ark Med Soc 2005;101(12):362–4.
[88] Lupinski RW, Shankar S, Agasthian T, et al. Primary cardiac paraganglioma. Ann Thorac Surg 2004;78(3):e43–4.
[89] McGann C, Tazelaar H, Cho SR, et al. In vivo detection of encapsulated intracardiac paraganglioma by delayed gadolinium enhancement magnetic resonance imaging. J Cardiovasc Magn Reson 2005;7(2):371–5.
[90] Orr LA, Pettigrew RI, Churchwell AL, et al. Gadolinium utilization in the MR evaluation of cardiac paraganglioma. Clin Imaging 1997;21(6):404–6.
[91] Burke A, Johns JP, Virmani R. Hemangiomas of the heart. A clinicopathologic study of ten cases. Am J Cardiovasc Pathol 1990;3(4):283–90.
[92] Jougon J, Laborde MN, Parrens M, et al. Cystic lymphangioma of the heart mimicking a mediastinal tumor. Eur J Cardiothorac Surg 2002;22(3):476–8.
[93] Kaji T, Takamatsu H, Noguchi H, et al. Cardiac lymphangioma: case report and review of the literature. J Pediatr Surg 2002;37(10):E32.
[94] Best AK, Dobson RL, Ahmad AR. Best cases from the AFIP: cardiac angiosarcoma. Radiographics 2003;23 Spec No:S141–5.
[95] Araoz PA, Eklund HE, Welch TJ, et al. CT and MR imaging of primary cardiac malignancies. Radiographics 1999;19(6):1421–34.
[96] Kim EE, Wallace S, Abello R, et al. Malignant cardiac fibrous histiocytomas and angiosarcomas: MR features. J Comput Assist Tomogr 1989;13(4):627–32.
[97] Bruna J, Lockwood M. Primary heart angiosarcoma detected by computed tomography and magnetic resonance imaging. Eur Radiol 1998;8(1):66–8.
[98] Kaminaga T, Takeshita T, Kimura I. Role of magnetic resonance imaging for evaluation of tumors in the cardiac region. Eur Radiol 2003;13(Suppl 6):L1–L10.
[99] Chalabreysse L, Berger F, Loire R, et al. Primary cardiac lymphoma in immunocompetent patients: a report of three cases and review of the literature. Virchows Arch 2002;441(5):456–61.
[100] Montalbetti L, Della Volpe A, Airaghi ML, et al. Primary cardiac lymphoma. A case report and review. Minerva Cardioangiol 1999;47(5):175–82.
[101] Dorsay TA, Ho VB, Rovira MJ, et al. Primary cardiac lymphoma: CT and MR findings. J Comput Assist Tomogr 1993;17(6):978–81.
[102] Kubo S, Tadamura E, Yamamuro M, et al. Primary cardiac lymphoma demonstrated by delayed contrast-enhanced magnetic resonance imaging. J Comput Assist Tomogr 2004;28(6):849–51.
[103] Glancy DL, Roberts WC. The heart in malignant melanoma. A study of 70 autopsy cases. Am J Cardiol 1968;21(4):555–71.
[104] Mukai K, Shinkai T, Tominaga K, et al. The incidence of secondary tumors of the heart and pericardium: a 10-year study. Jpn J Clin Oncol 1988;18(3):195–201.

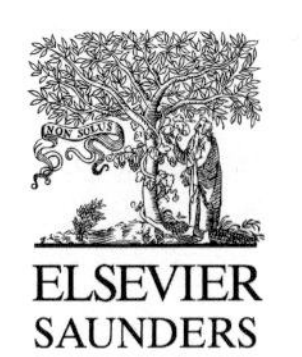

ELSEVIER
SAUNDERS

Cardiol Clin 25 (2007) 141–170

CARDIOLOGY
CLINICS

Coronary Magnetic Resonance Imaging

Warren J. Manning, MD[a,b,*], Reza Nezafat, PhD[a], Evan Appelbaum, MD[a], Peter G. Danias, MD, PhD[c], Thomas H. Hauser, MD[a], Susan B. Yeon, MD, JD[a]

[a]*Departments of Medicine and Radiology, Cardiovascular Division, Harvard-Thorndike Laboratory, Beth Israel Deaconess Medical Center and Harvard Medical School, Boston, MA, USA*

[b]*Department of Medicine, Cardiovascular Division, Harvard-Thorndike Laboratory, Beth Israel Deaconess Medical Center and Harvard Medical School, Boston, MA, USA*

[c]*Department of Medicine, St. Elizabeth's Hospital and Tufts University Medical School, Boston, MA, USA*

Despite ongoing progress in prevention and early diagnosis, coronary artery disease (CAD) remains the leading cause of death for men and women in the United States [1] and throughout the Western world. Catheter-based, invasive radiograph coronary angiography remains the gold standard for diagnosing significant ($\geq$50% diameter stenosis) CAD, with over a million catheter-based radiograph coronary angiograms performed annually in the United States [1] and higher volume in Europe. Although numerous noninvasive tests are available to help discriminate among those with and without significant angiographic disease, up to 35% of patients referred for catheter-based radiograph coronary angiography are found to have no significant stenoses [2]. Despite the absence of disease, these individuals remain exposed to the cost, inconvenience, and potential morbidity of radiograph angiography [3]. Data also suggest that in selected high-risk populations, such as those patients who have aortic valve stenosis, the incidence of subclinical stroke associated with retrograde catheter crossing of the stenotic valve may exceed 20% [4].

Although percutaneous intervention in single-vessel disease is performed commonly, the greatest impact on mortality occurs with mechanical intervention among patients who have left main (LM) and multivessel CAD. Thus, it would be desirable to have a noninvasive method that allowed direct visualization of the proximal/midnative coronary vessels for the accurate identification/exclusion of LM/multivessel CAD.

Over the last decade, coronary MRI has evolved as a potential replacement for catheter-based radiograph angiography among patients who have suspected anomalous CAD and coronary artery aneurysms. MRI has reached sufficient maturity such that it obviates the need for catheter-based radiograph angiography in the discrimination of patients with multivessel disease. This article highlights the technical challenges and general imaging strategies for coronary MRI. This is followed by a review of the clinical results for the assessment of anomalous CAD, coronary artery aneurysms, native vessel integrity, and coronary artery bypass graft disease using the more commonly applied MRI methods. It concludes with a brief discussion of the advantages/disadvantages and clinical results comparing coronary MRI with multidetector CT (MDCT) coronary angiography.

Coronary MRI—technical challenges and solutions

Technical challenges

Despite the routine clinical use of MRI for the evaluation of similar size vessels, coronary MRI is more technically challenging because of several

* Corresponding author. Department of Medicine, Cardiovascular Division, Harvard-Thorndike Laboratory, Beth Israel Deaconess Medical Center and Harvard Medical School, 330 Brookline Avenue, Boston, MA 02215.

E-mail address: wmanning@bidmc.harvard.edu (W.J. Manning).

doi:10.1016/j.ccl.2007.02.008

unique issues including small caliber (3 to 6 mm diameter), near constant motion during both the respiratory and the cardiac cycles, high level of tortuosity, and the surrounding signal from adjacent epicardial fat and myocardium.

Cardiac motion

Bulk epicardial motion is a major impediment to coronary MRI, and this can be separated into motion related to direct cardiac contraction/relaxation during the cardiac cycle and that caused by superimposed diaphragmatic and chest wall motion occurring during respiration. The magnitude of motion from each component may exceed the coronary artery diameter greatly, thereby leading to blurring artifacts in the absence of motion-suppressive methods. To compensate for bulk cardiac motion, a regular rhythm and accurate ECG synchronization and QRS detection are absolute requirements [5,6]. Alternative cardiac gating strategies using peripheral pulse detection methods lead to inferior coronary MRI because of the inconsistent relationship between the R wave and the peripheral pulse detection. Real-time cardiac magnetic resonance implementations [7] have inadequate spatial and temporal resolution for coronary MRI.

Both catheter based radiograph angiography [8,9] and MRI [10–12] methods have characterized coronary motion during the cardiac cycle. Both the proximal/mid-right coronary artery (RCA) and the left anterior descending (LAD) coronary arteries display a triphasic pattern (Fig. 1), with the magnitude of in-plane motion nearly twice as great for the RCA. During isovolumic relaxation, approximately 350 to 400 milliseconds after the R wave, and again at mid-diastole (immediately before atrial systole), coronary motion is minimal. The duration of the mid-diastolic diastasis period is related inversely to heart rate and dictates the data acquisition interval. The LAD diastasis is also longer than the RCA [12]. Compared with MDCT, where acquisition interval is limited by gantry rotation, in coronary MRI, the acquisition interval can be adapted to the individual patient's coronary motion. Although the use of a heart rate dependent formula for identifying the mid-diastolic diastasis period is effective in many subjects, there may be considerable intersubject variation [13,14]. Thus, use of a patient-specific diastasis period is recommended; this can be identified readily by the acquisition of high temporal resolution cine dataset orthogonal to the long axis of the proximal/mid RCA and

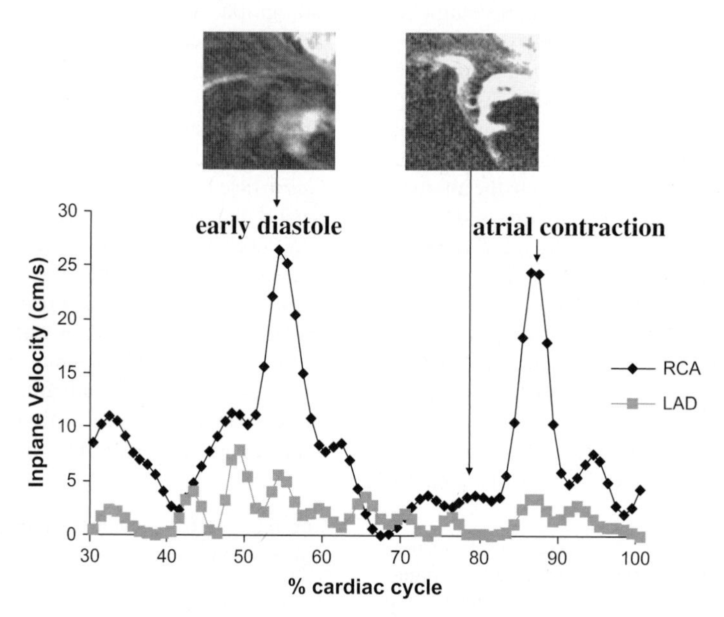

Fig. 1. Graph of in-plane right coronary artery (RCA) and left anterior descending coronary artery motion during the cardiac cycle. The *x axis* displays time as a percentage of the R-R interval. Note the improved image quality of the RCA cross section when acquired during mid-diastole as compared with early diastole (*From* Kim WY, Danias PG, Stuber M, et al. Impact of cardiac motion on right coronary MR angiography and vessel wall imaging. J Magn Reson Imaging 2001;14(4):383–90; with permission.)

of the LAD (using the same respiratory motion suppression method as used for the subsequent coronary MRI). For patients with a heart rate of 60 to 70 beats per minute, a coronary MRI acquisition duration of approximately 80 milliseconds during each cardiac cycle results in improved image quality [15]. With higher heart rates, the duration must be minimized (eg, <50 milliseconds), while with bradycardia, the acquisition interval can be expanded to 150 milliseconds or longer. The use of patient-specific acquisition windows serves to reduce overall scan time [13,14], and correction for heart rate variability improves image quality [16]. Semiautomated tools to identify the optimal data acquisition window are in development [17].

Because the intraluminal signal in gradient-echo coronary MRI depends on the inflow of unsaturated protons, mid-diastole has been identified as the preferred period for image acquisition. It corresponds to a period of minimal coronary motion and rapid (approximately 30 cm/s) coronary blood flow. The addition of sublingual nitrates before coronary MRI increases blood flow and causes measurable coronary vasodilation [18,19]. Steady-state free precession (SSFP) coronary MRI sequences are less sensitive to inflow effects and thus have advantages for systolic acquisitions.

Box 1. Respiratory suppression methods

Breath holding

Sustained end-expiratory breath hold

- Hyperventilation
- Supplemental oxygen

Free breathing

Multiple averages

Chest wall bellows

Magnetic resonance navigators

Navigator location:

Right hemidiaphragm

Left hemidiaphragm

- Basal left ventricle
- Coronary artery of interest
- Anterior thorax

Prone versus supine imaging

Single versus multiple navigators

Prospective versus retrospective navigator triggering

Navigator triggering versus navigator gating with real-time motion correction

Respiratory motion

The second major challenge for coronary MRI is compensation for respiratory motion. With inspiration, the diaphragm may descend up to 30 mm, and the chest wall expands, resulting in an inferior displacement and anterior rotation of the heart [20,21]. Minimizing respiratory motion artifacts can be achieved with several approaches (Box 1), including sustained end-expiratory breath holding, chest wall bellows, and the use of magnetic resonance navigators. Comparison of single breath hold with multiple breath-hold and navigator-gated respiratory methods suggests that free-breathing navigator methods are similar to a single breath hold [22]. Preliminary data on self-gating scans are encouraging [23], but remain to be explored better.

Breath-hold methods. Although dependent on patient cooperation, initial two-dimensional coronary MRI methods used prolonged (15- to 20-second) end-expiratory breath holds to suppress respiratory motion [24]. Although breath holding offers the advantage of relatively ease of implementation in compliant subjects, it severely limits sequence design with regards to temporal acquisition window and image spatial resolution. Both slice registration errors (because of variability in end-expiratory diaphragmatic position) and diaphragmatic drift during the breath hold are common [21,22,24,25]. The use of supplemental oxygen and hyperventilation (alone or in combination) can prolong the breath-hold duration [26,27], but these methods may not be appropriate for all patients, and both diaphragmatic drift and slice registration errors persist [27].

Free-breathing methods. Early free-breathing coronary MRI used signal averaging or chest wall bellows to reduce motion artifacts [28–30]. These quickly were supplanted by more accurate, flexible, and elegant magnetic resonance navigators.

Magnetic resonance navigators—triggering alone. Diaphragmatic MR navigators, first proposed by Ehman and Felmlee [31] for abdominal MRI, serve to overcome the time constraints and patient cooperation requirements imposed by multiple breath holds and offer superior spatial resolution opportunities. Magnetic resonance navigator implementation varies among the different vendors. The navigator can be positioned at any interface (see Box 1) that accurately reflects respiratory motion, including the dome of the right hemidiaphragm (Fig. 2) [25,30,32], the left hemidiaphragm, the anterior chest wall, the anterior free wall of the left ventricle [29], or even through the coronary artery of interest. The navigator should be located temporally immediately preceding the imaging portion of the sequence (Fig. 3) with data accepted (used for image reconstruction) only when the navigator indicates that the interface (eg, diaphragm) falls within a user defined window (usually 3 to 5 mm). For simplicity and ease in set-up, the dome of the right hemidiaphragm has become the preferred location [29,32–34]. Because of increased susceptibility at the lung–liver interface at higher field strengths (3T), a more central navigator position has been advocated [35]. With navigator triggering alone (ie, without correction/tracking), a 3 mm end-expiratory diaphragmatic gating window often is used with resultant 25% to 33% navigator efficiency (accepted/total) [29].

Magnetic resonance navigators—gating and slice tracking. From magnetic resonance studies of cardiac border position during the respiratory cycle, Wang and colleagues [20] observed that the overwhelming impact of respiration on cardiac position is in the superior–inferior direction. At end expiration, the ratio between cardiac and diaphragmatic displacement is approximately 0.6 for the RCA and approximately 0.7 for the left coronary artery [20], although there is variability [21,36]. This relatively fixed relationship offers the opportunity for prospective navigator gating with real-time tracking [35,36]. during which the position of the interface (diaphragm) is determined. The slice position coordinates then can be shifted in real-time (before the data collection) to appropriately adjust spatial coordinates [26,32,37]. Such an approach allows for the use of wider gating windows and shorter scan times (ie, increased navigator efficiency). With real-time tracking implementations, a 5 mm diaphragmatic gating window often is used with a navigator efficiency approaching 50% [36–38]. Coronary MRI with real-time navigator tracking has been shown to minimize registration errors (as compared with breath holding) with maintained or improved image quality [29,36,37]. Although the authors use a fixed superior–inferior correction factor of 0.6 (with no left–right or anterior–posterior correction) [38], others have observed significant individual variability in this relationship [21] and advocate for patient-specific algorithms. More sophisticated affine motion models that account for displacement in all three coordinates may offer advantages [39,40]. Using a navigator to monitor epicardial fat also has been proposed [41,42]. Prone positioning [43] and abdominal or

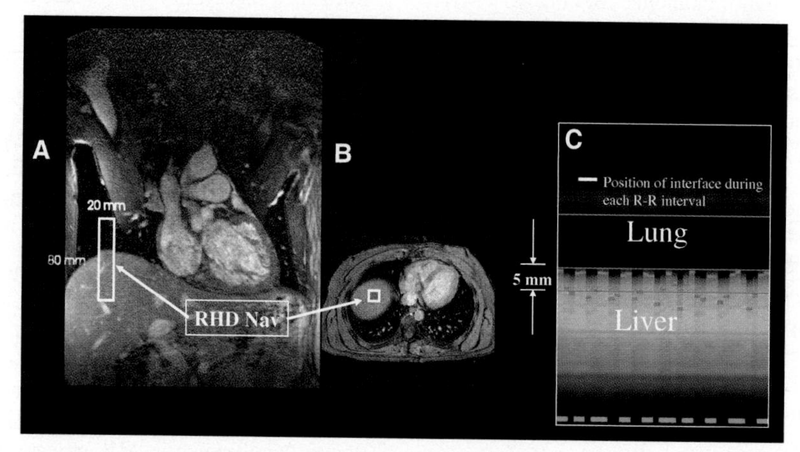

Fig. 2. Coronal (*A*) and transverse (*B*) thoracic image with identification of the navigator at the dome of the right hemidiaphragm (RHD NAV). (*C*) Respiratory motion of the lung–diaphragm interface recorded using a two-dimensional selective navigator with the lung (superior) and liver (inferior) interface. The maximum excursion between end-inspiration and end-expiration in this example is approximately 11 mm. The broken line in the middle of (*C*) indicates the position of the lung–liver interface at each R-R interval. Data are only accepted if the lung-liver interface is within the acceptance window of 5 mm. Data acquired with the navigator outside of the window are rejected. Accepted data are indicated by the broken line at the bottom of (*C*).

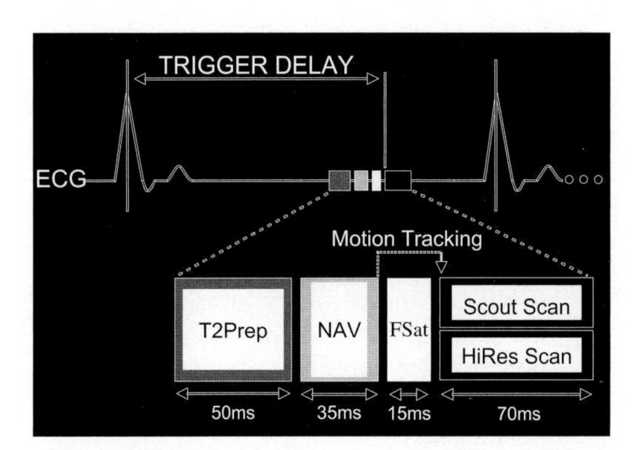

Fig. 3. Schematic of the coronary MRI pulse sequence for scout scanning (Scout Scan) and subsequent higher-resolution coronary MRI (HiRes-Scan). The elements of the sequence (T2-prep navigator [NAV], fat saturation prepulse [FSat], and the three-dimensional imaging sequence) are shown in temporal relationship to the ECG and trigger delay. Note that the ECG timing and respiratory suppression for the Scout Scan and higher resolution coronary MRI are consistent.

thoracic banding [44] additionally may impact image quality.

Finally, the authors have found that coronary MRI quality is improved by using consistent ECG timing and respiratory suppression methodology for all scout and imaging studies [45].

Spatial resolution

If not for limitations of signal to noise (SNR) and acquisition duration, isotropic coronary MRI spatial resolution approximating the 500 μ resolution data of MDCT would be used. Spatial resolution requirements for clinical coronary MRI depend on whether the goal is to simply identify the origin and proximal course of the coronary artery (eg, issues of anomalous coronary disease), or to identify focal stenoses in the proximal and middle segments. Fig. 4 displays a projection radiograph coronary angiogram at 300 μ, 500 μ, 1000 μ, and 2000 μ spatial resolution. At 500 μ and 1000 μ resolutions, focal disease is readily visible, while at resolutions greater than 1000 μ, only the course of the artery is apparent. Phantom studies confirm these observations [46].

Suppression of signal from surrounding tissue

The intrinsic contrast between the coronary blood pool and adjacent myocardium and epicardial fat can be manipulated using the in-flow effect for gradient echo sequences and by the application of MRI prepulses. Fat has a relatively short T1. Frequency-selective prepulses can be applied to saturate signal from fat tissue, thereby allowing visualization of the underlying coronary arteries [24,28,47].

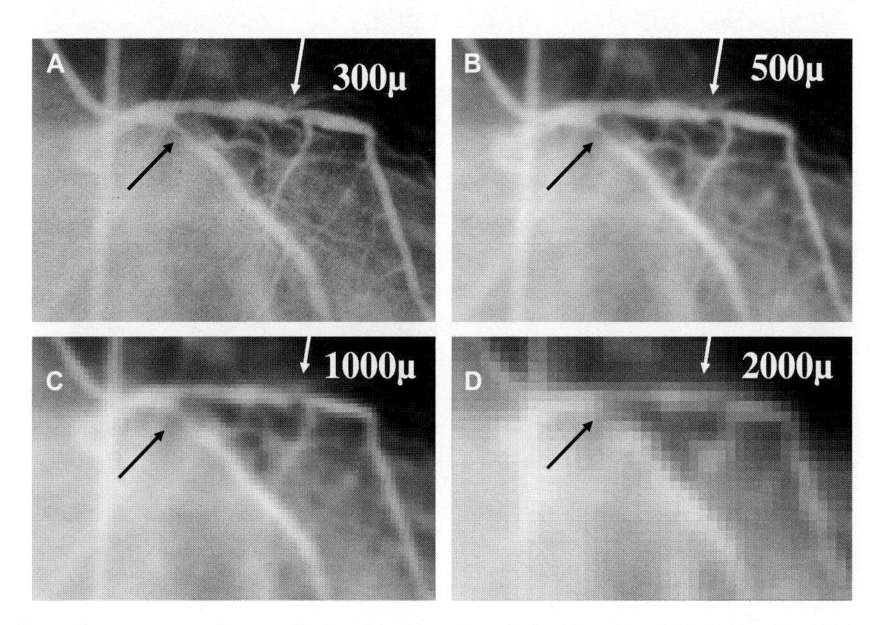

Fig. 4. Radiograph coronary angiogram displayed at 300 μ (*panel A*), 500 μ (*panel B*), 1000 μ (*panel C*), and 2000 μ (*panel D*) in-plane spatial resolution. The focal coronary stenoses of the proximal left circumflex coronary artery (*black arrow*) and the proximal left anterior descending coronary artery (*white arrow*) are appreciated with image resolution of less than 1000 μ. (*Courtesy of* Daniel Sodickson, MD, PhD.)

The coronary arteries also run in close proximity to the epi–myocardium. Myocardium and blood have relatively similar T1 relaxation values, but different T2 relaxation. Two methods that can enhance the contrast between the coronary lumen and underlying myocardium are T2 preparation prepulses [15,48,49] and magnetization transfer contrast [28,50]. The former often is used for coronary MRI, as it also suppresses deoxygenated venous blood, while the latter is used for coronary vein MRI [51]. The incremental impact of ECG triggering, respiratory gating, and T2 preparation prepulses is displayed in Fig. 5.

Coronary MRI acquisition sequences

Over the past two decades, coronary MRI sequences have continued to evolve with recent interest in 3T and parallel imaging implementations. The sequences can be conceptualized as being composed of the following building block components:

- Cardiac (eg, vector ECG) triggering to suppress bulk cardiac motion
- Respiratory motion suppression (eg, breath hold, navigators)
- Prepulses to enhance contrast-to-noise ratio (CNR) of the coronary arterial blood (eg, fat saturation, T2 preparation, magnetization transfer contrast, selective labeling of blood in the aortic root, exogenous MR contrast agents)
- Image acquisition that optimizes coronary arterial SNR (Fig. 6).

The imaging sequences (Box 2) may include black blood (fast spin echo and dual inversion), bright blood (segmented k space gradient echo and SSFP), all implemented as two-dimensional (typically breath-hold) or 3D (prolonged breath hold or free-breathing navigator) acquisitions.

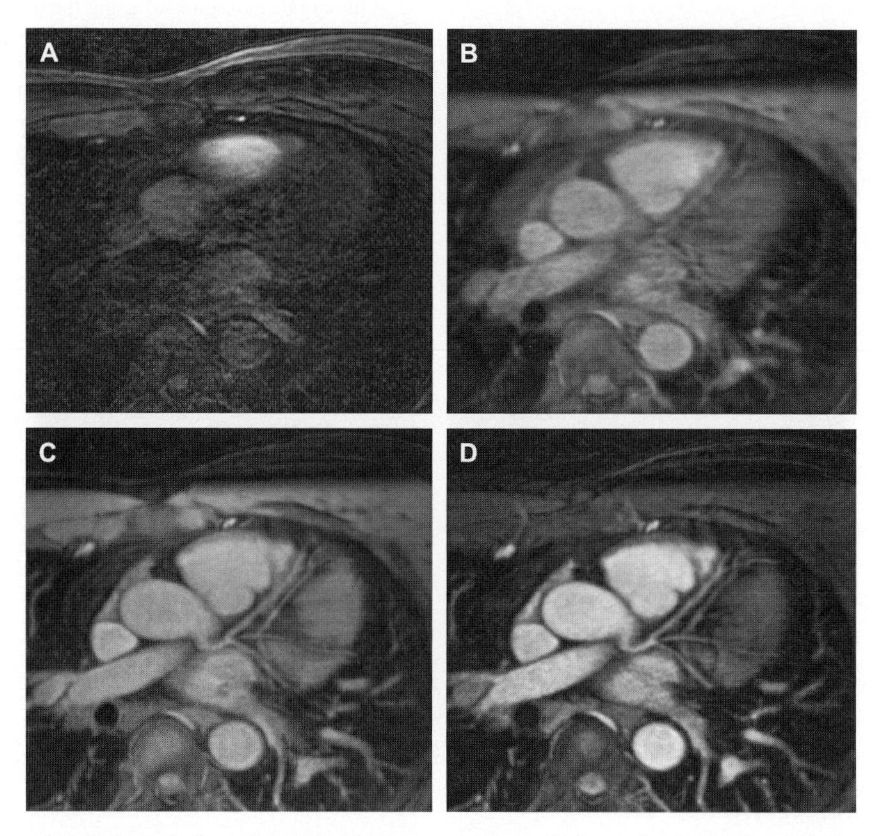

Fig. 5. Transverse image at the level of the left main coronary artery and left anterior descending coronary artery in the same subject (*A*) in the absence of cardiac and respiratory gating. The incremental value of (*B*) ECG triggered with mid-diastolic data acquisition, (*C*) navigator gating with real-time motion correction, and (*D*) T2 prepulse are readily apparent. (*Courtesy of* Matthias Stuber, PhD.)

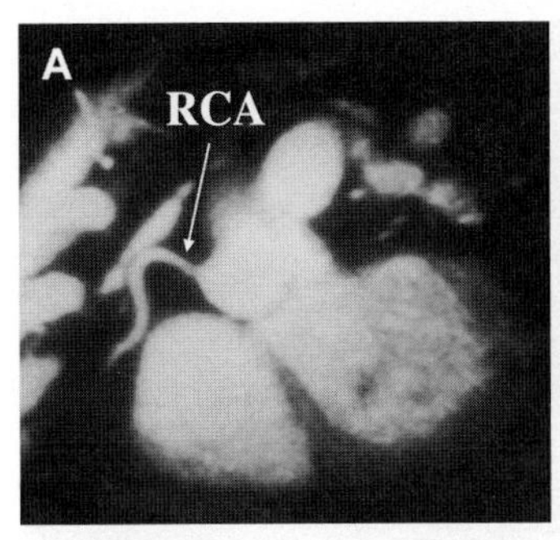

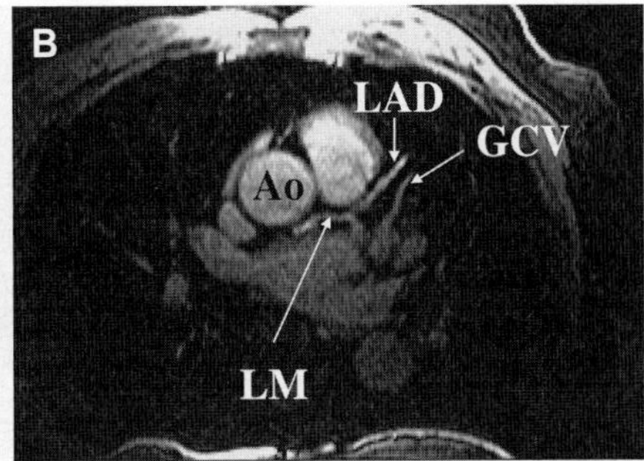

Fig. 6. (*A*) Breath hold transverse two-dimensional coronary MRI in a healthy subject at the level of the take-off of the right coronary artery (*white arrow*). (*B*) Breath hold two-dimensional transverse coronary MRI of the left main coronary artery and left anterior descending (LAD) coronary artery. Signal from the great cardiac vein is seen parallel with the LAD. (*Adapted from* Manning WJ, Li W, Boyle N, et al. Fat-suppressed breath-hold magnetic resonance coronary angiography. Circulation 1993;87(1):94–104; with permission.)

Conventional spin-echo coronary MRI

Early attempts to image the coronary arteries using conventional ECG-gated spin-echo approaches were met with limited success. Lieberman and colleagues [52] used ECG-gated spin-echo cardiovascular magnetic resonance (CMR) and was able to visualize portions of the native coronary arteries in only 30% of 23 subjects, while Paulin and colleagues [53] studied six patients using ECG-gated spin-echo imaging. Despite data acquisition during ventricular systole, the absence of respiratory motion suppression, and data acquisition over several minutes, the origin of the LM coronary artery was seen in all (100%) subjects and the ostium of the RCA in over half. No stenoses were visualized in either report. In the authors' experience, current axial T1 weighted fast spin-echo imaging of the thorax often will depict the origin of the right and left coronary artery.

Box 2. Coronary MRI methods

Black Blood
Spin Echo
Dual Inversion fast spin echo

Bright Blood
Segmented k space gradient echo
- Two-dimensional breath hold
- Three-dimensional free breathing [or breath hold]

Steady state free precession; balanced FFE, trueFISP, FIESTA
Contrast-enhanced coronary MRI
Extracellular and intravascular agents
Aortic root tagging methods

Parallel imaging techniques
Cartesian versus spiral versus radial acquisitions
High field (3T)

Two-dimensional segmented k space gradient echo coronary MRI

The first robust approach to coronary MRI was an ECG-triggered, breath hold, two-dimensional segmented k space gradient echo acquisition described over 15 years ago [24] and still applicable today on older magnetic resonance systems or situations in which anomalous CAD may be the clinical question. Data were acquired within a 112 millisecond temporal resolution (repetition time 14 milliseconds) during a sustained 16 heart beat breath hold with 1.9×0.9 mm in-plane spatial resolution) [54,55]. A series of 10 to 15 overlapping transverse or oblique images (each requiring a single breath hold) was acquired at the level of the origin of the RCA and left coronary arteries (see Fig. 6). Because of variability in the diaphragmatic position among breath holds, the acquisition of repetitive images with the same spatial coordinates displays adjacent coronary regions. The number of breath holds can be reduced by the combination of breath holds with navigator correction [29,37,38]. The combination of higher-resolution two-dimensional gradient echo imaging with free breathing navigators is highly reproducible and can detect coronary vasodilation in response to nitroglycerin [56].

Similar breath hold two-dimensional segmented k space gradient echo acquisitions also may be used to image the larger diameter coronary artery bypass grafts (Fig. 7). Reverse saphenous

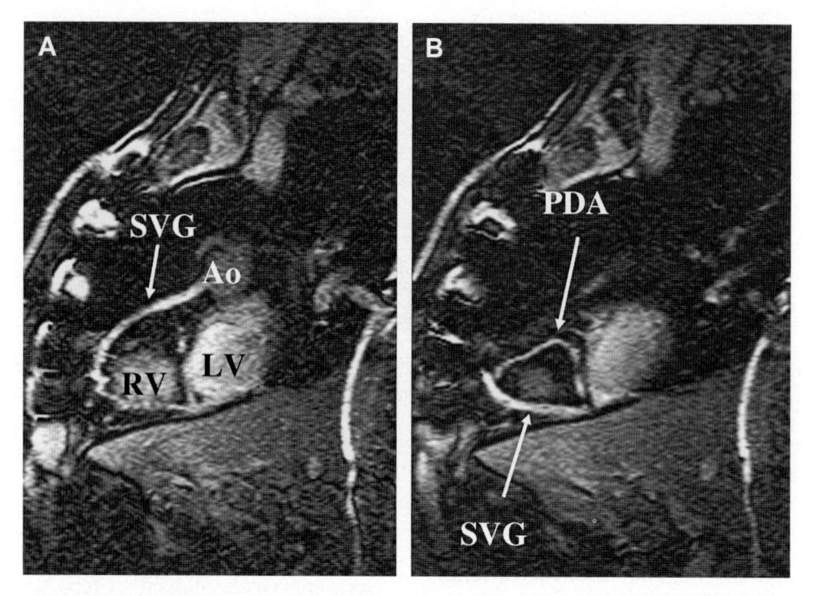

Fig. 7. Oblique breath-hold two-dimensional coronary MRI of a patent saphenous vein bypass graft (SVG). (*A, B*) Two adjacent images show the SVG (*arrows*) extending from its aortic origin (Ao) to the distal touchdown on the posterior descending coronary artery (PDA). RV, right ventricle; LV, left ventricle.

vein grafts are larger in diameter, and both saphenous vein grafts and internal mammary bypass grafts are less mobile than the native coronary arteries, with predominant flow during ventricular systole. This facilitates data acquisition during a longer period (150 to 200 milliseconds) within each R-R interval and with less rigorous respiratory motion criterion. Susceptibility artifacts from stainless steel bypass graft markers and vascular clips pose an impediment to bypass graft coronary MRI (Fig. 8).

Three-dimensional coronary MRI methods

The postprocessing capabilities of three-dimensional coronary MRI have made it the predominant approach for the past decade. The associated respiratory suppression approach has varied from prolonged breath hold with lower spatial resolution [47,57] to higher spatial resolution methods in combination with free breathing/navigator methods [15,28,58].

Because data from a volume of tissue surrounding the coronary arteries are acquired, the set-up of three-dimensional coronary MRI is less demanding of the patient and magnetic resonance technologist than repetitive two-dimensional breath-hold acquisitions. After obtaining thoracic scout (nine transverse, nine coronal, and nine sagittal interleaved acquisitions), the navigator is positioned at the dome of the right hemidiaphragm (see Fig. 2). A second scout, consisting of an ECG-triggered three-dimensional fast gradient echo-EPI scout then is acquired with diaphragmatic navigator gating of a volume that includes the coronary arteries, beginning at the cardiac base and extending inferiorly. A free breathing or breath-hold cine (consistent with the subsequent coronary MRI sequence) then is acquired perpendicular to the proximal/mid RCA to define the optimal delay and acquisition period (period of minimal in-plane motion). For LM, LAD, and left circumflex (LCX) imaging, a three-dimensional volume is prescribed interactively in the transverse plane centered about the LM coronary artery (identified in the second scout) using the same ECG delay and navigator parameters as the scout. Typically, a 30 mm slab with 20 overlapping slices is acquired using a segmented k space gradient echo acquisition with submillimeter in-plane spatial resolution (0.7×1.0 mm) and a temporal acquisition of 56 to 84 milliseconds/heart beat (Fig. 9) [15,58]. For imaging of the RCA, transverse images from the second scout depicting the proximal, mid, and distal RCA are identified. Using a three-point planscan software tool [58], the imaging plane passing through all three coordinates of the RCA is identified, and the targeted three-dimensional coronary sequence is repeated in

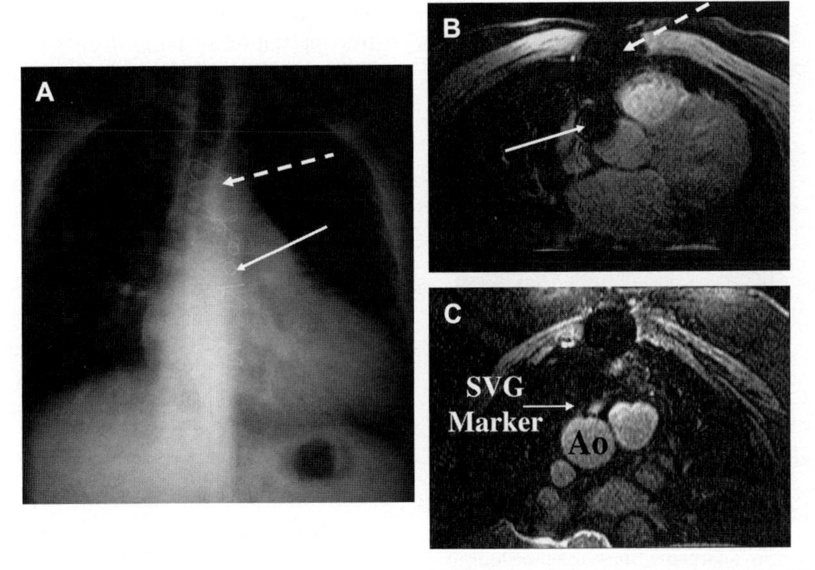

Fig. 8. (*A*) Posterior–anterior (PA) chest radiograph in a patient with coronary artery bypass grafts. Note the sternal wires (*dashed arrow*) and the coronary artery bypass graft markers (*solid arrow*). (*B*) Transverse coronary MRI in the same patient. Note the large local artifacts (signal voids) related to the sternal wires (*dashed arrow*) and bypass graft markers (*solid arrows*). The size of the artifacts are related to the type of graft marker used. (*C*) barium and tantalum markers (*arrow*) result in the smallest artifacts. The size of the artifacts are reduced somewhat with spin-echo/black-blood MRI.

this orientation (Figs. 10–12). For CMR systems that lack a three-point planscan interactive software tool, an imaging plane parallel with the right and left atrioventricular (AV) groove is suggested. Each submillimeter three-dimensional segmented gradient echo acquisition is typically 8 to10 minutes in duration (assuming a navigator efficiency of 40-55%). A similar approach has been applied for the coronary artery bypass grafts [59].

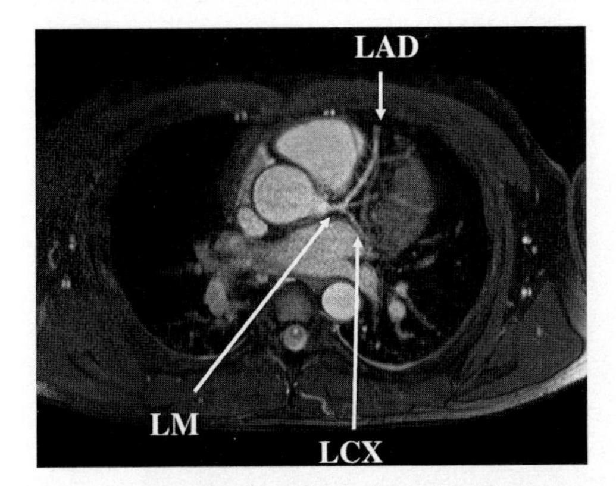

Fig. 9. Targeted thee-dimensional reformatted coronary MRI of the left coronary system acquired using free breathing and real-time navigator gating with motion correction in a healthy adult subject. The transverse acquisition displays the left main coronary artery, left anterior descending coronary artery,. and the left circumflex. The in-plane spatial resolution is 0.7 × 1.0 mm.

Segmented k space gradient echo coronary MRI methods are heavily dependent on the inflow of unsaturated protons. If coronary flow is slow/stagnant, saturation effects will cause a local signal loss that often is relatively exaggerated as compared with the lumen stenosis. SSFP (eg, trueFISP, balanced FFE, FIESTA) applications offer superior SNR with a 50% to 100% improvement in blood SNR and blood–myocardium CNR as compared with gradient echo methods [60] with reduced sensitivity to inflow effects. As a result, SSFP methods increasingly are used for both breath-hold [61–63] and free breathing coronary MRI [60,64,65]. They offer specific advantages for systolic imaging [44]. Fat saturation and T2 prepulses still are used. Reproducibility of free breathing targeted three-dimensional coronary approaches appears to be excellent [66]. As with the segmented k space gradient echo approach, (Fig. 13), both targeted breath-hold three-dimensional volumes [60,61,67] and whole-heart approaches [64, 65,68] analogous to MDCT approaches have been described. For the whole-heart approach,

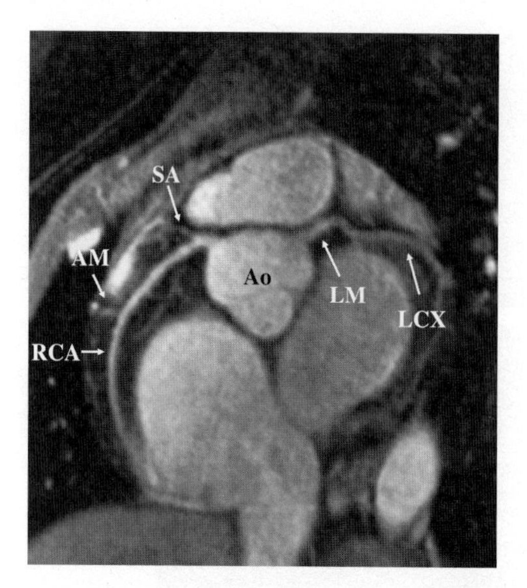

Fig. 10. Multiplanar reformatted targeted three-dimensional T2 preparation gradient echo coronary MRI depicting the right coronary artery (RCA), left main coronary artery, and left circumflex. The in-plane spatial resolution is 0.7 × 1.0 mm. The sinus node branch (SA) and an acute marginal (AM) branch of the RCA also are seen. Ao. aorta. (*Adapted from* Stuber M, Botnar RM, Danias PG, et al. Double-oblique free-breathing high-resolution three-dimensional coronary magnetic resonance angiography. J Am Coll Cardiol 1999;34(2): 524–31; with permission.)

a three-dimensional volume incorporating the entire heart is prescribed from coronal scouts [64]. The latter provides for visualization of more distal segments of the coronary arteries [64] and is more conducive to advanced postprocessing methods (Fig. 14). Isotropic voxels are also possible [69]. The higher SNR of SSFP imaging also allows for the application of parallel imaging (eg, SMASH (SiMultaneous Acquisition of Spatial Harmonics) [70,71] and SENSE (SENSitivity Encoding) [72,73] applications to reduce scan time) [62,63,74].

Coronary MRI—advanced methods

Despite ongoing advances, SNR and the speed of data acquisition remain limiting for coronary MRI. To overcome these hurdles, several laboratories continue with the development and implementation of novel approaches including spiral acquisitions, magnetic resonance contrast agents, and higher field (3T) imaging.

Spiral and radial coronary MRI

Alternative k space acquisitions, including spiral and radial coronary MRI, have received attention. Meyer and colleagues [57] first reported on the use of spiral coronary MRI. Advantages of spiral acquisitions include a more efficient filling of k space (Fig. 15), enhanced SNR [60,75], and favorable flow properties. Spirals have more complex reconstruction algorithms. Though a single-shot k space trajectory can be employed, interleaved spiral imaging is preferred because of reduced artifacts [57,75–77]. Such an approach may be implemented with a breath hold (two-dimensional) or with free breathing/navigator gating [60,75,76,78]. Data suggest single spiral acquisitions (per R-R interval) afford a near threefold improvement in SNR as compared with conventional Cartesian approaches (see Fig. 13) [60,75]. Acquiring two spirals during each R-R interval will halve the acquisition time,

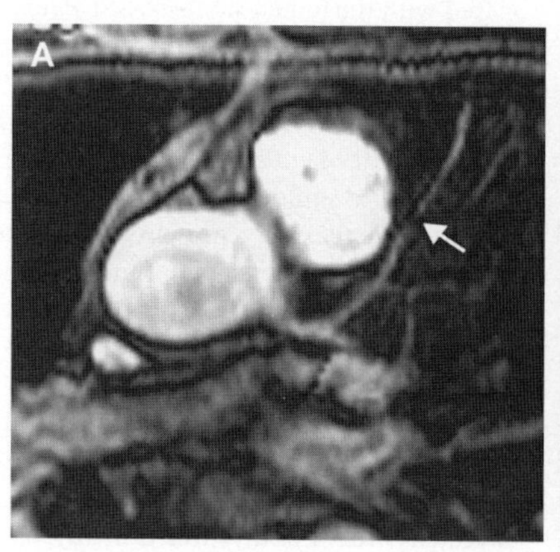

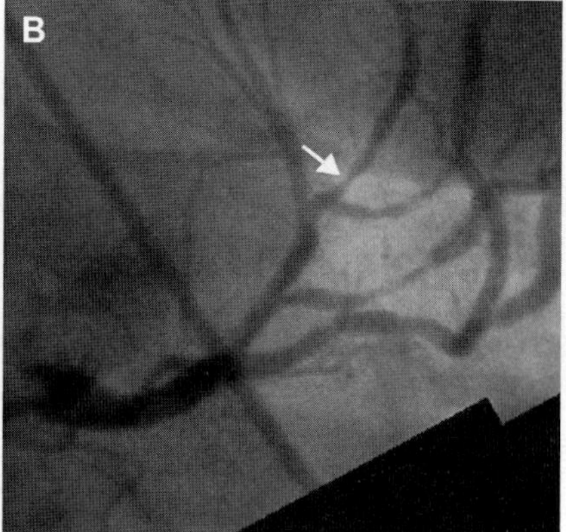

Fig. 11. Reconstruction from (*A*) breath hold targeted three-dimensional steady-state free precession (SSFP) coronary MRI demonstrating focal stenoses (*arrows*) in the mid left anterior descending coronary artery with (*B*) corresponding radiograph angiography. (*Courtesy of* Debiao Li, PhD.)

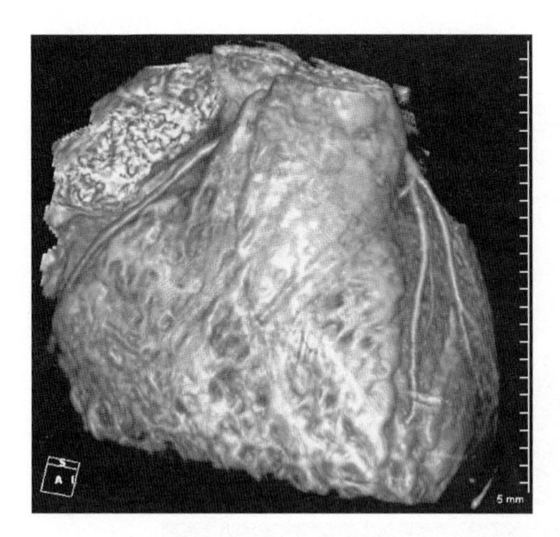

Fig. 12. Three-dimensional reconstruction of a whole-heart steady-state free precession (SSFP) coronary MRA following computer-assisted image segmentation enable major coronary vessels to be visualized. (*Courtesy of* Oliver Weber, PhD.)

while maintaining superior SNR (versus Cartesian acquisition) and CNR.

Radial approaches also offer the benefit of more rapid acquisitions with decreased sensitivity to motion. Data in healthy subjects appear promising [60,77–79] and may be particularly beneficial for coronary wall imaging [47,80].

Contrast-enhanced coronary MRI

With contrast-enhanced MRI methods, blood signal contrast is based on the intravascular T1 relaxation rate, potentially allowing for true lumen imaging. Contrast-enhanced magnetic resonance angiography (MRA) is employed widely for carotid, aortic, renal, and peripheral vascular applications, but the previously described unique timing constraints for coronary MRI have limited coronary applications of clinically available extracellular agents.

Exogenous MR contrast agents can be subcategorized into extracellular (interstitial) and intravascular agents. Extracellular paramagnetic contrast agents (gadolinium chelates) have been used for first-pass breath-hold studies through the coronary bed [81–83]. As with aortic MRA, a test bolus often is employed. These agents have been shown to be of some value for first-pass/single breath-hold approaches [81–83], but clinical studies directly comparing contrast with noncontrast coronary MRI are lacking. The requirement for placement of an intravenous catheter, added expense for the contrast agent, and dependence of the acquisition on a single breath hold (like MDCT) and without an opportunity for repetition limit targeted three-dimensional high-resolution applications.

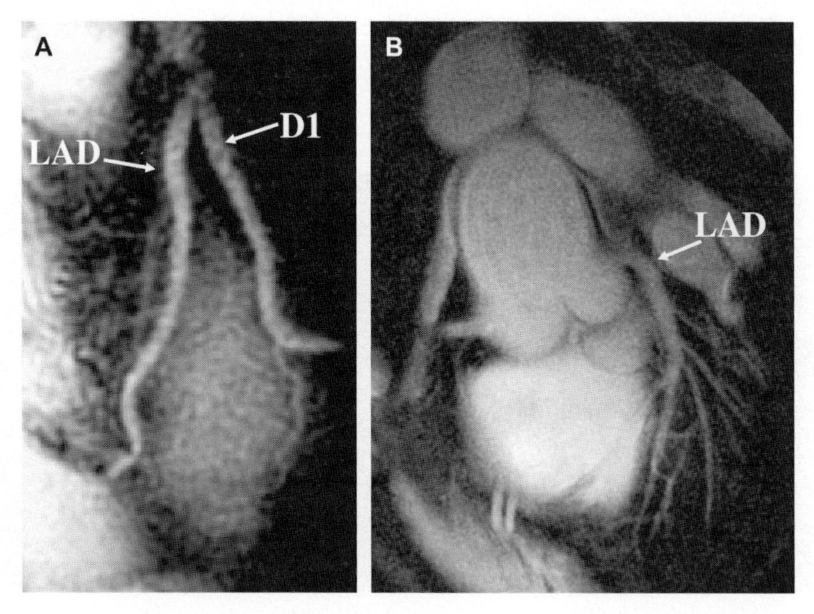

Fig. 13. Prolonged breath-hold three-dimensional spiral coronary MRI in two healthy subjects. (*A*) 0.8 mm spatial resolution demonstrating the left anterior descending (LAD) coronary artery and large first diagonal (D1). (*B*) 0.5 mm spatial resolution demonstrating the LAD and multiple branches. (*Courtesy of* Craig Meyer, PhD, and Bob Hu, MD.)

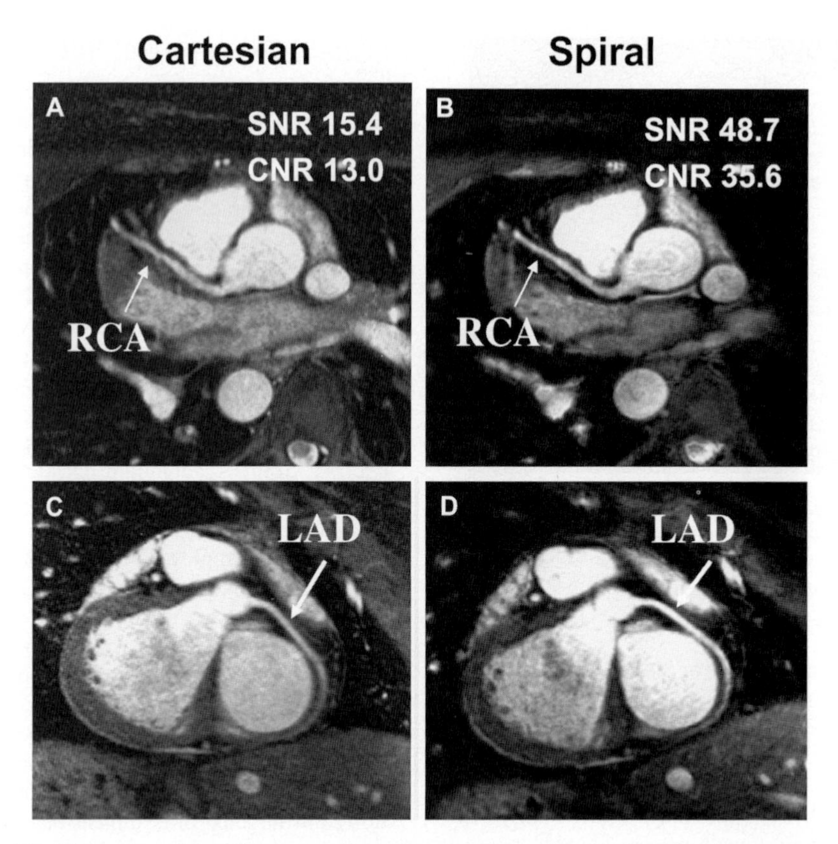

Fig. 14. Double oblique view of the left anterior descending coronary artery (*A, B*) and right coronary artery (*C, D*) acquired with a targeted three-dimensional fat- and muscle-suppressed (T2 preparation) Cartesian (*A, C*) and spiral (*B, D*) k space sampling technique. Because of more efficient k space sampling, the spiral technique results in a threefold signal-to-noise improvement compared with the conventional Cartesian segmented k space technique. (*Courtesy of* Peter Börnert, PhD.)

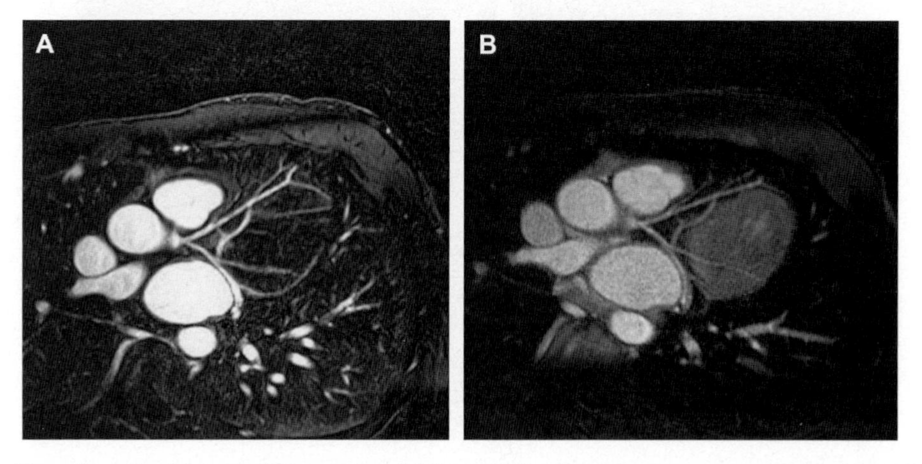

Fig. 15. Three-dimensional free-breathing coronary MRI using (*A*) an inversion recovery prepulse and novel intravascular contrast agent (B-22,956, Bracco Spa, Milan) and comparison with (*B*) conventional noncontrast T2 preparation coronary MRI. Note the improved contrast with the intravascular agent. (*Courtesy of* Eike Nagel, MD.)

Several novel intravascular (blood pool) magnetic resonance contrast agents are under development and being evaluated for coronary MRI, including gadolinium based [84–87] and ultrasmall particle superparamagnetic iron oxide-based [88–90] contrast agents. These intravascular agents afford longer scan times with free-breathing or repeated breath-hold methods. A 180-degree inversion prepulse often is used to highlight the marked T1 reduction with imaging when the longitudinal magnetization of myocardium crosses the null point (see Fig. 14) [85]. Improvements in CNR of 60% to 100% have been reported. One intravascular magnetic resonance contrast agent is available in Europe (Vasovist, Scherring AG, Germany), but none are approved for use in the United States.

3 T coronary MRI

The most exciting area of interest has been high-field, 3 T coronary MRI. SNR is related directly to field strength (B_0). Although most coronary MRI investigations have been performed on 1.5 T systems, commercial 3 T systems are increasingly available. Technical hurdles to address artifacts caused by field inhomogeneities, increased susceptibility artifacts, reduced T2* [35,91,92], T1 prolongation, and the amplified magnetohydrodynamic effect (see Fig. 1) [5] are being addressed. Free breathing navigator and breath-hold three-dimensional coronary MRI studies in healthy volunteers have demonstrated greater than 50% improvement in SNR with impressive image quality using both segmented k space gradient echo (Fig. 16), SSFP, spiral, and contrast-enhanced methods [35,93,94].

Special considerations: intracoronary stents

Improvements in long-term patency rates for percutaneous coronary interventions using conventional and drug-eluting intracoronary stents have resulted in their widespread use in over 80% of the growing number of percutaneous revascularizations. Typically made from high-grade stainless steel, these stents pose a particular imaging problem for CMR. Although the attractive force and local heating are negligible both at 1.5 T [95–100] and 3 T [101], and in the United States, both the Cypher (Cordis, Miami Lakes, Florida) and Taxus Liberte (Boston Scientific, Natick, Massachusetts) drug-eluding stents are approved for magnetic resonance scanning immediately after implantation, the local susceptibility artifact that leads to signal voids/artifacts at the site of the stent can be substantial (Fig. 17). The signal void depends on both the stent material [102] and the MRI sequence. There appear to be relatively small artifacts with tantalum stents [103] and very prominent artifacts with stainless steel stents. Artifacts are also relatively larger with gradient echo methods. This signal void/artifact precludes direct evaluation of intrastent and peri-stent coronary integrity, although assessment of blood flow/direction proximal and distal to the stent using

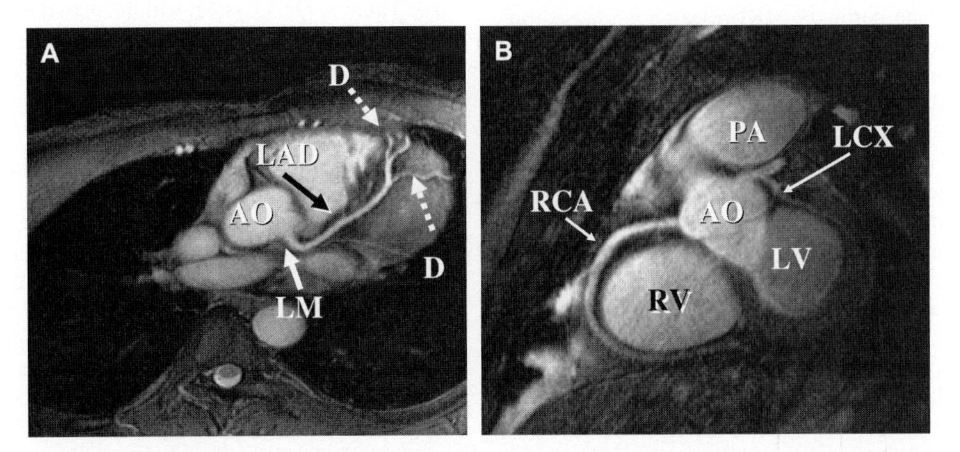

Fig. 16. Three-dimensional free-breathing left coronary MRI obtained in a healthy subject at 3T. The increased signal to noise afforded by the higher field strength allows for enhanced (0.6 × 0.6 mm) spatial resolution. (*A*) The left main (LM), left anterior descending, and diagonal (D) branches are seen readily. (*B*) Oblique of the right coronary artery. The LM and left circumflex also are seen. (*From* Stuber M, Botnar RM, Fischer SE, et al. Preliminary report on in vivo coronary MRA at 3 Tesla in humans. Magn Reson Med 2002;48(3):425–9; with permission.)

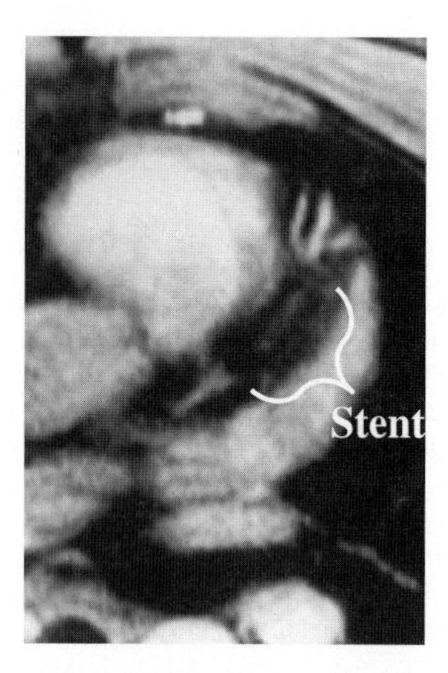

Fig. 17. Transverse, two-dimensional breath hold gradient-echo coronary MRI at the level of the left anterior descending coronary artery in a patient with a patent stent. Note the signal void (*black marker*) corresponding to the site of the stent. (*Courtesy of* Christopher Kramer, MD.)

magnetic resonance flow methods or spin-labeling methods may provide indirect evidence of a patency by documentation of antegrade flow. Recently, animal studies using novel magnetic resonance lucent stent materials have been reported [103]. Mechanical properties, biocompatibility, and long-term patency rates for these novel stents are unknown.

Future technical developments

Current coronary MRI research is focused on improving motion correction algorithms and advancing the imaging methods previously described in this article. The goal is to provide a noninvasive imaging tool that will allow for early identification/exclusion of proximal and midsized coronary arteries. Although once thought unlikely, several groups now have imaged the coronary vessel wall and plaque successfully [47,80,104–107], including subclinical wall thickening among patients without severe stenoses referred for radiograph angiography [80]. Intracoronary visualization of thrombus also has been described using novel fibrin-binding contrast agents [108]. These novel approaches will continue to bring intense interest and enthusiasm to the coronary MRI arena for many years to come. The birth of interventional cardiac MRI also is taking place, including real-time approaches with direct injection of conventional and novel magnetic resonance contrast agents into the coronary artery of interest [109–112], as well as intracoronary stent placement under real-time magnetic resonance guidance [103].

Coronary MRI—clinical studies

Since the mid-1980s, many investigators have contributed to the understanding of the clinical assessment of coronary MRI in comparison with catheter-based radiograph angiography. More recently, comparisons with MDCT have been published are presented here.

Coronary MRI of normal coronary arteries

Although ECG-gated spin-echo MRI often demonstrate the origins of the coronary arteries, it was the relatively low spatial resolution (1.5 $\times$ 2.0 mm) breath-hold two-dimensional segmented k space gradient echo approach [24] that first offered a clinically robust approach for native vessel coronary MRI. As implemented across all vendor platforms, the LM, LAD and RCA are visualized in most compliant subjects (Table 1) [55,113–118] with proximal coronary artery diameter in healthy subjects similar to values obtained by radiograph angiography and pathology [119] and coronary vasodilation demonstrated in response to nitroglycerin [18,19,56]. Targeted three-dimensional segmented k space gradient echo and whole-heart SSFP coronary MRI are the dominant imaging protocols, with reported successful visualization of all the major vessels in nearly every subject (see Table 1) [28,33,58,64] with increased contiguous visualization length as compared with two-dimensional approaches.

Anomalous coronary artery identification

The ability of coronary MRI to reliably identify the major coronary arteries immediately provides for its use for the identification and characterization of anomalous CAD. Although unusual (<1% of the general population [120,121]) and usually benign, congenital coronary anomalies in which the anomalous segment courses anterior to the aorta and posterior to the pulmonary artery are a well-recognized cause of myocardial ischemia and sudden cardiac death, especially among young adults [122]. These adverse events commonly occur during or immediately following intense exercise and are thought to be related to compression of the anomalous segment, vessel kinking, or the presence of eccentric stenoses [122]. Projection

Table 1
Successful visualization of the native coronary arteries using two- and three-dimensional segmented K space gradient echo coronary MRI

Investigator	Technique	Respiratory compensation	Number of subjects	RCA	LM	LAD	LCX
Manning, 1993 [55]	2D GRE	BH	25	100%	96%	100%	76%
Pennell, 1993 [113]	2D GRE	BH	26	95%	95%	91%	76%
Duerinckx, 1994 [114]	2D GRE	BH	20	100%	95%	86%	77%
Sakuma, 1994 [115]	2D GRE cine	BH	18	100%	100%	100%	67%
Masui, 1995[116]	2D GRE	BH	13	85%	92%	100%	92%
Davis, 1996 [117]	2D GRE	BH	33[a]	100%	100%	100%	100%
Li, 1993 [28]	3D GRE	Multiple averages	14	100%	100%	86%	93%
Post, 1996 [33]	3D GRE	Retro Nav G	20	100%	100%	100%	100%
Wielopolski, 1998 [118]	3D Seg EPI	BH	32	100%	100%	100%	100%
Botnar, 1999 [15]	3D GRE	Pro Nav G/C	13	97%	100%	100%	97%
Weber, 2003 [64]	3D SSFP	Pro Nav G/C	12	100%	100%	100%	100%

Abbreviations: BH, breath hold; GRE, gradient echo; LAD, left anterior descending coronary artery; LCX, left circumflex coronary artery; LM, left main coronary artery; Pro Nav G/C, prospective navigator gating with correction; RCA, right coronary artery; Retro Nav, retrospective navigator gating; Seg EPI, segmented EPI; SSFP, steady state free precession; 3D, three-dimensional; 2D, two-dimensional.

[a] Including 18 heart transplant recipients.

radiograph angiography traditionally has been the imaging test of choice for diagnosing and characterizing these anomalies. The presence or absence of an anomalous vessel sometimes only is suspected after the procedure, however, particularly in a situation where there was unsuccessful engagement or visualization of a coronary artery. In addition, the declining routine use of a pulmonary artery catheter has made characterization of the anterior versus posterior trajectory of the anomalous vessels more difficult to appreciate on the projection views.

Coronary MRI has several advantages in the diagnosis of coronary anomalies. In addition to being noninvasive and not requiring ionizing radiation (likely to be an important consideration among adolescents and younger adults with suspected anomalous coronary artery disease) or iodinated contrast agents, coronary MRI provides a clear three-dimensional roadmap of the mediastinum. With three-dimensional coronary MRI, one subsequently can acquire and/or reconstruct an image in any orientation (Fig. 18). Most early studies used a two-dimensional breath-hold segmented k space gradient echo approach [123–125], although most centers now use targeted three-dimensional or whole-heart free breathing navigator coronary MRI because of superior reconstruction capabilities afforded by three-dimensional datasets with similar results.

Early reports of coronary MRI to visualize anomalous coronary arteries included case report confirmation of radiograph angiographic data. Subsequently, there have been at least six published series [123–128] of patients who underwent a blinded comparison of coronary MRI data with radiograph angiography. These studies uniformly have reported excellent accuracy, including several instances in which coronary MRI was determined to be superior to radiograph angiography (Table 2). Preliminary data for anomalous coronary disease recently have been extended to the whole-heart approach at both 1.5 T and 3 T [129,130]. At experienced CMR centers, clinical coronary MRI is now the preferred test for patients in whom anomalous disease is suspected, known anomalous disease needs to be further clarified, or if the patient has another cardiac anomaly associated with coronary anomalies (eg, Tetralogy of Fallot). Although MDCT also has been demonstrated to be efficacious for this indication [131,132], coronary MRI would be preferred because of the absence of ionizing radiation or need for intravenous access.

In a somewhat analogous fashion, two-dimensional breath-hold coronary MRI also has been used to define the altered coronary artery orientation in the cardiac transplant population [117]. Among cardiac transplant recipients, coronary MRI has documented a 25° anterior (clockwise) ostial rotation, likely explaining the more complex coronary engagement during radiograph angiography.

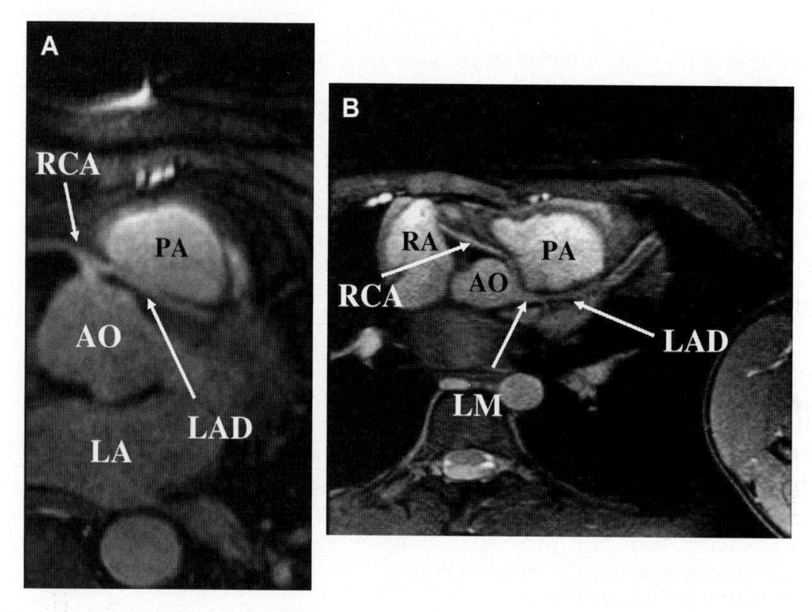

Fig. 18. Free-breathing targeted three-dimensional coronary MRI using T2 prepulse navigator gating with real-time motion correction. (*A*) Transverse orientation depicting a malignant-type anomalous left anterior descending coronary artery originating from the right coronary artery (RCA). (*B*) Transverse image in another patient with a malignant-type anomalous origin of the RCA from the left coronary cusp. Ao, aorta; PA, pulmonary artery; LA, left atrium; RA, right atrium.

Coronary artery aneurysms/Kawasaki's disease

Though relatively uncommon, coronary artery aneurysms are receiving increasing attention for assessment by coronary MRI. In the absence of a percutaneous intervention, most acquired coronary aneurysms are felt to be caused by mucocutaneous lymph node syndrome (Kawasaki's disease), a generalized vasculitis of unknown etiology usually occurring in children under 5 years. Infants and children with this syndrome may show evidence of myocarditis and/or pericarditis, with nearly 20% developing coronary artery aneurysms. These aneurysms are the source of both short- and long-term morbidity and mortality [133]. Fortunately, half of the children with coronary aneurysms during the acute phase of the disease have normal-appearing coronary lumen on catheter-based radiograph angiography 2 years later [133,134]. Among children, transthoracic echocardiography is usually adequate for diagnosing and following aneurysms, but echocardiography is deficient after adolescence and in obese children. These young adults therefore often are referred for serial catheter- based radiograph coronary angiography. Coronary MRI data from two series of adolescents and young adults with coronary artery aneurysms (Fig. 19) have confirmed the high accuracy of coronary MRI for both the identification and the characterization (diameter/length) of these aneurysms [135–137]. Although not specifically examined, these data suggest that coronary aneurysms can be followed effectively with serial coronary MRI studies. Similar data have been reported for ectatic coronary vessels [138].

Table 2
Anomalous coronary MRI

Investigator	Number of patients	Correctly classified anomalous vessels
McConnell, 1995 [123]	15	14 (93%)
Post, 1995 [124]	19	19 (100%)[a]
Vliegen, 1997 [125]	12	11 (92%)[b]
Taylor, 2000 [126]	25	24 (96%)
Bunce, 2003 [127]	26	26 (100%)[c]
Razmi, 2001 [128]	12	12 (100%)

[a] Including three patients originally misclassified by radiograph angiography.

[b] Including five patients unable to be classified by radiograph angiography.

[c] Including 11 patients unable to be classified by radiograph angiography.

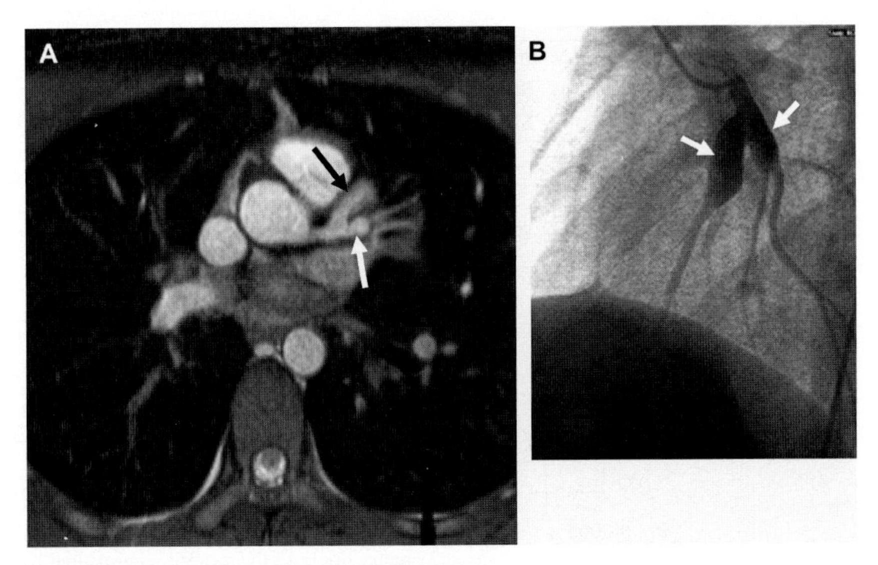

Fig. 19. (*A*) Transverse targeted three-dimensional T2 prepulse coronary MRI of a subject with a left coronary artery aneurysm and (*B*) corresponding radiograph angiogram, demonstrating good correlation of coronary MRI findings.

Coronary MRI for identification of native vessel coronary stenoses

Although data support a broad clinical role for coronary MRI in the assessment of suspected anomalous CAD (and coronary artery bypass graft patency), data are not yet sufficient to support clinical coronary MRI for routine identification of coronary artery stenoses among patients presenting with chest pain or for screening purposes of even high-risk patients. Increasing data, however, suggest a role for coronary MRI among patients referred for catheter-based radiograph angiography and especially for the discrimination of ischemic versus nonischemic cardiomyopathy [139].

As previously discussed, gradient echo sequences demonstrate flow in the coronary lumen with rapidly moving laminar blood flow appearing bright, while areas of stagnant flow and/or focal turbulence appear dark because of local saturation (stagnant flow) or dephasing (turbulence) (Fig. 20). Areas of focal stenoses appear as varying severity of signal voids in the coronary

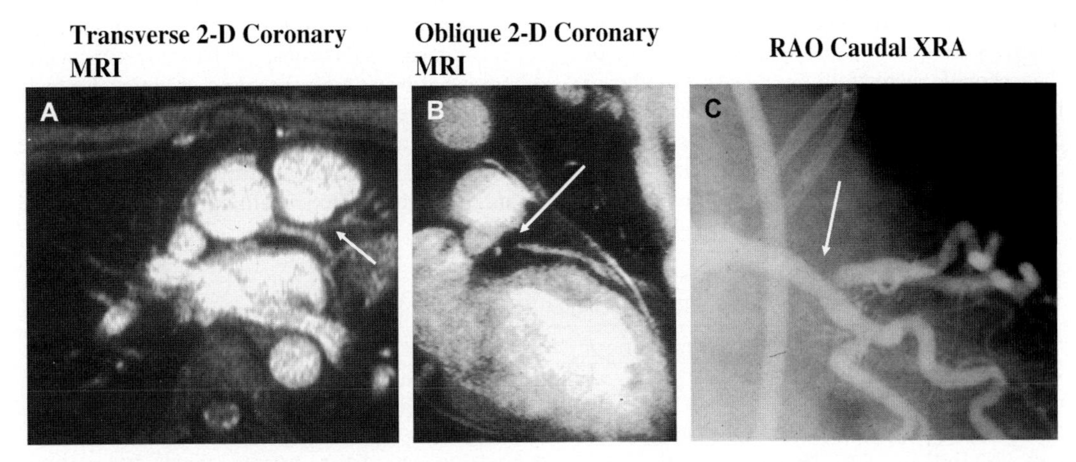

Fig. 20. Transverse (*A*) and oblique (*B*) two-dimensional breath-hold coronary MRI. In panel A, a 45 year-old woman with atypical chest pain demonstrates a signal void (*arrows*) in the proximal left anterior descending coronary artery (LAD). Visualization of the more distal LAD and diagonal vessel are seen in the image, as well as the proximal left circumflex. Panel C demonstrates the corresponding right anterior oblique (RAO) caudal radiograph angiogram (XRA) confirming the tight ostial LAD stenosis (*arrow*) seen by MRI.

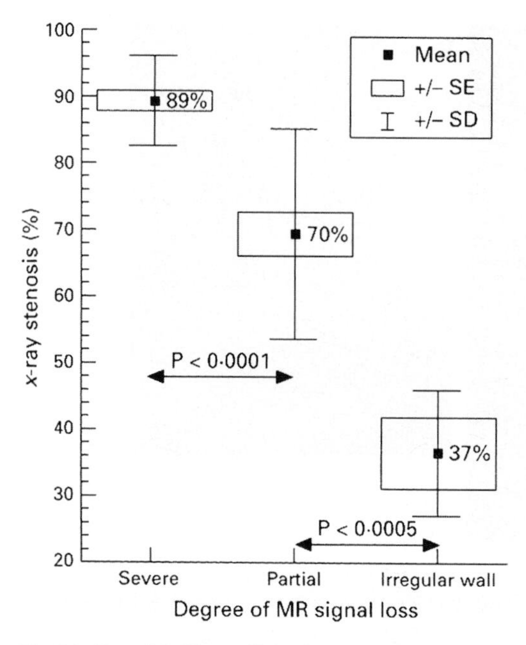

Fig. 21. Breath-hold two-dimensional segmented k space gradient echo coronary MRI comparison of focal magnetic resonance signal loss versus radiograph coronary artery diameter stenosis. Note the strong correlation between the severity of signal loss by coronary MRI and the degree of radiograph angiographic stenosis. (*From* Pennell DJ, Bogren HG, Keegan J, et al. Assessment of coronary artery bypass stenosis by magnetic resonance imaging. Heart 1996;75(2):127–33; with permission.)

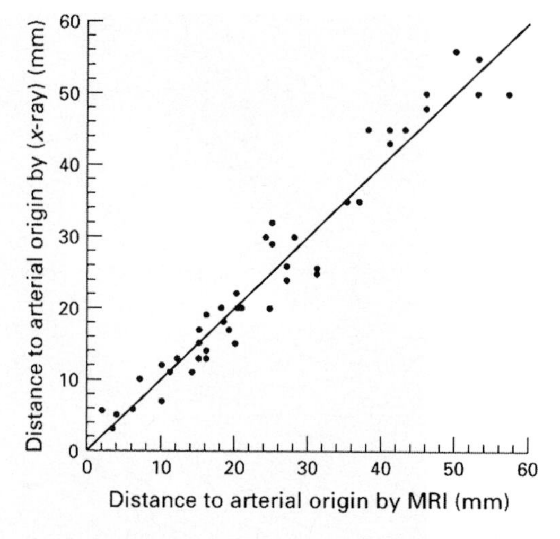

Fig. 22. Scatterplot comparing the distance from the coronary origin to the stenosis as measured by radiograph and magnetic resonance coronary angiography. (*From* Pennell DJ, Bogren HG, Keegan J, et al. Assessment of coronary artery bypass stenosis by magnetic resonance imaging. Heart 1996;75(2):127–33; with permission.)

MRI, with the severity of the signal loss related to the angiographic stenosis (Fig. 21) [140]. Because of time constraints of a breath hold, two-dimensional breath-hold coronary MRI has relatively limited in-plane spatial resolution, but the technique successfully has demonstrated proximal coronary stenoses in several clinical studies (Table 3) [54,114,140,141]. When reported, the distance from the vessel origin to the focal stenosis on coronary MRI correlates closely with radiograph angiography (Fig. 22) [140]. Unfortunately, there have been wide variations in reported sensitivity and specificity, which are likely caused by technical issues/methodology, including the wide variation in patient selection, presence of arrhythmias, prevalence of disease and technical (magnetic resonance vendor, echo time, receiver coils, timing of the acquisition, acquisition duration, breath hold maneuvers) issues, and the need for somewhat exhausting 20 to 40 breath holds to complete a study. To date, no multicenter two-dimensional coronary MRI study using a uniform hardware, software, and scanning protocol has been reported.

With the increasing availability of magnetic resonance navigators, many CMR centers have migrated to a free-breathing three-dimensional

Table 3
Two-dimensional Breath hold coronary MRI for identification of ≥50% diameter focal coronary stenoses

Investigator	Number of subjects	# (%) Vessels	Sensitivity	Specificity
Manning, 1993 [54]	39	52 (35%)	90% (71% 100%)	92% (78% 100%)
Duerinckx, 2004 [114]	20	27 (34%)	63% (0% 73%)	– (37% to 82%)
Pennell, 1996 [140]	39	55 (35%)	85% (75% 100%)	—
Post, 1997 [141]	35	35 (28%)	63% (0% to 100%)	89% (73% to 96%)
Nitatori, 1995 [142]	57[a]	—	87%	94%
	13[b]	—	43%	90%

[a] With ≥90% diameter stenosis.
[b] With 50% to 75% diameter stenosis.

gradient echo coronary MRI for ease in patient acceptance (free breathing) and for improved SNR with facilitated multiplanar reconstructions. As with two-dimensional gradient echo methods, a focal stenosis/turbulence appears as a signal void along the course of the vessel (Fig. 23). Data from several single-center sites now have been published using both retrospective navigators and prospective navigators with real-time correction (Table 4) [143–146]. Early studies using retrospective navigators used relatively prolonged acquisition times (260 milliseconds) [33,147,148] with subsequent studies using acquisition intervals of less than 120 milliseconds [149–151]. These single-center reports are very encouraging, with overall sensitivity and specificity of up to 90% for proximal coronary disease [151]. Although assessment of stenosis sensitivity was been found to be similar for both source and projection images [149], the authors' strong preference is to make diagnoses with the source images. They then use the projection images to visually convey their findings to the referring physician.

Subsequently, single-center studies using more sophisticated prospective navigators with real-time motion correction have shown improved results, especially for the proximal coronary segments and in subjects with high image-quality scans (see Table 4) [152–157]. An international multicenter, free breathing three-dimensional volume- targeted coronary MRI study of 109 patients without prior radiograph angiography using common hardware and software demonstrated high sensitivity (although only modest specificity) and negative predictive value of coronary MRI for the identification of coronary disease (≥50% diameter stenosis by quantitative coronary angiography) (Table 5) [139]. The sensitivity and negative predictive value were particularly high for the identification of LM or multivessel disease. These data demonstrate a clinical role for coronary MRI if the concern is multivessel disease. Accordingly, the authors have found coronary MRI to be especially valuable for patients who present with a dilated cardiomyopathy in the absence of clinical infarction. Coronary MRI is highly accurate, and superior to delayed enhancement methods for determining the etiology (ischemic versus nonischemic) of the cardiomyopathy [158].

Limited data are known regarding breath-hold three-dimensional SSFP coronary MRI. One small study [157] that used relatively low spatial resolution breath-hold three-dimensional coronary MRI for the 40% of their subjects with inadequate free breathing images reported low overall results (sensitivity 65%, specificity 73%).

Increasing data are now available on whole-heart SSFP coronary MRI methods. Although using an inferior in-plane spatial resolution, data appear to be at least as accurate as free-breathing methods (see Table 4) [44,68,159].

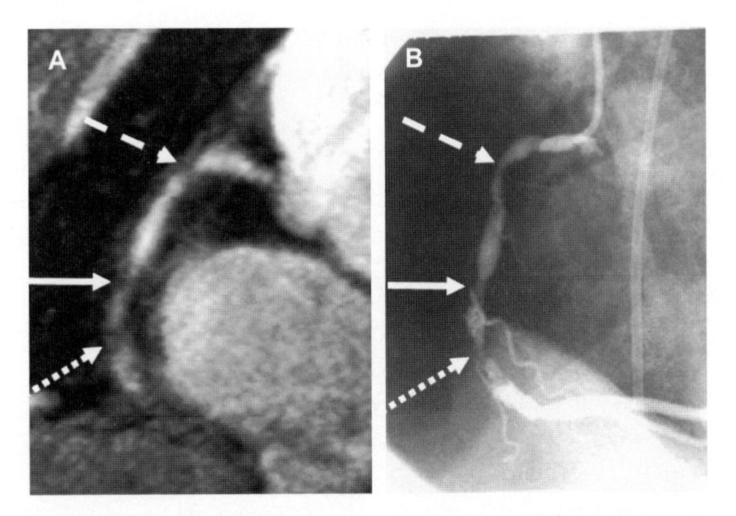

Fig. 23. (*A*) Free-breathing targeted three-dimensional T2 prepulse coronary MRI with navigator gating and real-time motion correction and (*B*) corresponding radiograph angiography in a patient with proximal (*dashed arrow*) and mid-RCA stenoses (*solid and dotted arrows*). (*From* Stuber M, Botnar RM, Fischer SE, et al. Preliminary report on in vivo coronary MRA at 3 Tesla in humans. Magn Reson Med 2002;48(3):425–9; with permission.)

Table 4
Free-breathing three-dimensional gradient echo coronary MRI using retrospective and prospective navigators for identification of focal ≥50% diameter coronary stenoses

			For ≥50% diameter stenosis		
Investigator	Number of subjects	# (%) Vessels	Sensitivity	Specificity	
Retrospective navigator gating targeted three-dimensional coronary MRI					
Post, 1996 [33]	20	21 (27%)	38% (0% to 57%)	95% (85% to 100%)	
Muller, 1997 [147]	35	—	83%[a]	94%[a]	
Woodard, 1998 [148]	10	10 (100%)	70%	—	
Sandstede, 1999 [143]	30	30 (100%)	81%[b]	89%[b]	
Van Geuns, 1999 [149]	32	—	50% (50% to 55%)[c]	91%[c](73% to 95%)	
Huber, 1999 [150]	40	20 (50%)	73% (25% to 100%)	50% (25% to 82%)	
Sardanelli, 2000 [151]	42	40% of segments	82% (57% to 100%)	89% (72% to 100%)	
			90% proximal	90% proximal	
Prospective navigators with real-time correction-targeted three-dimensional coronary MRI					
Bunce, 2001 [152]	34	—	—	88%	72%
Moustapha, 2001 [153]	25	—	—	92%	55%
	—	—	—	90% (proximal)	92% (proximal)
Sommer, 2002 [154]	112	—	—	74%	63%
	—	—	—	88% (good quality)	91% (good quality)
Bogaert, 2003 [155]	19	—	—	85–92%	50–83%
Plein, 2002 [156]	10	—	—	75%	85%
Ozgun, 2004 [144]	14	—	TFE	91%	57%
	—	—	SSFP	76%	85%
Dewey, 2006 [157]	15[d]	30	SSFP	86%	98%
Maintz, 2004 [60]	—	—	TFE	92%	67%
	—	un	SSFP	81%	82%
Ozgun, 2005 [145]	20	—	SSFP	82%	82%
Jahnke, 2004 [146]	21	—	SSFP	79%	91%
Prospective navigator with real-time correction whole-heart SSFP					
Sakuma, 2005 [68]	101	—	—	82%	91%
Jahnke, 2005 [159]	55	—	—	78%	91%
Sakuma, 2006 [44]	106	—	—	82%	90%

Abbreviations: SSFP, steady state free precession; TFE, turbo field echo; W/, with.
[a] Excluding five patients for "lack of cooperation" and 15 segments for being uninterpretable.
[b] Based on 23 (77%) with high-quality scans.
[c] Based on 74% of coronary artery segments analyzable by MRI.
[d] Based on 60% of patients with good free breathing coronary MRI images.

Comparison of coronary MRI with multidetector CT

Single-center data comparing MDCT with coronary MRI generally have shown equivalence with MDCT. The first direct study by Gerber and colleagues [160] compared free-breathing targeted three-dimensional coronary MRI with four-slice MDCT. This demonstrated a slight superiority

Table 5
Free breathing three-dimensional navigator coronary MRI: multicenter trial results

	Patient	Left main/3VD
Sensitivity	93%	100%
Specificity	59%	85%
Prevalence	42%	15%
Positive Predictive Value	70%	54%
Negative Predictive Value	81%	100%

Data from Kim WY, Danias PG, Stuber M, et al. Coronary magnetic resonance angiography for the detection of coronary stenoses. N Engl J Med 2001; 345(26):1863–9.

of coronary MRI for overall accuracy (Table 6) [161,162]. A follow-up study in 52 patients by the same group with 16-slice MDCT demonstrated equivalence with visual analysis [163]. Another 16-slice MDCT comparative study showed a superiority for MDCT [164] for sensitivity, but the coronary MRI technique was the inferior combined free-breathing and breath-hold approach [157]. Interestingly, the patient coronary MRI sensitivity (74%) was improved between their two studies, suggesting a learning curve for coronary MRI. Patients did express a preference for MDCT [157], with an advantage of MDCT being very rapid and simplified protocols at the expense of substantial radiation exposure and need for iodinated contrast.

Coronary MRI for coronary artery bypass graft assessment

Compared with the native coronary arteries, reverse saphenous vein and internal mammary artery grafts are relatively easy to image because of their relatively minimal motion during the cardiac and respiratory cycle and the larger lumen of reverse saphenous vein grafts. Furthermore, their predictable and less convoluted course has allowed imaging of bypass grafts even with less sophisticated MRI techniques.

With schematic knowledge of the origin and touchdown site of each graft, conventional free breathing ECG-gated two-dimensional spin-echo [165–168] and two-dimensional gradient-echo [169–172] magnetic resonance in the transverse plane have been used to reliably assess bypass graft patency (Fig. 24) (see Table 6). Patency is determined by visualizing a patent graft lumen in at least two contiguous transverse images along its expected course (presenting as signal void for spin-echo techniques and bright signal for gradient-echo approaches). If signal consistent with flow is identified in the area of the graft lumen, it is very likely to be patent. If a patent lumen is seen only at one level (eg, for spin-echo techniques, a signal void is seen at only one level), a graft is considered indeterminate. If a patent graft lumen is not seen at any level, the graft is considered occluded. Combining spin-echo and gradient-echo imaging in the same patient does not appear to improve accuracy [170]. Three-dimensional noncontrast [173] and contrast-enhanced coronary MRI also have been described for assessing graft patency [174,175], with slightly improved results (see Table 6). The accuracy of ECG-gated SSFP sequences appears to be similar to that of spin-echo and gradient-echo approaches [176].

Limitations of coronary MRI bypass graft assessment include difficulties related to local signal loss/artifact caused by implanted metallic objects (hemostatic clips, ostial stainless steel graft markers, sternal wires, coexistent prosthetic valves and supporting struts or rings, and graft stents) (Table 7) (see Figs. 10 and 24). The inability to

Table 6
Comparative studies of coronary MRI and multidetector CT

Investigator	Imaging method	Sensitivity	Specificity	PPV
Gerber, 2005 [160]	MRI:FB-SSFP	62%	84%[b]	49%
	Four-slice multidetector CT (MDCT)	79%[a]	71%	40%
Kefer, 2005 [163]	MRI:FB-SSFP	88%	50%	77%
	16-slice MDCT	92%	67%	84%
Dewey, 2006 [164]	MRI-BH/FB	74%[b]	75%	95%
	16-slice MDCT	92%	79%	95%

Abbreviations: BH, breath hold; FB-SSFP, free breathing steady state free precession; PPV, positive predictive value.
[a] $P < .05$.
[b] $P < .001$.

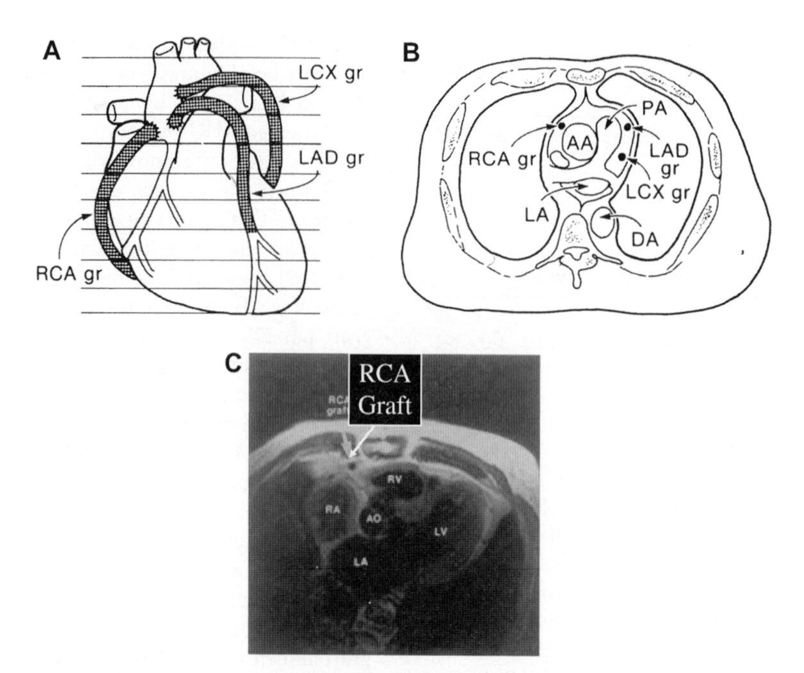

Fig. 24. (*A*) Coronal and (*B*) transverse schematic of the anatomic location of coronary artery bypass grafts (right coronary artery graft, left anterior descending coronary artery gr, left circumflex gr) originating from the aortic root and anastomosing with the distal native coronary arteries with location of contiguous transverse slices. (*C*) Transverse ECG-gated conventional spin echo coronary MRI image demonstrating flow (*arrow*) in an anatomic area corresponding to the graft indicating graft patency at that level. (*Adapted from* Aurigemma GP, Reichek N Axel L, et al. Noninvasive determination of coronary artery bypass graft patency by cine magnetic resonance imaging. Circulation 1989;80(6):1595–602.)

Table 7
Sensitivity, specificity, and accuracy of coronary MRI for assessment of coronary artery bypass graft patency

Investigator	Technique	Number of grafts	Patency	Sensitivity	Specificity	Accuracy
White, 1987 [168]	2D spin-echo	72	69%	86%	59%	78%
Rubinstein, 1987 [161]	2D spin-echo	47	62%	90%	72%	83%
Jenkins, 1988 [162]	2D spin-echo	41	63%	89%	73%	83%
Galjee, 1996 [170]	2D spin-echo	98	74%	98%	85%	89%
White, 1988 [169]	2D GRE	28	50%	93%	86%	89%
Aurigemma, 1989 [171]	2D GRE	45	73%	88%	100%	91%
Galjee, 1996 [170]	2D GRE	98	74%	98%	88%	96%
Engelmann, 2000 [172]	2D GRE	55	100% (IMA)	100%	—	100%
	—	—	66% (SVG)	92%	85%	89%
Molinari, 2000 [173]	3D GRE	51	76.5%	91%	97%	96%
Engelmann, 2000 [172]	CE-3D GRE	96 SVG	66%	92%	85%	89%
	—	37 IMA	100%	100%	—	100%
Wintersperger, 1998 [174]	CE-3D GRE	39	87%	97%	100%	97%
Vrachliotis, 1997 [175]	CE-3D GRE	45	67%	93%	97%	95%

Abbreviations: CE, contrast enhanced; GRE, gradient echo; IMA, internal mammary artery graft; SVG, saphenous vein graft; 3D, three-dimensional; 2D, two-dimensional.

Data from Kim WY, Danias PG, Stuber M, et al. Coronary magnetic resonance angiography for the detection of coronary stenoses. N Engl J Med 2001;345(26):1863–9.

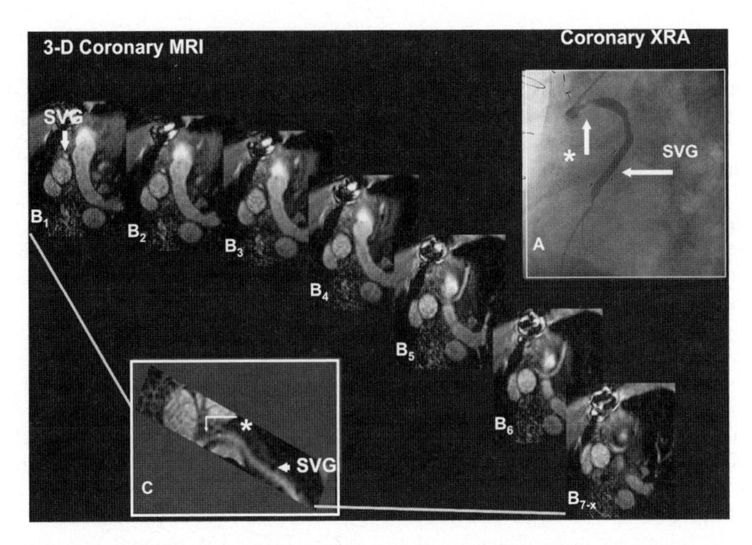

Fig. 25. Radiograph angiogram of saphenous vein graft to the left anterior descending coronary artery with a 56% proximal stenosis (*). (*B1-7*) Individual slices of the MRI obtained in the oblique plane. (*C*) MPR of the three-dimensional scan demonstrating the loss of graft lumen (tapering graft contour) corresponding to the radiograph angiographic stenosis (*arrow*). (*Adapted from* Langerak SE, Vliegen HW, de Roos A, et al. Detection of vein graft disease during high-resolution magnetic resonance angiography. Circulation 2002;105(3):328–33; with permission.)

identify severely diseased yet patent grafts is also a hindrance to clinical utility and acceptance. Langerak and colleagues [59], however, found free-breathing navigator three-dimensional gradient echo coronary MRI to be quite accurate for assessing saphenous vein graft stenoses (Fig. 25), with very good agreement between quantitative radiograph angiography for assessing graft occlusion and graft stenoses (Table 8). This group also has advocated assessment of rest and adenosine stress coronary artery flow assessment using phase velocity magnetic resonance techniques [177,178] and suggests superior results for flow assessment.

Table 8
Diagnostic accuracy of submillimeter coronary MRI for saphenous vein graft disease

	Sensitivity	Specificity
Graft occlusion	83% (36% to 100%)	100% (92% to 100%)
Graft stenosis ≥50%	82% (57% to 96%)	88% (72% to 97%)
Graft stenosis ≥70%	73% (39% to 94%)	80% (64% to 91%)

Data from Langerak SE, Vliegen HW, de Roos A, et al. Detection of vein graft disease during high-resolution magnetic resonance angiography. Circulation 2002;105(3):328–33.

Summary

Over the past 15 years, coronary MRI has been transformed from a scientific curiosity to a clinically useful imaging tool in selected populations, including the identification and characterization of anomalous coronary arteries, characterization of aneurysms, and assessment of coronary artery bypass graft patency. Coronary MRI also appears to be of clinical value for assessing native vessel integrity in selected patients, especially those patients with suspected left main/multivessel disease. A normal coronary MRI strongly suggests the absence of severe multivessel disease. Technical and methodological advances in motion suppression, along with increasing experience and development on 3 T platforms and intravascular contrast agents no doubt will facilitate improved accuracy and increased clinical use. As with MDCT, data from multicenter trials will continue to define the clinical role of coronary MRI.

References

[1] Heart disease and stroke statistics - 2006 update. Dallas (TX): American Heart Association; 2007.

[2] Budoff MJ, Georgiou D, Brody A, et al. Ultrafast computed tomography as a diagnostic modality in the detection of coronary artery disease: a multicenter study. Circulation 1996;93(5):898–904.

[3] Davidson CJ, Mark DB, Pieper KS, et al. Thrombotic and cardiovascular complications related to nonionic contrast media during cardiac catheterization: analysis of 8,517 patients. Am J Cardiol 1990;65(22):1481–4.

[4] Omran H, Schmidt H, Hackenbroch M, et al. Silent and apparent cerebral embolism after retrograde catheterisation of the aortic valve in valvular stenosis: a prospective, randomised study. Lancet 2003; 361(9365):1241–6.

[5] Polson MJ, Barker AT, Gardiner S. The effect of rapid rise time magnetic fields on the ECG of the rat. Clin Phys Physiol Meas 1982;3(3):231–4.

[6] Fischer SE, Wickline SA, Lorenz CH. Novel real-time R wave detection algorithm based on the vectorcardiogram for accurate gated magnetic resonance acquisitions. Magn Reson Med 1999; 42(2):361–70.

[7] Kaji S, Yang PC, Kerr AB, et al. Rapid evaluation of left ventricular volume and mass without breath holding using real-time interactive cardiac magnetic resonance imaging system. J Am Coll Cardiol 2001;38(2):527–33.

[8] Paulin S. Coronary angiography. A technical, anatomic, and clinical study. Acta Radiol Diagn (Stockh) Suppl 1964;54:1–215.

[9] Wang Y, Vidan E, Bergman GW. Cardiac motion of coronary arteries: variability in the rest period and implications for coronary MR angiography. Radiology 1999;213(3):751–8.

[10] Hofman MB, Wickline SA, Lorenz CH. Quantification of in-plane motion of the coronary arteries during the cardiac cycle: implications for acquisition window duration for MR flow quantification. J Magn Reson Imaging 1998;8(3):568–76.

[11] Kim WY, Danias PG, Stuber M, et al. Impact of bulk cardiac motion on right coronary MR angiography and vessel wall imaging. J Magn Reson Imaging 2001;14(4):383–90.

[12] Jahnke C, Paetsch I, Achenbach S, et al. Coronary MR imaging: breath-hold capability and patterns, coronary artery rest periods, and beta blocker use. Radiology 2006;239(1):71–8.

[13] Jahnke C, Gebker R, Schnackenburg B, et al. Comparison of individually adapted breath-hold and free-breathing coronary MRA using steady-state free precession [abstract]. J Cardiovasc Magn Reson 2004;6:166–7.

[14] Plein S, Jones TR, Ridgway JP, et al. Three-dimensional coronary MR angiography performed with subject-specific cardiac acquisition windows and motion-adapted respiratory gating. AJR Am J Roentgenol 2003;180(2):505–12.

[15] Botnar RM, Stuber M, Danias PG, et al. Improved coronary artery definition with T2 weighted, free-breathing, three-dimensional coronary MRA-Circulation 1999;99(24):3139–48.

[16] Leiner T, Katsimaglis G, Yeh EN, et al. Correction for heart rate variability improves coronary magnetic resonance angiography. J Magn Reson Magn Imaging 2005;22:577–82.

[17] Bi X, Chung YC, Weale P, et al. Automatic data acquisition window determination for coronary MRA [abstract]. J Cardiovasc Magn Reson 2007; 9(2):234–5.

[18] Pepe A, Lombardi M, Takacs I, et al. Nitrate-induced coronary vasodilation by stress–magnetic resonance imaging: a novel noninvasive test of coronary vasomotion. J Magn Reson Imaging 2004; 20(3):390–4.

[19] Terachima M, Meyer CH, Keeffe BG, et al. Noninvasive assessment of coronary vasodilation using magnetic resonance angiography. J Am Coll Cardiol 2005;45(1):104–10.

[20] Wang Y, Riederer SJ, Ehman RL. Respiratory motion of the heart: kinematics and the implications for the spatial resolution in coronary imaging. Magn Reson Med 1995;33(5):713–9.

[21] Taylor AM, Jhooti P, Wiesmann F, et al. MR navigator echo monitoring of temporal changes in diaphragm position: implications for MR coronary angiography. J Magn Reson Imaging 1997;7(4): 629–36.

[22] Fischer RW, Botnar RM, Nehrke K, et al. Analysis of residual coronary artery motion for breath-hold and navigator approaches using real-time coronary MRI. Magn Reson Med 2006;55(3):612–8.

[23] Uribe SA, Muthurangu V, Boubertakh R Sr. et al. Whole-heart cine MRI using real-time respiratory self-gating [abstract]. J Cardiovasc Magn Reson 2007;9(2):207–8.

[24] Edelman RR, Manning WJ, Burstein D, et al. Coronary arteries: breath-hold MR angiography. Radiology 1991;181(3):641–3.

[25] Huber S, Bornstedt A, Schnackenburg B, et al. The impact of different positions and thoraicial restrains on respiratory-induced cardiac motion. J Cardiovasc Magn Reson 2006;8(3):483–8.

[26] Holland AE, Goldfarb JW, Edelman RR. Diaphragmatic and cardiac motion during suspended breathing: preliminary experience and implications for breath-hold MR imaging. Radiology 1998; 209(2):483–9.

[27] Danias PG, Stuber M, Botnar RM, et al. Navigator assessment of breath-hold duration: impact of supplemental oxygen and hyperventilation. AJR Am J Roentgenol 1998;171(2):395–7.

[28] Li D, Paschal CB, Haacke EM, et al. Coronary arteries: three-dimensional MR imaging with fat saturation and magnetization transfer contrast. Radiology 1993;187(2):401–6.

[29] McConnell MV, Khasgiwala VC, Savord BJ, et al. Comparison of respiratory suppression methods and navigator locations for MR coronary angiography. AJR Am J Roentgenol 1997;168(5): 1369–75.

[30] Oshinski JN, Hofland L, Mukundan S Jr, et al. Two-dimensional coronary MR angiography

without breath holding. Radiology 1996;201(3): 737–43.
[31] Ehman RL, Felmlee JP. Adaptive technique for high-definition MR imaging of moving structures. Radiology 1989;173(1):255–63.
[32] Stuber M, Botnar RM, Danias PG, et al. Submillimeter three-dimensional coronary MR angiography with real-time navigator correction: comparison of navigator locations. Radiology 1999; 212(2):579–87.
[33] Post JC, van Rossum AC, Hofman MB, et al. Three-dimensional respiratory-gated MR angiography of coronary arteries: comparison with conventional coronary angiography. AJR Am J Roentgenol 1996;166(6):1399–404.
[34] Li D, Kaushikkar S, Haacke EM, et al. Coronary arteries: three-dimensional MR imaging with retrospective respiratory gating. Radiology 1996;201(3): 857–63.
[35] Stuber M, Botnar RM, Fischer SE, et al. Preliminary report on in vivo coronary MRA at 3 Tesla in humans. Magn Reson Med 2002;48(3): 425–9.
[36] Nagel E, Bornstedt A, Schnackenburg B, et al. Optimization of real-time adaptive navigator correction for 3D magnetic resonance coronary angiography. Magn Reson Med 1999;42(2):408–11.
[37] Danias PG, McConnell MV, Khasgiwala VC, et al. Prospective navigator correction of image position for coronary MR angiography. Radiology 1997; 203(3):733–6.
[38] Danias PG, Stuber M, Botnar RM, et al. Relationship between coronary artery and diaphragmatic respiratory motion: lessons from real-time cardiac MR imaging. AJR Am J Roentgenol 1999;172(4): 1061–5.
[39] McConnell MV, Khasgiwala VC, Savord BJ, et al. Prospective adaptive navigator correction for breath-hold MR coronary angiography. Magn Reson Med 1997;37(1):148–52.
[40] Manke D, Nehrke K, Bornert P, et al. Respiratory motion in coronary magnetic resonance angiography: a comparison of different motion models. J Magn Reson Imaging 2002;15(6):661–71.
[41] Manke D, Nehrke K, Boernert P. Novel prospective respiratory motion correction approach for free-breathing coronary MR angiography using a patient-adapted affine motion model. Magn Reson Med 2003;50:122–31.
[42] Nguyen TD, Nuval A, Mulukutla S, et al. Direct monitoring of coronary artery motion with cardiac fat navigator echoes. Magn Reson Med 2003;50: 235–41.
[43] Stuber M, Danias PG, Botnar RM, et al. Superiority of prone position in free-breathing 3D coronary MRA in patients with coronary disease. J Magn Reson Imaging 2001;13(2):185–91.
[44] Sakuma H, Ichikawa Y, Chino S, et al. Detection of coronary artery stenosis with whole-heart coronary magnetic resonance angiography. J Am Coll Cardiol 2006;48(10):1946–50.
[45] Spuentrup E, Stuber M, Botnar RM, et al. The impact of navigator timing parameters and navigator spatial resolution on 3D coronary magnetic resonance angiography. J Magn Reson Imaging 2001; 14(3):311–8.
[46] Schar M, Kim W, Stuber M. The impact of spatial resolution and respiratory motion on MR imaging of atherosclerotic plaque. J Magn Reson Imaging 2003;17(5):538–44.
[47] Park J, Larson AC, Zhang Q, et al. 4D Radial coronary artery imaging within a single breath hold: cine angiography with phase-sensitive fat suppression (CAPS). Magn Reson Med 2005;54(5): 833–40.
[48] Brittain JH, Hu BS, Wright GA, et al. Coronary angiography with magnetization-prepared T2 contrast. Magn Reson Med 1995;33(5):689–96.
[49] Shea SM, Deshpande VS, Chung YC, et al. Three-dimensional true-FISP imaging of the coronary arteries: improved contrast with T2-preparation. J Magn Reson Imaging 2002;15(5): 597–602.
[50] Balaban RS, Ceckler TL. Magnetization transfer contrast in magnetic resonance imaging. Magn Reson Q 1992;8(2):116–37.
[51] Nezsafat R, Yeon S, Wylie JV, et al. MR coronary vein imaging in cardiac resynchronization therapy: initial experience [abstract]. J Cardiovasc Magn Reson 2007;9(2):139–40.
[52] Lieberman JM, Botti RE, Nelson AD. Magnetic resonance imaging of the heart. Radiol Clin North Am 1984;22(4):847–58.
[53] Paulin S, von Schulthess GK, Fossel E, et al. MR imaging of the aortic root and proximal coronary arteries. AJR Am J Roentgenol 1987;148(4): 665–70.
[54] Manning WJ, Li W, Edelman RR. A preliminary report comparing magnetic resonance coronary angiography with conventional angiography. N Engl J Med 1993;328(12):828–32.
[55] Manning WJ, Li W, Boyle N, et al. Fat-suppressed breath-hold magnetic resonance coronary angiography. Circulation 1993;87(1):94–104.
[56] Keegan J, Horkaew P, Buchanan TJ, et al. Intra- and interstudy reproducibility of coronary artery diameter measurements in magnetic resonance coronary angiography. J Magn Reson Imaging 2004; 20(1):160–6.
[57] Meyer CH, Hu BS, Nishimura DG, et al. Fast spiral coronary artery imaging. Magn Reson Med 1992;28(2):202–13.
[58] Stuber M, Botnar RM, Danias PG, et al. Double-oblique free-breathing high-resolution three-dimensional coronary magnetic resonance angiography. J Am Coll Cardiol 1999;34(2):524–31.
[59] Langerak SE, Vliegen HW, de Roos A, et al. Detection of vein graft disease using high-resolution

magnetic resonance angiography. Circulation 2002;105(3):328–33.

[60] Maintz D, Aepfelbacher FC, Kissinger KV, et al. Coronary MR angiography: comparison of quantitative and qualitative data from four techniques. AJR Am J Roentgenol 2004;182(2): 515–21.

[61] Deshpande VS, Shea SM, Laub G, et al. 3D magnetization-prepared true-FISP: a new technique for imaging coronary arteries. Magn Reson Med 2001;46(3):494–502.

[62] Park J, McCarthy R, Li D. Feasibility and performance of breath-hold 3D TRUE-FISP coronary MRAQ using self-calibrating parallel acquisition. Magn Reson Med 2004;52(1):7–13.

[63] Niendorf T, Saranathan M, Lingamneni A, et al. Short breath-hold volumetric coronary MR angiography employing steady-state free precession in conjunction with parallel imaging. Magn Reson Med 2005;53(4):885–94.

[64] Weber OM, Martin AJ, Higgins CB. Whole-heart steady-state free precession coronary artery magnetic resonance angiography. Magn Reson Med 2003; 50(6):1223–8.

[65] Stehning C, Boernert P, Nehrke K, et al. Free-breathing 3D balanced FFE coronary magnetic resonance angiography with prolonged cardiac acquisition windows and intra-RR motion correction. Magn Reson Med 2005;53(3):719–23.

[66] Greil GF, Desai MY, Fenchel M, et al. Reproducibility of free-breathing cardiovascular magnetic resonance coronary angiography. J Cardiovasc Magn Reson 2007;9(1):49–56.

[67] Spuentrup E, Boernert P, Botnar RM, et al. Navigator-gated free-breathing three-dimensional balanced fast field echo (TrueFISP) coronary magnetic resonance angiography. Invest Radiol 2002;37(11):637–42.

[68] Sakuma H, Ichikawa Y, Suzawa N, et al. Assessment of coronary arteries with total study time of less than 30 minutes using whole-heart coronary MR angiography. Radiology 2005; 237(1):316–21.

[69] Botnar RM, Stuber M, Kissinger KV. Free-breathing 3D coronary MRA: the impact of isotropic image resolution. J Magn Reson Imaging 2000;11(4): 389–93.

[70] Sodickson DK, Manning WJ. Simultaneous acquisition of spatial harmonics (SMASH): fast imaging with radiofrequency coil arrays. Magn Reson Med 1997;38(4):591–603.

[71] Niendorf T, Hardy CJ, Giaquinto RO. Toward single breath hold whole-heart coverage coronary MRA using highly accelerated parallel imaging with a 32-channel MR system. Magn Reson Med 2006;56(1):167–76.

[72] Pruessmann KP, Weiger M, Scheidegger MB, et al. SENSE: sensitivity encoding for fast MRI. Magn Reson Med 1999;42(5):952–62.

[73] Weber O, Martin A, Higgins CB. Whole-heart coronary MRA using high SENSE factors [abstract]. J Cardiovasc Magn Reson 2004;6(1): 317–25.

[74] Park J, Larson AC, Zhang Q, et al. High-resolution steady-state free precession coronary magnetic resonance angiography within a breath hold: parallel imaging with extended cardiac data acquisition. Magn Reson Med 2005;54(5):1100–6.

[75] Bornert P, Stuber M, Botnar RM, et al. Direct comparison of 3D spiral vs. Cartesian gradient-echo coronary magnetic resonance angiography. Magn Reson Med 2001;46(4):789–94.

[76] Thedens DR, Irarrazaval P, Sachs TS, et al. Fast magnetic resonance coronary angiography with a three-dimensional stack of spirals trajectory. Magn Reson Med 1999;41(6):1170–9.

[77] Bornert P, Aldefeld B, Nehrke K. Improved 3D spiral imaging for coronary MR angiography. Magn Reson Med 2001;45(1):172–5.

[78] Weber OM, Pujadas S, Martin AJ, et al. Free-breathing, three-dimensional coronary artery magnetic resonance angiography: comparison of sequences. J Magn Reson Imaging 2004;20(3): 395–402.

[79] Leiner T, Katsimaglis G, Kissinger KV, et al. Comparison of Cartesian and radial balanced GTFE coronary MRA [abstract]. J Cardiovasc Magn Reson 2004;6(1):75.

[80] Botnar RM, Stuber M, Kissinger KV, et al. Noninvasive coronary vessel wall and plaque imaging with magnetic resonance imaging. Circulation 2000;102(12):2582–7.

[81] Zheng J, Li D, Bae KT, et al. Three-dimensional gadolinium-enhanced coronary magnetic resonance angiography: initial experience. J Cardiovasc Magn Reson 1999;1(1):33–41.

[82] Goldfarb JW, Edelman RR. Coronary arteries: breath-hold, gadolinium-enhanced, three-dimensional MR angiography. Radiology 1998;206(3): 830–4.

[83] Deshpande V, Li D. Contrast-enhanced coronary artery imaging using 3D TrueFISP. Magn Reson Med 2003;50(3):570–7.

[84] Paetsch I, Jahnke C, Barkhausen J, et al. Detection of coronary stenoses with contrast-enhanced, three-dimensional free-breathing coronary MR angiography using the gadolinium-based intravascular contrast agent gadocoletic acid (B-22956). J Cardiovasc Magn Reson 2006;8(3):509–16.

[85] Stuber M, Botnar RM, Danias PG, et al. Contrast agent-enhanced, free-breathing, three-dimensional coronary magnetic resonance angiography. J Magn Reson Imaging 1999;10(5):790–9.

[86] Huber ME, Paetsch I, Schnackenburg B, et al. Performance of a new gadolinium-based intravascular contrast agent in free-breathing inversion-recovery 3D coronary MRA. Magn Reson Med 2003;49(1): 115–21.

[87] Herborn CU, Barkhausen J, Paetsch I, et al. Coronary arteries: contrast-enhanced MR imaging with SH L 643A—experience in 12 volunteers. Radiology 2003;229(1):217–23.

[88] Knuesel PR, Nanz D, Wolfensberger U, et al. Multislice breath-hold spiral magnetic resonance coronary angiography in patients with coronary artery disease: effect of intravascular contrast medium. J Magn Reson Imaging 2002;16(6):660–7.

[89] Taylor AM, Panting JR, Keegan J, et al. Safety and preliminary findings with the intravascular contrast agent NC100150 injection for MR coronary angiography. J Magn Reson Imaging 1999; 9(2):220–7.

[90] Sandstede JJ, Pabst T, Wacker C, et al. Breath-hold 3D MR coronary angiography with a new intravascular contrast agent (feruglose)—first clinical experiences. Magn Reson Imaging 2001;19(2):201–5.

[91] Noeske R, Seifert F, Rhein KH, et al. Human cardiac imaging at 3 T using phased array coils. Magn Reson Med 2000;44(6):978–82.

[92] Atalay MK, Poncelet BP, Kantor HL, et al. Cardiac susceptibility artifacts arising from the heart–lung interface. Magn Reson Med 2001;45(2):341–5.

[93] Santos JM, Cunningham CH, Lustig M, et al. Single breath-hold whole-heart MRA using variable density spirals at 3T. Magn Reson Med 2006; 55(2):371–9.

[94] Bi X, Li D. Coronary arteries at 3.0T: contrast-enhanced magnetization-prepared three-dimensional breath-hold MR angiography. J Magn Reson Imaging 2005;21(2):133–9.

[95] Strohm O, Kivelitz D, Gross W, et al. Safety of implantable coronary stents during 1H-magnetic resonance imaging at 1.0 and 1.5 T. J Cardiovasc Magn Reson 1999;1(3):239–45.

[96] Kramer CM, Rogers WJ Jr, Pakstis DL. Absence of adverse outcomes after magnetic resonance imaging early after stent placement for acute myocardial infarction: a preliminary study. J Cardiovasc Magn Reson 2000;2(4):257–61.

[97] Gerber TC, Fasseas P, Lennon RJ, et al. Clinical safety of magnetic resonance imaging early after coronary artery stent placement. J Am Coll Cardiol 2003;42(7):1295–8.

[98] Hug J, Nagel E, Bornstedt, et al. Coronary arterial stents: safety and artifacts during MR imaging. Radiology 2000;216(3):781–7.

[99] Scott NA, Pettigrew RI. Absence of movement of coronary stents after placement in a magnetic resonance imaging field. Am J Cardiol 1994;73(12):900–1.

[100] Shellock FG, Shellock VJ. Metallic stents: evaluation of MR imaging safety. AJR Am J Roentgenol 1999;173(3):543–7.

[101] Shellock FG. MR safety at 3-Tesla: bare metal and drug-eluting coronary artery stents. Signals 2005; 53(2):26–7.

[102] Maintz DC, Botnar RM, Fischbach R, et al. Coronary magnetic resonance angiography for assessment of the stent lumen: a phantom study. J Cardiovasc Magn Reson 2002;4(3):359–67.

[103] Spuentrup E, Ruebben A, Schaeffter T, et al. Magnetic resonance–guided coronary artery stent placement in a swine model. Circulation 2002;105(7): 874–9.

[104] Meyer CH, Macovski A, Nishimura DG. Coronary vessel wall imaging [abstract]. Proc Inter Soc Magn Reson Med. Presented at the 6th Annual Meeting of the International Society of Magnetic Resonance in Medicine. Sydney, Australia, 1998. p. 15.

[105] Fayad ZA, Fuster V, Fallon JT, et al. Noninvasive in vivo human coronary artery lumen and wall imaging using black-blood magnetic resonance imaging. Circulation 2000;102(5):506–10.

[106] Botnar RM, Stuber M, Lamerichs R, et al. Initial experiences with in vivo right coronary artery human MR vessel wall imaging at 3Tesla. J Cardiovasc Magn Reson 2003;5(4):589–94.

[107] Koktzoglou I, Simonetti O, Li D. Coronary artery wall imaging: initial experience at 3 Tesla. J Magn Reson Imaging 2005;21(2):128–32.

[108] Botnar RM, Wiethoff AJ, Parsons EC Jr, et al. In vivo molecular MR imaging of acute coronary thrombosis using a fibrin-targeted contrast agent [abstract]J Cardiovasc Magn Reson 2004;6:109–10.

[109] Serfaty JM, Atalar E, Declerck J, et al. Real-time projection MR angiography: feasibility study. Radiology 2000;217(1):290–5.

[110] Green JD, Omary RA, Schirf BE, et al. Catheter-directed contrast-enhanced coronary MR angiography in swine using magnetization-prepared True-FISP. Magn Reson Med 2003;50(6):1317–21.

[111] Green JD, Schirf BE, Omary RA, et al. Projection imaging of the right coronary artery with an intravenous injection of contrast agent. Magn Reson Med 2004;52(4):699–703.

[112] Olsson LE, Chai CM, Axelsson O, et al. MR coronary angiography in pigs with intra-arterial injections of a hyperpolarized 13C substance. Magn Reson Med 2006;55(4):731–7.

[113] Pennell DJ, Keegan J, Firmin DN, et al. Magnetic resonance imaging of coronary arteries: technique and preliminary results. Br Heart J 1993;70(4): 315–26.

[114] Duerinckx AJ, Urman MK. Two-dimensional coronary MR angiography: analysis of initial clinical results. Radiology 1994;193(3):731–8.

[115] Sakuma H, Caputo GR, Steffens JC, et al. Breath-hold MR cine angiography of coronary arteries in healthy volunteers: value of multiangle oblique imaging planes. AJR Am J Roentgenol 1994;163(3): 533–7.

[116] Masui T, Isoda H, Mochizuki T, et al. MR angiography of the coronary arteries. Radiat Med 1995; 13(1):47–50.

[117] Davis SF, Kannam JP, Edelman RR, et al. Magnetic resonance coronary angiography in heart

transplant recipients. J Heart Lung Transplant 1996;15(6):580–6.
[118] Wielopolski PA, van Geuns RJ, de Feyter PJ, et al. Breath-hold coronary MR angiography with volume-targeted imaging. Radiology 1998;209(1): 209–19.
[119] Scheidegger MB, Hess OM, Boesiger P. Validation of coronary artery MR angiography: comparison of measured vessel diameters with quantitative contrast angiography [abstract]. Soc of Magnetic Reson: Book of Abstracts 1994;497.
[120] Engel HJ, Torres C, Page HL Jr. Major variations in anatomical origin of the coronary arteries: angiographic observations in 4250 patients without associated congenital heart disease. Cathet Cardiovasc Diagn 1975;1(2):157–69.
[121] Chaitman BR, Lesperance J, Saltiel J, et al. Clinical, angiographic, and hemodynamic findings in patients with anomalous origin of the coronary arteries. Circulation 1976;53(1):122–31.
[122] Angelini P. Coronary artery anomolies: an entity in search of an identity. Circulation 2007;115(10): 1296–305.
[123] McConnell MV, Ganz P, Selwyn A, et al. Identification of anomalous coronary arteries and their anatomic course by magnetic resonance coronary angiography. Circulation 1995;92(11):3158–62.
[124] Post JC, van Rossum AC, Bronzwaer, et al. Magnetic resonance angiography of anomalous coronary arteries. A new gold standard for delineating the proximal course? Circulation 1995;92(11): 3163–71.
[125] Vliegen HW, Doornbos J, de Roos A, et al. Value of fast gradient echo magnetic resonance angiography as an adjunct to coronary arteriography in detecting and confirming the course of clinically significant coronary artery anomalies. Am J Cardiol 1997;79(6):773–6.
[126] Taylor AM, Thorne SA, Rubens MB, et al. Coronary artery imaging in grown-up congenital heart disease: complementary role of magnetic resonance and x-ray coronary angiography. Circulation 2000; 101(14):1670–8.
[127] Bunce NH, Lorenz CH, Keegan J, et al. Coronary artery anomalies: assessment with free-breathing three-dimensional coronary MR angiography. Radiology 2003;227(1):201–8.
[128] Razmi RM, Chun W, Rathi VK, et al. Coronary magnetic resonance angiography (CMRA): the gold standard for determining the proximal course of anomalous coronary arteries [abstract]. J Am Coll Cardiol 2001;(37):380.
[129] Setser RM, Arruda J, Weaver JA, et al. Exclusion of coronary artery anomalies in patients with congenital cardiovascular abnormalities using whole-heart approach [abstract]. J Cardiovasc Magn Reson 2007;9(2):128–9.
[130] Gharib AM, Ho VB, Rosing DR, et al. Feasibility of using free-breathing 3D whole-heart coronary MR angiography at 3T to assess coronary artery anomalies and variants [abstract]. J Cardiovasc Magn Reson 2007;9(2):129–30.
[131] Schmid M, Achenbach S, Ludwig J, et al. Visualization of coronary artery anomalies by contrast-enhanced multidetector rows spiral computed tomography. Int J Cardiol 2006;111(3):430–5.
[132] Deibler AR, Kuzo RS, Vohringer M, et al. Imaging of congenital coronary anomalies with multislice computed tomography. Mayo Clin Proc 2004; 79(8):1017–23.
[133] Akagi T, Rose V, Benson LN, et al. Outcome of coronary artery aneurysms after Kawasaki disease. J Pediatr 1992;121(5 Pt 1):689–94.
[134] Kato H, Ichinose E, Yoshioka F, et al. Fate of coronary aneurysms in Kawasaki disease: serial coronary angiography and long-term follow-up study. Am J Cardiol 1982;49(7):1758–66.
[135] Greil GF, Stuber M, Botnar RM, et al. Coronary magnetic resonance angiography in adolescents and young adults with Kawasaki disease. Circulation 2002;105(8):908–11.
[136] Mavrogeni S, Papadopoulos G, Douskou M, et al. Magnetic resonance angiography is equivalent to x-ray coronary angiography for the evaluation of coronary arteries in Kawasaki disease. J Am Coll Cardiol 2004;43(4):649–52.
[137] Mavrogeni S, Papadopoulos G, Douskou M, et al. Magnetic resonance angiography, function and viability evaluation in patients with Kawasaki disease. J Cardiovasc Magn Reson 2006; 8(4):493–8.
[138] Mavrogeni S, Papadakis E, Foussas S, et al. Correlation between magnetic resonance angiography (MRA) and quantitative coronary angiography (QCA) in ectatic coronary vessels. J Cardiovasc Magn Reson 2004;6(1):17–23.
[139] Kim WY, Danias PG, Stuber M, et al. Coronary magnetic resonance angiography for the detection of coronary stenoses. N Engl J Med 2001;345(26): 1863–9.
[140] Pennell DJ, Bogren HG, Keegan J, et al. Assessment of coronary artery stenosis by magnetic resonance imaging. Heart 1996;75(2):127–33.
[141] Post JC, van Rossum AC, Hofman MB, et al. Clinical utility of two-dimensional magnetic resonance angiography in detecting coronary artery disease. Eur Heart J 1997;18(3):426–33.
[142] Nitatori T, Hanaoka H, Yoshino A, et al. Clinical application of magnetic resonance angiography for coronary arteries: correlation with conventional angiography and evaluation of imaging time. Nippon Igaku Hoshasen Gakkai Zasshi 1995;55(9): 670–6.
[143] Sandstede JJ, Pabst T, Beer M, et al. Three-dimensional MR coronary angiography using the navigator technique compared with conventional coronary angiography. AJR Am J Roentgenol 1999;172(1):135–9.

[144] Ozgun M, Quante M, Kouwenhoven M, et al. Comparison of spoiled TFE and balancedTFE coronary MR angiography [abstract]. J Cardiovasc Magn Reson 2004;6(1):268–9.
[145] Ozgun M, Hoffmeier A, Kouwenhoven M, et al. Comparison of 3D segmented gradient-echo and steady-state free precession coronary MRI sequences in patients with coronary artery disease. AJR Am J Roentgenol 2005;185(1):103–9.
[146] Jahnke C, Paetsch I, Schnackenburg B, et al. Coronary MR angiography with steady-state free precession: individually adapted breath-hold technique versus free-breathing technique. Radiology 2004;232(3):669–76.
[147] Muller MF, Fleisch M, Kroeker R, et al. Proximal coronary artery stenosis: three-dimensional MRI with fat saturation and navigator echo. J Magn Reson Imaging 1997;7(4):644–51.
[148] Woodard PK, Li D, Haacke EM, et al. Detection of coronary stenoses on source and projection images using three-dimensional MR angiography with retrospective respiratory gating: preliminary experience. AJR Am J Roentgenol 1998;170(4):883–8.
[149] van Geuns RJ, de Bruin HG, Rensing BJ, et al. Magnetic resonance imaging of the coronary arteries: clinical results from three dimensional evaluation of a respiratory gated technique. Heart 1999; 82(4):515–9.
[150] Huber A, Nikolaou K, Gonschior P, et al. Navigator echo-based respiratory gating for three-dimensional MR coronary angiography: results from healthy volunteers and patients with proximal coronary artery stenoses. AJR Am J Roentgenol 1999; 173(1):95–101.
[151] Sardanelli F, Molinari G, Zandrino F, et al. Three-dimensional, navigator echo MR coronary angiography in detecting stenoses of the major epicardial vessels, with conventional coronary angiography as the standard of reference. Radiology 2000; 214(3):808–14.
[152] Bunce NRS, Jhooti P, Lorenz C, et al. The assessment of coronary artery disease by combined magnetic resonance coronary arteriography and perfusion [abstract]. J Cardiovasc Magn Reson 2001;3(1):118.
[153] Moustapha AI, Muthupillai R, Wilson J, et al. Coronary magnetic resonance angiography using a free breathing, T2 weighted, three-dimensional gradient echo sequence with navigator respiratory and ECG gating used to detect coronary artery disease [abstract]. J Am Coll Cardiol 2001;37(Suppl):380.
[154] Sommer T, Hofer U, Meyer C, et al. Submillimeter 3D coronary MR angiography with real-time navigator correction inn 112 patients with suspected coronary artery disease [abstract]. J Cardiovasc Magn Reson 2002;4(1):28.
[155] Bogaert J, Kuzo R, Dymarkowski S, et al. Coronary artery imaging with real-time navigator three-dimensional turbo-field-echo MR coronary angiography: initial experience. Radiology 2003; 226(3):707–16.
[156] Plein S, Radjenovic A, Ridgway JP, et al. Coronary artery disease: assessment with a comprehensive MR imaging protocol—initial results. Radiology 2002;225(1):300–7.
[157] Dewey M, Teige F, Schnapauff D, et al. Combination of free-breathing and breath-hold steady-state free precession magnetic resonance angiography for detection of coronary artery stenoses. J Magn Reson Imaging 2006;23(5):674–81.
[158] Hauser TH, Yeon SB, Appelbaum E, et al. Discrimination of ischemic vs. nonischemic cardiomyopathy among patients with heart failure using combined coronary MRI and delayed enhancement MR [abstract]. J Cardiovasc Magn Reson 2005;7(1):94.
[159] Jahnke C, Paetsch I, Nehrke K, et al. Rapid and complete coronary arterial tree visualization with magnetic resonance imaging: feasibility and diagnostic performance. Eur Heart J 2005;26(21): 2313–9.
[160] Gerber BL, Coche E, Pasquet A, et al. Coronary artery stenosis: direct comparison of four section multidetector row CT and three-dimensional navigator MR imaging for detection-initial results. Radiology 2005;234(1):98–108.
[161] Rubinstein RI, Askenase AD, Thickman D, et al. Magnetic resonance imaging to evaluate patency of aortocoronary bypass grafts. Circulation 1987; 76(4):786–91.
[162] Jenkins JP, Love HG, Foster CJ, et al. Detection of coronary artery bypass graft patency as assessed by magnetic resonance imaging. Br J Radiol 1988; 61(721):2–4.
[163] Kefer J, Coche E, Legros G, et al. Head-to-head comparison of three-dimensional navigator-gated magnetic resonance imaging and 16-slice computed tomography to detect coronary artery stenosis in patients. J Am Coll Cardiol 2005;46(1):92–100.
[164] Dewey M, Teige F, Schnapauff D, et al. Noninvasive detection of coronary artery stenoses with multislice computed tomography or magnetic resonance imaging. Ann Intern Med 2006;145(6): 407–15.
[165] Goldman S, Copeland J, Moritz T, et al. Saphenous vein graft patency 1 year after coronary artery bypass surgery and effects of antiplatelet therapy. Results of a Veterans Administration cooperative study. Circulation 1989;80(5):1190–7.
[166] Fitzgibbon GM, Kafka HP, Leach AJ, et al. Coronary bypass graft fate and patient outcome: angiographic follow-up of 5065 grafts related to survival and reoperation in 1388 patients during 25 years. J Am Coll Cardiol 1996;28(3):616–26.
[167] van Geuns RJ, Wielopolski PA, de Bruin HG, et al. MR coronary angiography with breath-hold targeted volumes: preliminary clinical results. Radiology 2000;217(1):270–7.

[168] White RD, Caputo GR, Mark AS, et al. Coronary artery bypass graft patency: noninvasive evaluation with MR imaging. Radiology 1987;164(3):681–6.
[169] White RD, Pflugfelder PW, Lipton MJ, et al. Coronary artery bypass grafts: evaluation of patency with cine MR imaging. AJR Am J Roentgenol 1988;150(6):1271–4.
[170] Galjee MA, van Rossum AC, Doesburg T, et al. Value of magnetic resonance imaging in assessing patency and function of coronary artery bypass grafts. An angiographically controlled study. Circulation 1996;93(4):660–6.
[171] Aurigemma GP, Reichek N, Axel L, et al. Noninvasive determination of coronary artery bypass graft patency by cine magnetic resonance imaging. Circulation 1989;80(6):1595–602.
[172] Engelmann MG, Knez A, von Smekal A, et al. Noninvasive coronary bypass graft imaging after multivessel revascularisation. Int J Cardiol 2000; 76(1):65–74.
[173] Molinari G, Sardanelli F, Zandrino F, et al. Value of navigator echo magnetic resonance angiography in detecting occlusion/patency of arterial and venous, single and sequential coronary bypass grafts. Int J Card Imaging 2000;16(3):149–60.
[174] Wintersperger BJ, Engelmann MG, von Smekal A, et al. Patency of coronary bypass grafts: assessment with breath-hold contrast-enhanced MR angiography—value of a nonelectrocardiographically triggered technique. Radiology 1998;208(2): 345–51.
[175] Vrachliotis TG, Bis KG, Aliabadi D, et al. Contrast-enhanced breath-hold MR angiography for evaluating patency of coronary artery bypass grafts. AJR Am J Roentgenol 1997;168(4): 1073–80.
[176] Bunce NH, Lorenz CH, John AS, et al. Coronary artery bypass graft patency: assessment with true ast imaging with steady-state precession versus gadolinium-enhanced MR angiography. Radiology 2003;227(2):440–6.
[177] Langerak SE, Kunz P, Vliegen HW, et al. MR flow mapping in coronary artery bypass grafts: a validation study with Doppler flow measurements. Radiology 2002;222(1):127–35.
[178] Langerak SE, Vliegen HW, Jukema JW, et al. Value of magnetic resonance imaging for the noninvasive detection of stenosis in coronary artery bypass grafts and recipient coronary arteries-Circulation 2003;107(11):1502–8.

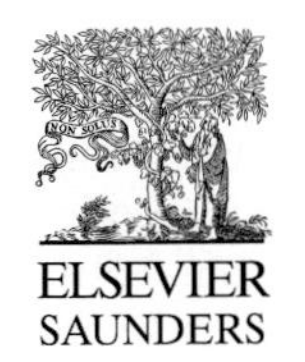

ELSEVIER
SAUNDERS

Cardiol Clin 25 (2007) 171–184

CARDIOLOGY
CLINICS

MRI of the Thoracic Aorta

Christopher J. François, MD, James C. Carr, MD*

Department of Radiology, Northwestern University Medical School and Northwestern Memorial Hospital, 676 St. Clair Street, Suite 800, Chicago, IL 60611, USA

Diseases of the thoracic aorta are a significant cause of morbidity and mortality and can result in potentially catastrophic consequences. Conventional digital subtraction angiography (DSA) has been the gold standard for imaging for many years; however, this is associated with well-recognized adverse effects [1] and provides only limited information about vessel morphology. DSA now is used primarily as a first-line investigation in the setting of trauma [2]. CT is now the most frequently used modality for evaluating the thoracic aorta and has high diagnostic accuracy for detecting aortic pathology, particularly with the advent of multidetector scanners [3,4]. CT has the advantage of being quick and readily available in most hospital settings; however it employs ionizing radiation [5] and potentially nephrotoxic contrast agents. Transesophageal echocardiography (TEE) also can be used to assess the thoracic aorta, particularly in the diagnosis of aortic dissection; however, it is relatively invasive and provides limited coverage of the entire vessel [6].

MRI increasingly is becoming the first-line investigation for evaluating diseases in the thoracic aorta [7,8]. MRI possesses the capability for multiplanar imaging; it uses a nontoxic contrast agent and does not involve ionizing radiation. With recent advances in gradient hardware, much shorter repetition times (TR) are now achievable, resulting in significant increases in acquisition speed. This has prompted the development of new pulse sequences and ultrafast magnetic resonance angiography (MRA) techniques. The principal challenge to universal implementation of MRI as a first-line imaging tool for the thoracic aorta remains its less widespread availability compared with CT.

Magnetic resonance imaging techniques

Most MRI strategies for assessing the thoracic aorta involve a technique to assess vessel morphology combined with contrast-enhanced MRA. Improvements in gradient strength have seen a resurgence of balanced steady-state free precession techniques (SSFP), also referred to by their commercial names of TrueFISP (Siemens, Malvern, Pennsylvania), FIESTA (GE, Waukesha, Wisconsin), and b-FFE (Philips, Bothell, Washington). In addition, shortened TRs allow ultrafast MRA to be implemented with subsecond temporal resolution. These newer techniques can be used to supplement the older well-established strategies, and in many cases, they have replaced them.

Steady-state free precession

Balanced SSFP techniques, such as TrueFISP, are gradient echo techniques that are used widely for cine imaging of the heart [9–14]. TrueFISP is T2* weighted and produces high signal from blood without the need for a contrast agent. Contrast to noise depends on T2/T1 differences, which, at short TR, are high for blood and soft tissues. To produce artifact-free images, TrueFISP must be implemented at short TR, and, as a result, they only can be used successfully used on scanners with high-performance gradients. The typical TR is 3.2 milliseconds with an echo time (TE) of 1.6 milliseconds. Signal intensity is maximal at a flip angle of 60 to 70°. A 256 imaging matrix is used, resulting in in-plane resolution of approximately $2.0 \times 1.5\ mm^2$.

* Corresponding author.
E-mail address: jcarr@radiology.nwu.edu (J.C. Carr).

0733-8651/07/$ - see front matter © 2007 Published by Elsevier Inc.
doi:10.1016/j.ccl.2007.02.005

TrueFISP can be implemented as a single-shot (Fig. 1), cine, or three-dimensional technique for imaging the thoracic aorta [15]. The single-shot strategy is an electrocardiographically (ECG) triggered two-dimensional acquisition. A trigger delay (approximately 200 to 400 ms) can be used to push the acquisition further into diastole, depending on the heart rate. The acquisition time per image is of the order of 450 milliseconds, resulting in one image per heartbeat. Because of the speed of acquisition, the technique is essentially independent of respiratory motion artifact. Consequently, imaging can be performed successfully without breath holding, which is particularly advantageous in critically ill patients. The aorta typically is covered in an interleaved manner in axial, coronal, and sagittal orientations.

Cine TrueFISP is a breath-hold ECG-triggered segmented k space acquisition. The imaging time is approximately 7 to 9 seconds per slice. Cine images typically are acquired at selected anatomic levels and orientations. A sagittal oblique candy-cane image through the upper chest is particularly useful for demonstrating the aortic arch. In cases of ascending aortic dissection, coronal and long axis images through the aortic valve are used to exclude significant aortic insufficiency.

Real-time TrueFISP, which does not require breath holding or ECG triggering, is a useful alternative cine technique in patients who cannot hold their breath [16,17]. Despite the lower spatial and temporal resolution with this technique, diagnostic images of the thoracic aorta and aortic valve usually can be obtained. Recently, three-dimensional TrueFISP techniques have been developed to image the coronary arteries and thoracic aorta. These sequences are performed using a nonselective, segmented acquistion with motion adaptive respiratory navigators to obtain isotropic three-dimensional data with very high spatial resolution.

Black blood techniques

Black blood techniques demonstrate the wall of the thoracic aorta and can be useful for evaluating various pathologies (Fig. 2), including acute aortic syndromes (intramural hematoma, penetrating ulcerative plaque, dissection), atherosclerosis, vasculitis, or neoplasms.

Numerous different strategies can be used. ECG-triggered breath-hold black blood turbo spin echo (TSE) [18], uses a double inversion technique to null the blood signal. The first 180° inversion recovery pulse is nonslice selective and occurs at the R wave trigger. It inverts the magnetization in the entire tissue volume, including the blood signal. This is followed immediately by a slice-selective reversion 180° pulse, which regenerates the magnetization in the slice to be imaged. At a specific inversion time (TI), the blood signal is nulled completely. Blood flowing into the slice is nulled from the first 180° inversion pulse, resulting in a black blood appearance. Imaging occurs during diastole. Approximately 12 to 16 lines of k space are acquired in each heart beat, and the center of k space is acquired at the TI. The entire image is acquired over several heartbeats.

ECG-triggered black blood HASTE uses a black blood preparation to null signal from blood [19]. This is a single-shot technique, with the entire image being acquired in a single heart

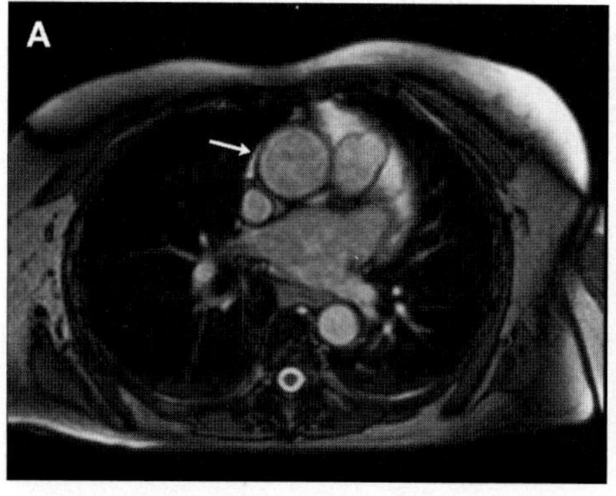

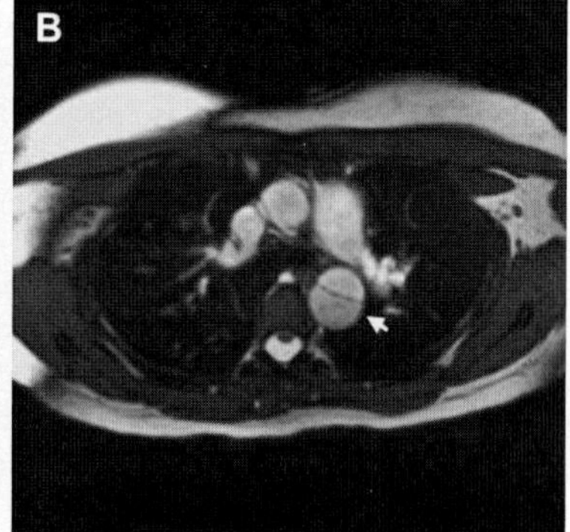

Fig. 1. Balanced steady-state free precession (SSFP). (*A*) Axial SSFP images through the middle chest in a patient who had a dilated ascending aorta (*long arrow*) and (*B*) in a second patient who had a descending thoracic aortic dissection (Fig. 1 B *from* Cynthia Rigsby, MD, Children's Memorial Hospital, Chicago.)

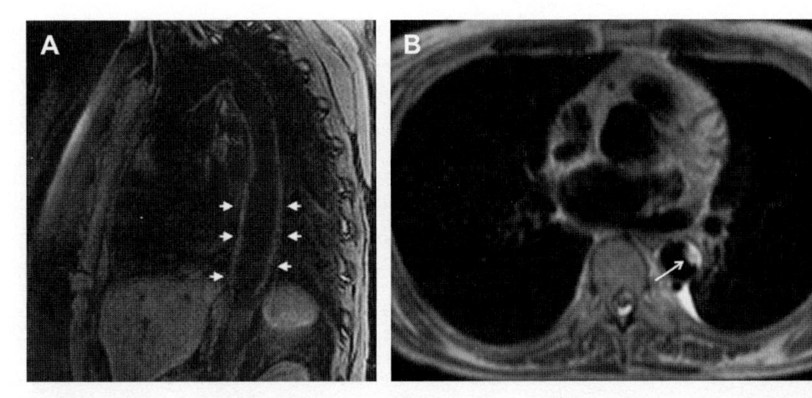

Fig. 2. Black blood imaging. (*A*) Left-anterior oblique black blood image of the thoracic aorta in a patient who had Takayasu aortitis demonstrating diffuse thickening of the wall of the aorta (*small arrows*). (*B*) Axial T2-weighted black blood image in a different patient who had primary intimal sarcoma of the descending thoracic aorta (*long arrow*).

beat. This is a useful alternative in patients who cannot hold their breath.

Recently, a fast diffusion-prepared (DP) balanced SSFP-based magnetic resonance technique that allows for three-dimensional dark blood imaging has been described. Because the three-dimensional DP-SSFP technique relies on blood motion (rather than inflow) to suppress magnetic resonance signal from blood, it can be of use for time-efficient dark blood MRI of the entire thoracic aorta when set to acquire in a sagittal–oblique plane. In addition, because this is a three-dimensional technique, the images offer improved slice resolution and more intuitive visualization of the thoracic aorta relative to two-dimensional methods.

T1-weighted gradient echo fat-saturated imaging

T1 gradient echo fat-saturated (GRE-FS) imaging before and after contrast injection is used routinely in evaluating pathology in the chest and also provides an overview of the entire thoracic aorta and surrounding structures [20]. It is particularly helpful in demonstrating intramural abnormalities, and it may replace black blood techniques in many situations. A two-dimensional breath-hold gradient echo pulse sequence with fat saturation is used to cover the thorax in an interleaved manner. The entire thoracic aorta is covered in axial and either coronal or sagittal orientations before and after contrast injection. The postcontrast set of images usually is obtained following the MRA.

Contrast-enhanced magnetic resonance angiography

Temporally resolved subsecond contrast-enhanced magnetic resonance angiography

Advances in gradient strength have resulted in much shorter TRs than were previously achievable. Much shorter acquisition times are now possible, allowing contrast-enhanced MRA (CE-MRA) to be implemented with subsecond temporal resolution (Fig. 3) [21,22]. This is particularly advantageous in the thoracic aorta, where high temporal resolution is useful for evaluating high-flow vascular lesions such as shunts and dissections. Subsecond CE-MRA is also accurate in detecting other pathology in the thoracic aorta and may replace conventional CE-MRA completely in many situations.

The basic pulse sequence is a three-dimensional gradient echo acquisition, similar to conventional CE-MRA. Asymmetric k-space scanning is used in all three axes, to further shorten the acquisition time. A TR of 1.6 milliseconds and a TE of 0.8 milliseconds are used. The flip angle is typically 20 to 25°. The three-dimensional slab thickness is 80 mm, with four partitions actually acquired. A 256 matrix size is used, yielding in-plane resolution of 2.0×1.5 mm^2; 6 mL of gadolinium is injected at 6 mL/s by means of an 18 G cannula placed in an antecubital vein. The contrast injection and magnetic resonance acquisition are started simultaneously, and patients are asked to breath hold in inspiration. Approximately 24 three-dimensional volumes typically are acquired in a single breath hold. The first three-dimensional set serves as a mask, and subtraction occurs in line. Maximum

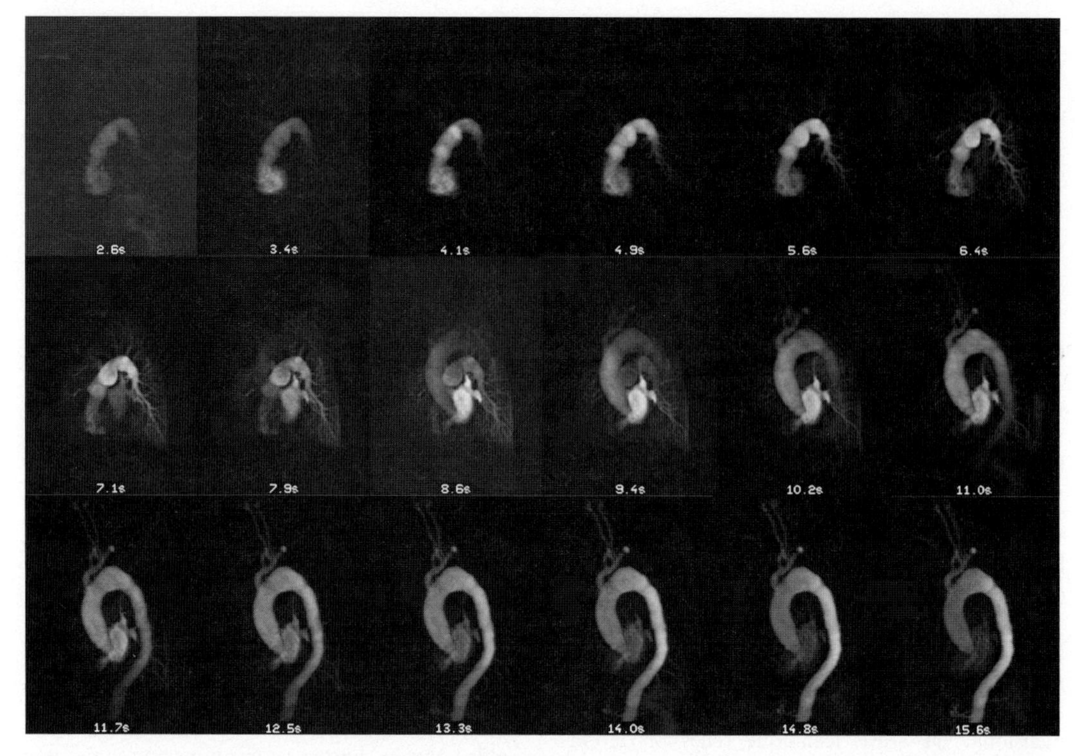

Fig. 3. Subsecond magnetic resonance angiography (MRA). Left anterior oblique maximum intensity projection images from a dynamic, time-resolved MRA with subsecond temporal resolution. The patient has an aneurysm of the aortic arch.

intensity projection (MIP) images are produced automatically. The entire series can be viewed as a cine loop with a frame time of 900 milliseconds or less.

To reduce the acquisition time per three-dimensional volume to a minimum, through-plane resolution is sacrificed resulting in near-projectional MRA. The main objective is to depict high-flow vascular abnormalities in the plane of the scan with as high temporal resolution as possible and, as a result, through-plane information is less important. In-plane resolution is reduced only moderately and is sufficient for diagnosing most thoracic aortic pathology. Because of the rapid frame rates, there does not appear to be an appreciable reduction in image quality in patients who cannot hold their breath, and therefore, this technique is particularly advantageous in critically ill individuals. Above all, because of the light contrast load, subsecond CE-MRA can be repeated numerous times in combination with conventional CE-MRA to provide a comprehensive assessment of vascular abnormalities.

Conventional contrast-enhanced magnetic resonance angiography

Conventional CE-MRA [23–27] is performed for comprehensive evaluation of the thoracic aorta; however, most abnormalities are already evident from the subsecond CE-MRA images. Conventional CE-MRA provides better spatial resolution, particularly in the z direction, and may produce better depiction of abnormalities such as penetrating atherosclerotic ulcers. Conventional CE-MRA can be performed without or with ECG triggering. CE-MRA performed without ECG triggering requires less time to acquire and is useful in patients who have difficulty holding their breath. Non-ECG triggered CE-MRA, however, is less useful for assessing the ascending thoracic aorta, which is degraded commonly by motion artifact from cardiac pulsation or obscured by overlapping vascular structures. In patients who require high-resolution images of the aortic root and ascending aorta, ECG trig gering is employed. Image data are acquired only during the same phase of the cardiac cycle with each heartbeat, usually end diastole. As a result, the images are not degraded by cardiac motion, but they do require a longer breath hold.

The basic pulse sequence for conventional CE-MRA is a standard three-dimensional gradient echo acquisition. The contrast transit time is calculated from the subsecond CE-MRA. A 512 matrix size is used, yielding a typical voxel size of $1.5 \times 0.8 \times 1.5$ mm^3; 40 mL of gadolinium is injected at 2.5 mL/s by means of an 18 G cannula placed in an antecubital vein. Images are acquired during breath holding. Subtracted three-dimensional sets are calculated from the raw data, and these are subjected to a MIP postprocessing algorithm.

Phased contrast magnetic resonance angiography

Phased contrast MRA (PC-MRA) is most useful when CE-MRA shows an aortic stenosis or when an aortic valve stenosis is suspected [28,29].

PC-MRA uses velocity differences or phase shifts in moving spins to produce image contrast in vessels. Phase shifts for moving spins are generated by applying magnetic field gradients of opposite polarity. The velocity encoding (VENC) value controls the amplitude of the magnetic gradient and is typically 150 to 200 cm/s in the aorta. If the VENC is too low, aliasing will occur, resulting in mismapping or dropout of signal from the center of the lumen. PC-MRA results in two sets of data (ie, phase images and magnitude images). The sequence can be ECG-triggered or retrospectively gated. It is important that the two-dimensional slice is orientated perpendicular to the vessel of interest and that the region of interest is positioned in the center of the magnetic field to avoid artifact from eddy currents.

Time flow and time–velocity curves can be generated from the PC-MRA data, and peak flow and peak velocity values are calculated. Analysis of curve shape and slope helps decide whether stenoses are significant. These measurements can be particularly useful for routine follow-up of stenoses.

Other techniques

The speed at which CE-MRA is performed is limited primarily by the time it takes to acquire phase-encoding steps. This, in turn, depends on the performance of the gradient hardware. As gradient technology improves, this information is acquired more rapidly only at the expense of producing unwanted neuromuscular stimulation caused by rapid gradient switching.

Numerous techniques have evolved that attempt to improve temporal resolution by changing the way data are acquired and processed. With the SMASH (simultaneous acquisition of spatial harmonics) [30,31] and SENSE (sensitivity encoding) [32,33] techniques, component coil signals in a radiofrequency coil array are used to encode spatial information partially by substituting for phase-encoding gradient steps that have been omitted. This allows some of the magnetic resonance image to be acquired in parallel taking some of the strain off the gradients. Up to fourfold accelerations have been demonstrated in people. With three-dimensional TRICKS (time-resolved imaging of contrast kinetics) [34], the high spatial frequencies are sampled less frequently than the low spatial frequencies. As a result, high contrast information is acquired preferentially. Data sharing and temporal interpolation also are employed to further improve temporal resolution. All of these newly developed techniques can be combined with conventional three-dimensional CE-MRA pulse sequences, and they have the potential to produce unprecedented improvements in temporal resolution (Fig. 4).

Abnormalities of the thoracic aorta

Aortic dissection

Aortic dissection results from the passage of blood out of the true lumen through a defect in the vessel wall into the tunica media, separating media from intima [35–37]. This results in the creation of a true and false lumen separated by an intimal flap. Aortic dissections typically are caused by poorly controlled hypertension but also may be associated with other entities such as aortic coarctation, iatrogenic injury, or valvular disease. The adverse effects result from either proximal or distal migration of the dissection to involve and occlude branch vessels of the aorta. When the dissection migrates proximally to involve the coronary arteries and aortic valve, the consequences are catastrophic. Aortic dissections are classified as Stanford Type A, involving the ascending thoracic aorta (Fig. 5) or Stanford Type B, without involvement of the ascending thoracic aorta (Fig. 6). Type A dissections are surgical emergencies, whereas type B dissections are treated medically. Therefore, the main objective of

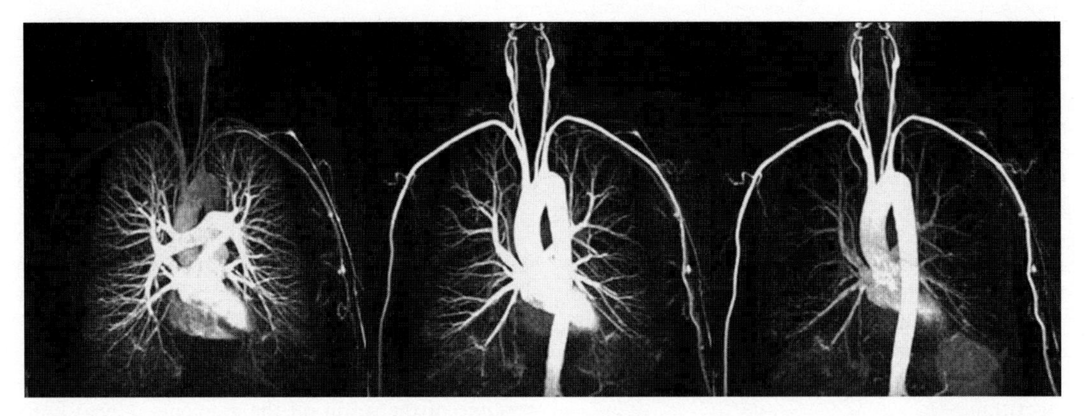

Fig. 4. Time-resolved contrast enhanced magnetic resonance angiography (CE-MRA). Coronal maximum-intensity projection (MIP) images from a time-resolved, dynamic CE-MRA of the chest. Each image took 3 seconds to acquire.

imaging is not only to identify the presence of a dissection but also to distinguish type A from type B.

MRI has high sensitivity and specificity for detection of dissection and now is regarded as the gold standard for assessment of this abnormality [3,20,27]. Single-shot TrueFISP recently has been shown to be highly accurate for diagnosis and classification of aortic dissection (see Figs. 5 and 6) [15]. Because of the inherent high signal to noise from blood, both true and false lumen and dissection flap are clearly visible. In fact, the diagnosis is made on the TrueFISP localizers in many instances. Moreover, the technique can be imple mented without breath holding in a total imaging time of less than 2 minutes. This is ideally suited to critically ill patients who cannot hold their breath. Breath-hold cine TrueFISP can be used to evaluate aortic insufficiency and hemopericardium in type A dissections; however these patients are rarely fit enough to hold their breath. In these situations, non-ECG-triggered real-time TrueFISP, although of lower spatial resolution, can be a useful alternative [16,17]. T1 GRE-FS imaging before and after contrast is essential for detecting intramural hematoma or thrombosed false lumen associated with a dissection. Recent intramural hemorrhage will appear hyperintense on noncontrast images. It may be more difficult to detect older hemorrhage, however, which may appear isointense or hypointense to surrounding structures. It may be very difficult to distinguish intramural hematoma from a thrombosed false lumen of an aortic dissection. CE-MRA is also accurate in diagnosing aortic dissections; however, the

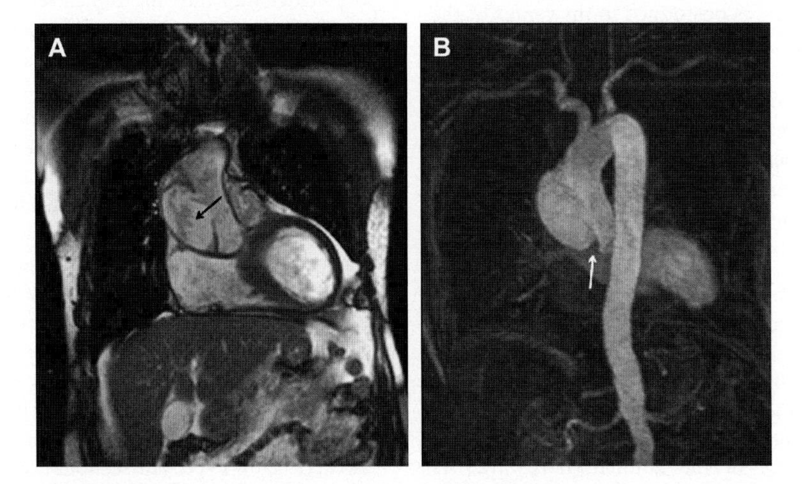

Fig. 5. Aortic dissection. Coronal balanced steady-state free precession technique (*A*) and maximum intensity projection (*B*) images from a patient who had a dissection of the ascending aorta (*arrows*).

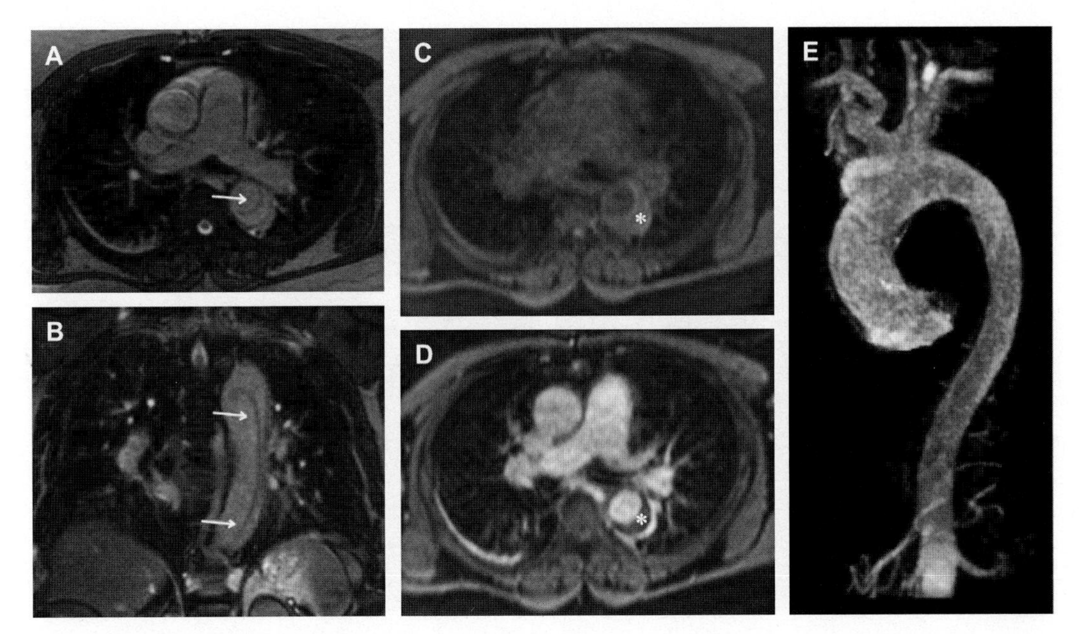

Fig. 6. Aortic dissection. (*A*) Axial and (*B*) coronal balanced steady-state free precession technique images from a patient with a descending aortic dissection (*arrows*). Axial fat-suppressed T1-weighted gradient echos without (*C*) and with (*D*) contrast demonstrate thrombosis of the false lumen (*asterisks*) that does not fill with contrast on the contrast-enhanced magnetic resonance angiography (*E*).

diagnosis usually is made already on the TrueFISP images. CE-MRA is useful for assessing the proximal and distal extent of the dissection and its involvement of branch vessels. A separate CE-MRA study of the abdomen may be required to assess distal dissections extending into the abdominal aorta, particularly to evaluate involvement of the renal and mesenteric vasculature. Subsecond CE-MRA can demonstrate sequential filling of the true and false lumen and may help identify the entry and exit points of the dissection. In addition, subsecond CE-MRA can demonstrate pseudoaneurysms or intramural hematomas clearly.

Intramural hematoma and penetrating atherosclerotic ulceration

There is considerable clinical and imaging overlap between intramural hematoma, thrombosed false lumen in a localized dissection, and penetrating atherosclerotic ulcer [38–43]. In fact, intramural hematoma may arise from either a thrombosed false lumen or a penetrating ulcer. In all cases, the intramural blood is detected on T1 GRE-FS or black blood techniques. Penetrat ing atherosclerotic ulcers are depicted well on postcontrast T1 GRE-FS images or the partition images from a conventional CE-MRA [44].

Aneurysms

Aneurysms of the thoracic aorta are relatively common and are important because of their potentially reversible lethal consequences [45]. The most common cause is atherosclerosis, where aneurysms most commonly affect the descending aorta. Less common causes include trauma, congenital abnormalities, connective tissue disorders such as Erhlers-Danlos and Marfan's syndrome, and rare infections such as syphilis. MRI is ideally suited to evaluate aneurysms because of its ability for multiplanar imaging [7,46]. All of the previously mentioned techniques are accurate in detecting aneurysms; however CE-MRA is most useful for depicting location, extent, and exact diameter. MRI is used frequently as a follow-up tool for monitoring the progression of disease;therefore, to produce consistent results, vessel dimensions should be measured at the same anatomic locations each time. It is important to remember that MIP images represent a cast of the lumen; therefore measurements should be obtained from source images where the vessel wall is visible (Fig. 7). Another advantage of MRI is the ability to use multiple pulse sequences, allowing more comprehensive evaluation of pathology. Where aneurysms involve the ascending aorta or sinuses

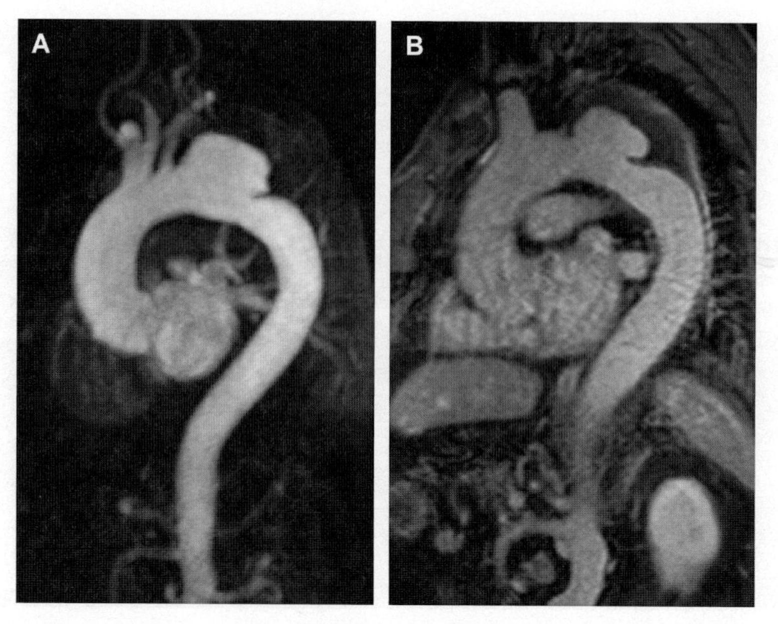

Fig. 7. (*A*) Sagittal-oblique maximum intensity projection image from a contrast-enhanced magnetic resonance angiography (CE-MRA) study in a patient who had a saccular aneurysm of the distal aortic arch. (*B*) Sagittal-oblique T1-weighted gradient echo image obtained after the administration of intravenous contrast demonstrates a large amount of intra-aneurysmal thrombus and the true size of the aneurysm compared with the size that would be measured from the MRA.

of Valsalva, concomitant aortic valve disease can be evaluated using cine imaging of the heart.

Aortic stenosis

Stenoses in the thoracic aorta are caused commonly by atherosclerosis but are usually multifocal and rarely flow-limiting. Coarctation of the aorta causes a more severe stenosis at the junction of the aortic arch and descending aorta and may be focal (usually incidental finding in adults) or diffuse (usually symptomatic in infants) (Fig. 8). It usually is associated with multiple chest wall collaterals. Residual coarctation can present later in life following a previous coarctation repair. Pseudocoarctation resembles a true coarctation but is caused by aortic kinking just distal to the origin of the left subclavian artery. It is not hemodynamically flow-limiting and therefore is not associated with multiple collaterals. Less common causes of aortic stenosis include extrinsic compression from tumor or rare inflammatory conditions such as Takayasu's aortitis.

CE-MRA is the most useful technique for evaluating stenoses in the thoracic aorta. Temporally resolved subsecond CE-MRA will depict aortic stenoses accurately, but it is particularly useful in hemodynamically significant lesions such as coarctations, where it demonstrates gradual filling of chest wall collaterals. The addition of TrueFISP or T1 GRE-FS will exclude an adjacent mass causing extrinsic compression. PC-MRA can be used to measure velocity and flow, both proximal and distal to a stenosis, and it helps assess the significance of a stenosis [47]. It may be more useful in monitoring disease progression over time; however, it is important to obtain measurements in similar anatomic locations to produce accurate and consistent results.

Congenital abnormalities

Numerous congenital abnormalities affect the thoracic aorta, including right-sided aortic arch, aberrant subclavian artery, aortic coarctation (see Fig. 8), patent ductus arteriosis (PDA, Fig. 9), double aortic arch (Fig. 10), and aortic hypoplasia (Fig. 11). All of these conditions are visualized best using CE-MRA [48,49]. With congenital abnormalities, three-dimensional postprocessing techniques can be used to great effect, allowing the abnormality to be viewed from different orien tations (Fig. 12). Cine imaging of the heart always

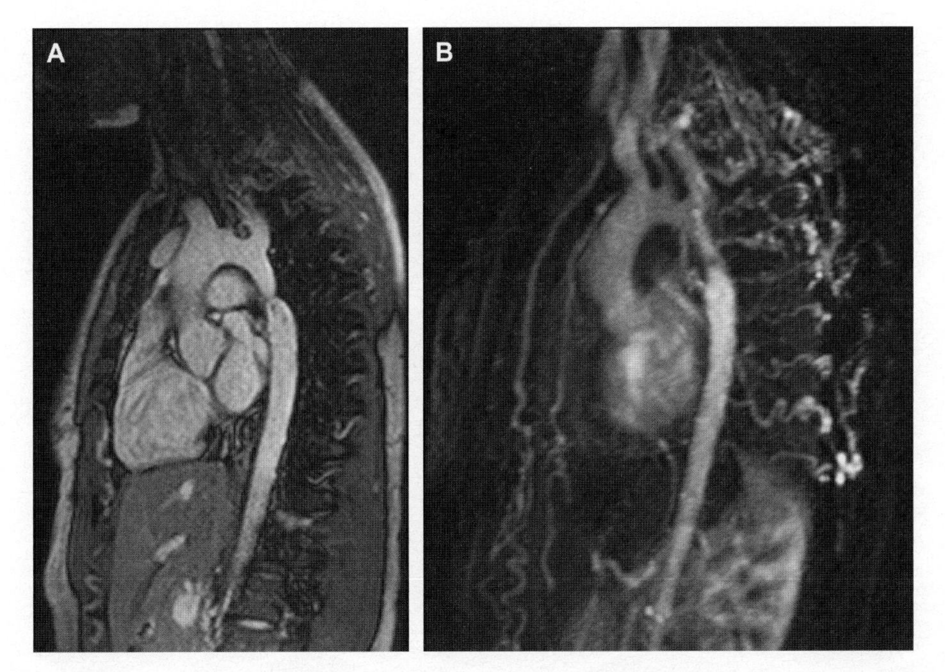

Fig. 8. Coarctation of the aorta. Left anterior oblique steady-state free precession technique (*A*) and contrast-enhanced magnetic resonance angiography (*B*) images from a patient who had an untreated coarctation of the aorta and numerous enlarged collateral arteries.

should accompany an assessment for congenital abnormalities of the aorta to detect accompanying lesions in the heart.

Aortic coarctations and PDAs usually are evaluated using a combination of CE-MRA, balanced SSFP, and PC techniques (see Fig. 9). Because of the high spatial resolution of three-dimensional CE-MRA, this technique is used for accurate morphological assessment of these abnormalities. Using a computer workstation, accurate orthogonal measurements of the aorta can be made at multiple locations proximal and distal to the coarctation or across the PDA. PC-MRA is used to quantify flow rates and flow velocities through the abnormality also. In patients who have aortic coarctation, the

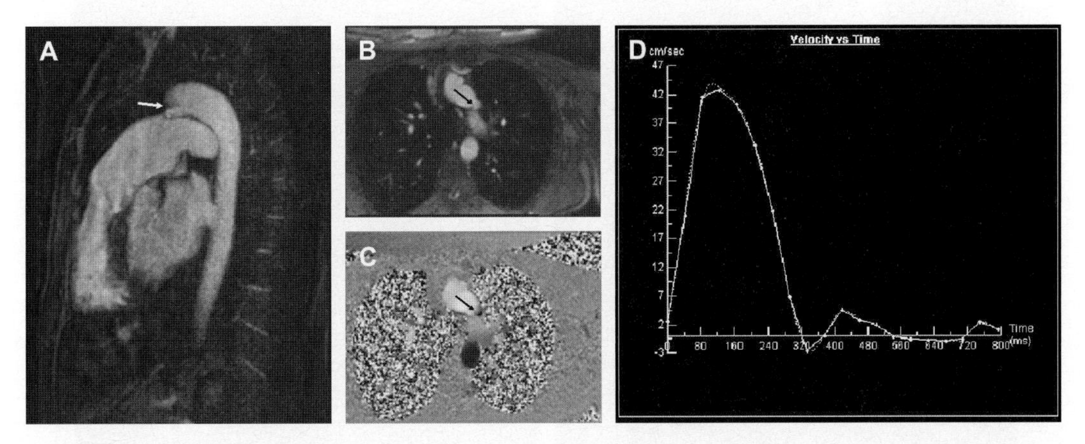

Fig. 9. Patent ductus arteriosus (PDA). Maximum intensity projection image (*A*) from a contrast-enhanced magnetic resonance angiograph shows a large PDA. (*B*) Magnitude and (*C*) phase contrast images obtained at the level of the PDA (*arrow on image A*). By placing regions of interest over the vessel on the images throughout the cardiac cycle and measuring the velocity at each phase, it is possible to generate velocity–time or flow–time curves (*D*).

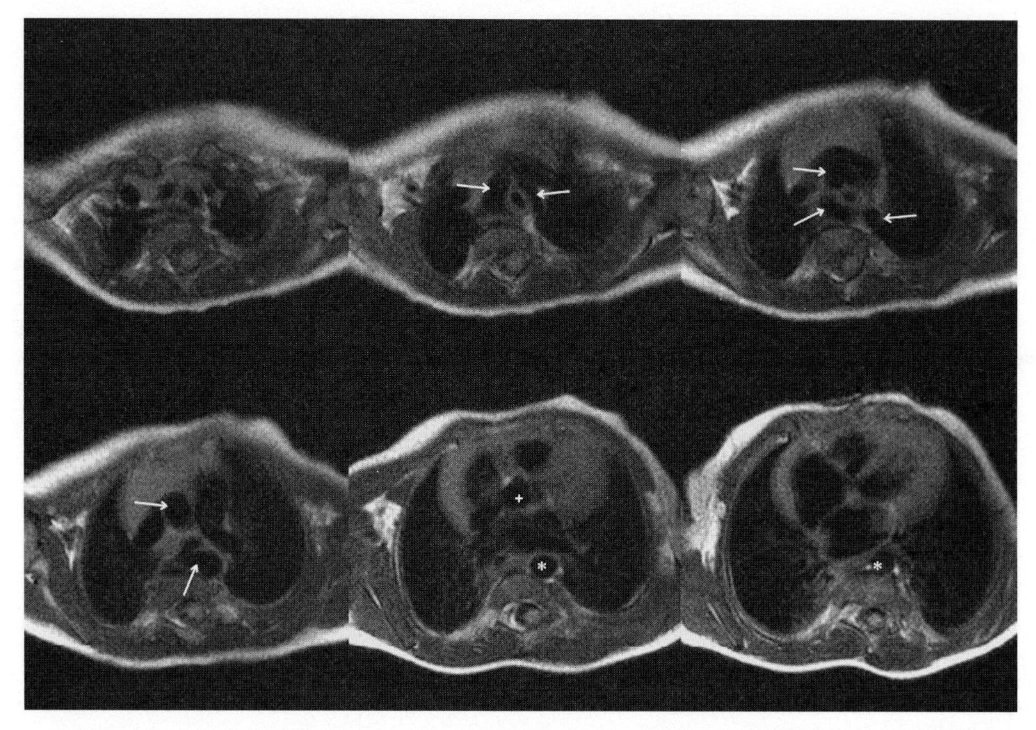

Fig. 10. Double aortic arch. Black-blood images in an infant who had a double aortic arch (*arrows*). * represents the descending aorta. + represents the ascending aorta. (*From* Cynthia Rigsby, MD, Children's Memorial Hospital, Chicago.)

minimal cross-sectional area and the mean deceleration of flow in the descending aorta have been found to be highly predictive of a moderate or severe coarctation gradient ($\geq$20 mmHg), when compared with pressure measurements made with catheter angiography. These measurements can be used to follow patients before and after treatment.

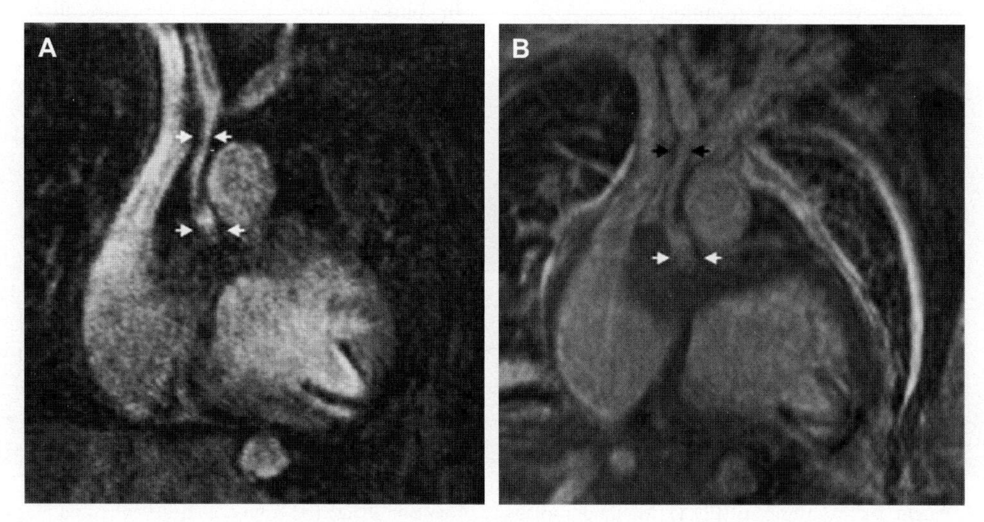

Fig. 11. Aortic hypoplasia. Multiplanar reformatted images from (*A*) contrast-enhanced magnetic resonance angiography (CE-MRA) and (*B*) three-dimensional whole-chest steady-state free precession technique MRA reveal severe narrowing of the entire ascending aorta (*arrows*).

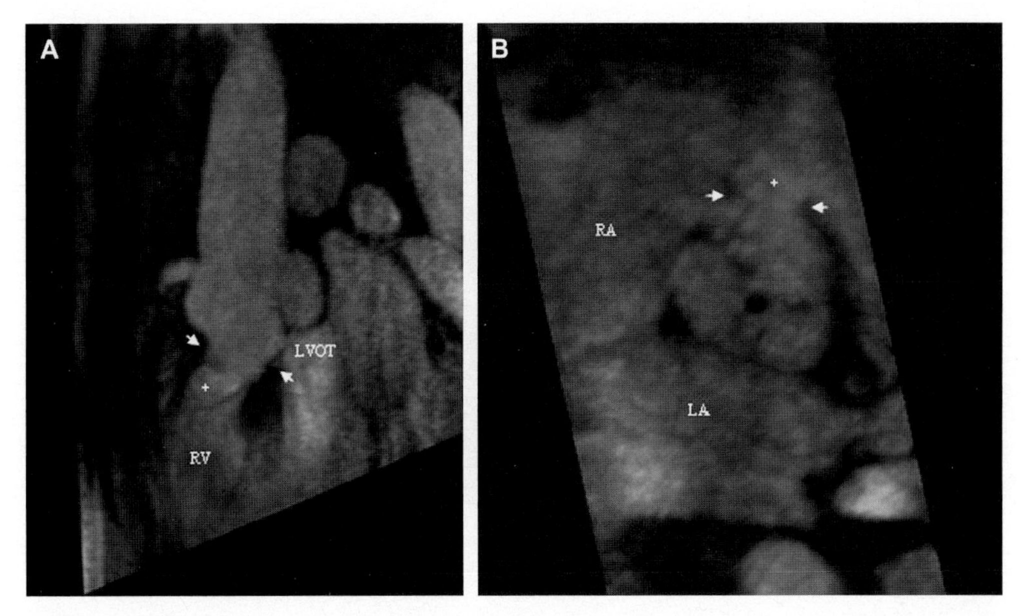

Fig. 12. Membranous ventricular septal defect (VSD). Multiplanar reformatted images from a contrast-enhanced magnetic resonance angiography (CE-MRA) study in a patient who had a membranous VSD. CE-MRA also confirms an aneurysm (+) of the right coronary sinus that prolapses through the VSD (*short arrows*). *Abbreviations:* LA, left atrium; RV, right ventricle; LVOT, left ventricular outflow tract; RA, right atrium.

Vasculitis

Because of the high spatial and contrast resolution offered by newer MRI techniques, which permit assessment of the aortic wall, rheumatologists routinely include MRI in the work-up of patients who have vasculitis, particularly in patients who have vasculitis affecting larger vessels—giant cell arthritis and Takayasu's arthritis (Fig. 13) [50,51]. MRA of patients who have Takayasu's arthritis, in addition to demon strating the degree of luminal narrowing, will

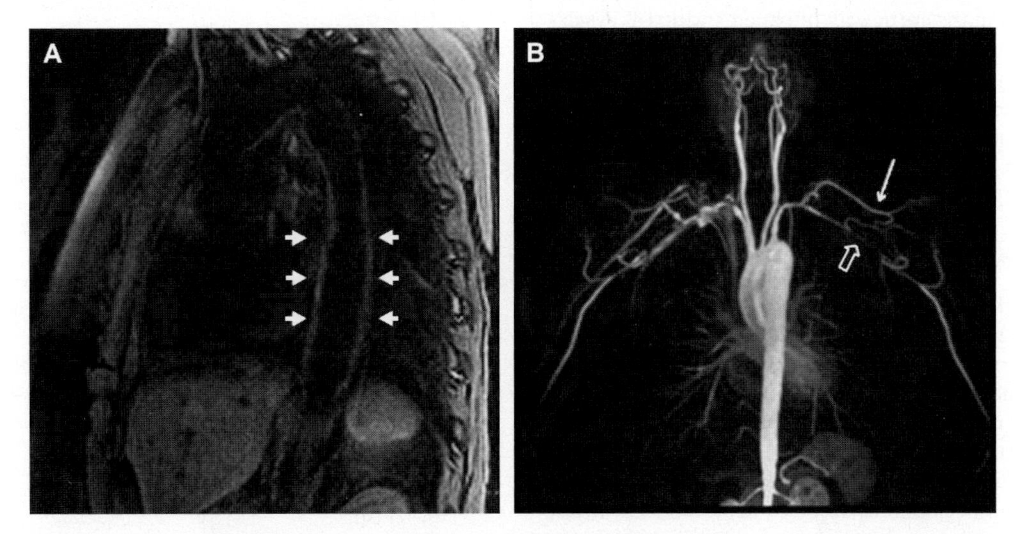

Fig. 13. Takayasu's aortitis. (*A*) Left anterior oblique dark-blood steady-state free precession technique demonstrates diffuse thickening of the wall of the aorta (*short arrows*). (*B*) Contrast-enhanced magnetic resonance angiography demonstrates occlusion of the left subclavian artery (*open arrow*). Large collateral arteries have developed to provide flow to the left upper extremity (*long arrow*).

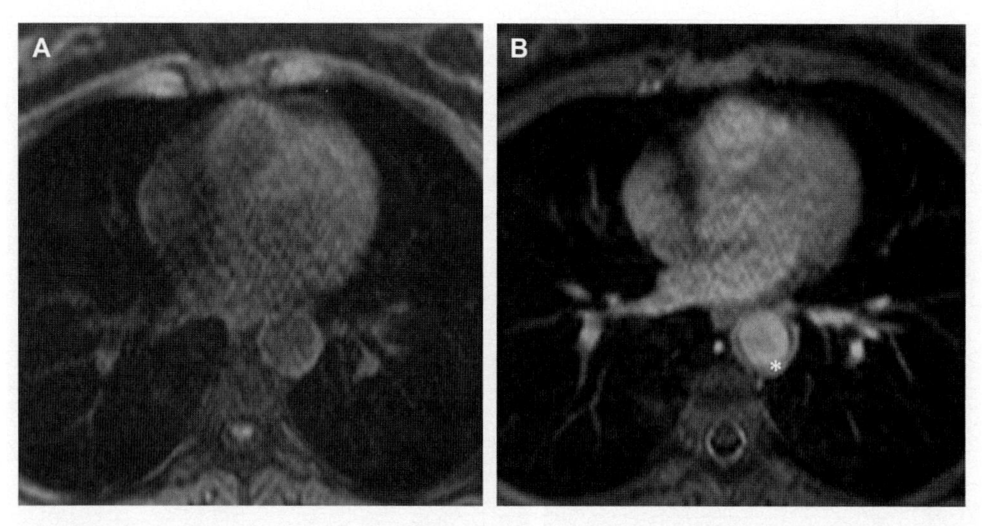

Fig. 14. Takayasu's aortitis. Fat-suppressed T1-weighted gradient echo images obtained without (*A*) and with (*B*) contrast demonstrate enhancement of the thickened wall of the aorta (*asterisk*).

demonstrate segmental thickening of the vessel wall, mural thrombus, inflammatory changes in the periaortic fat, vascular dilatation, and vascular stenoses. The examination usually includes dark blood sequences to visualize the vessel wall before and after the administration of intravenous contrast material (Fig. 14) in addition to CE-MRA sequences. Recently, delayed contrast-enhanced MRI techniques, similar to those used to assess myocardial viability in the heart, have been used to characterize the degree of inflammation in the aortic wall of patients with Takayasu's arthritis [50]. MRI with cine imaging of the heart also can be used to evaluate the effect of the disease on cardiovascular function. In addition to imaging at the time of presentation, MRA can be used to assess patient response to therapy.

Summary

There are numerous pulse sequences available for evaluating the diverse pathology, which affects the thoracic aorta. Preliminary imaging using TrueFISP and pre- and postcontrast T1 GRE-FS usually is required to assess morphology of the aorta and adjacent structures. CE-MRA is the mainstay in the investigative approach. The addition of temporally resolved subsecond CE-MRA is particularly useful for assessing high-flow vascular lesions such as shunts, while at the same time not adding much to the overall contrast load. PC-MRA may help further characterize stenotic lesions and can be useful for monitoring progression of disease.

References

[1] Waugh JR, Sacharias N. Arteriographic complications in the DSA era. Radiology 1992;182:243–6.
[2] Mirvis SE, Pais SO, Gens DR. Thoracic aortic rupture: advantages of intra-arterial digital subtraction angiography. AJR Am J Roentgenol 1986;146:987–991.
[3] Hartnell GG. Imaging of aortic aneurysms and dissections: CT and MRI. J Thorac Imaging 2001;16:35–46.
[4] Rubin GD. Helical CT angiography of the thoracic aorta. J Thorac Imaging 1997;12:128–49.
[5] Hidajat N, Maurer J, Schroder R, et al. Radiation exposure in spiral computed tomography—dose distribution and dose reduction. Invest Radiol 1999;34:51–7.
[6] Scott CH, Keane MG, Ferrari VA. Echocardiographic evaluation of the thoracic aorta. Semin Roentgenol 2001;36:325–333.
[7] Roberts DA. Magnetic resonance imaging of thoracic aortic aneurysm and dissection. Semin Roentgenol 2001;36:295–308.
[8] Fattori R, Nienaber CA. MRI of acute and chronic aortic pathology: preoperative and postoperative evaluation. J Magn Reson Imaging 1999;10:741–50.
[9] Oppelt A, Graumann R, Barfuss H. FISP—a new fast MRI sequence. Electromedica 1986;54:15–8.
[10] Fang W, Pereles FS, Bundy J, et al. Evaluating left ventricular function using real-time TrueFISP:

a comparison with conventional techniques. Proceedings of the ISMRM 2000;1:308.
[11] Deimling M, Heid O. Magnetization-prepared TrueFISP imaging. Proceedings of the Society of Magnetic Resonance 1994;1:495.
[12] Carr J, Simonetti O, Bundy J, et al. Cine MR angiography of the heart with segmented true fast imaging with steady-state precession. Radiology 2001;219: 828–34.
[13] Bundy J, Simonetti O, Laub G, et al. Segmented TrueFISP imaging of the heart. Proceedings of the ISMRM 1999;2:1282.
[14] Barkhausen J, Ruehm S, Goyen M, et al. MR evaluation of ventricular function: true fast imaging with steady-state precession versus fast low-angle shot cine MR imaging: feasibility study. Radiology 2001;219:264–9.
[15] Pereles FS, McCarthy RM, Baskaran V, et al. Thoracic aortic dissection and aneurysm: evaluation with nonenhanced TrueFISP MR angiography in less than 4 minutes. Radiology 2002;223: 270–4.
[16] Barkhausen J, Goyen M, Ruhm SG, et al. Assessment of ventricular function with single breath hold real-time steady-state free precession cine MR imaging. AJR Am J Roentgenol 2002;178:731–5.
[17] Lee VS, Resnick D, Bundy JM, et al. Cardiac function: MR evaluation in one breath hold with real-time true fast imaging with steady-state precession. Radiology 2002;222:835–42.
[18] Simonetti OP, Finn JP, White RD, et al. Black-blood T2-weighted inversion–recovery MR imaging of the heart. Radiology 1996;199:49–57.
[19] Stehling MK, Holzknecht NG, Laub G, et al. Single-shot T1- and T2-weighted magnetic resonance imaging of the heart with black blood: preliminary experience. MAGMA 1996;4:231–40.
[20] Summers RM, Sostman HD, Spritzer CE, et al. Fast spoiled gradient-recalled MR imaging of thoracic aortic dissection: preliminary clinical experience at 1.5T. Magn Reson Imaging 1996;14:1–9.
[21] Carr J, McCarthy R, Laub G, et al. Subsecond, contrast-enhanced 3D MR angiography: a new technique for dynamic imaging of the vasculature. Presented at the Proceedings of the 9th meeting of the International Society for Magnetic Resonance in Medicine. Glasgow, Scotland; April 21–27, 2001.
[22] Finn JP, Baskaran V, Carr J, et al. Low-dose, contrast-enhanced 3D MR angiography of the thorax with sub-second temporal resolution. Radiology 2002;224:896–904.
[23] Prince M. Gadolinium-enhanced MR aortography. Radiology 1994;191:155–64.
[24] Prince MR, Narasimham DL, Stanley JC, et al. Breath-hold Gadolinium-enhanced MR angiography of the abdominal aorta and its major branches. Radiology 1995;197:785–92.
[25] Krinsky GA, Reuss PM, Lee VS, et al. Thoracic aorta: comparison of single-dose breath-hold and double-dose non-breath-hold gadolinium-enhanced three-dimensional MR angiography. AJR Am J Roentgenol 1999;173:145–50.
[26] Krinsky GA, Rofsky NM, DeCorato DR, et al. Thoracic aorta: comparison of gadolinium-enhanced three-dimensional MR angiography with conventional MR imaging. Radiology 1997;202: 183–93.
[27] Prince MR, Narasimham DL, Jacoby WT, et al. Three-dimensional gadolinium-enhanced MR angiography of the thoracic aorta. AJR Am J Roentgenol 1996;166:1387–97.
[28] Dumoulin CL, Yucel EK, Vock P, et al. Two and three dimensional phase contrast MR angiography of the abdomen. J Comput Assist Tomogr 1990;14: 779–84.
[29] Lundin B, Cooper TG, Meyer RA, et al. Measurement of total and unilateral renal blood flow by oblique-angle velocity-encoded 2D cine magnetic resonance angiography. Magn Reson Imaging 1993;11:51–9.
[30] Sodickson D, Manning WJ. Simultaneous acquisition of spatial harmonics (SMASH): fast imaging with radiofrequency coil arrays. Magn Reson Med 1997;38:591–603.
[31] Sodickson D, McKenzie C, Li W, et al. Contrast-enhanced 3D MR angiography with simultaneous acquisition of spatial harmonics: a pilot study. Radiology 2000;217:284–9.
[32] Weiger M, Pruessmann K, Kassner K, et al. Contrast-enhanced 3D MRA using SENSE. J Magn Reson Imaging 2000;12:671–7.
[33] Weiger M, Pruessmann K, Boesiger P. Cardiac real-time imaging using SENSE. Magn Reson Med 2000; 43:177–84.
[34] Korosec FRFR, Grist TM, Mistretta CA. Time-resolved contrast-enhanced 3D MR angiography. Magn Reson Med 1996;36:345–51.
[35] DeSanctis RW, Doroghazi RM, Austen WG, et al. Aortic dissection. N Engl J Med 1987;317: 1060–7.
[36] DeBakey ME, Henly WS, Cooley DA, et al. Surgical management of dissecting aneurysms of the aorta. J Thorac Cardiovasc Surg 1965;49:130–48.
[37] Nienaber CA, Con Kodolitsch Y, Nicolas V, et al. The diagnosis of aortic dissection by non-invasive imaging procedures. N Engl J Med 1993;328:1–9.
[38] Wolff KA, Herold CJ, Tempany CM, et al. Aortic dissection: atypical patterns seen at MR imaging. Radiology 1991;181:489–95.
[39] Harris JA, Bis KG, Glover JL, et al. Penetrating atherosclerotic ulcers of the aorta. J Vasc Surg 1994;19: 90–8.
[40] Stanson AW, Kazimer FJ, Orszulak TA, et al. The penetrating aortic ulcer: pathologic manifestations, diagnosis and management. Mayo Clin Proc 1988; 63:718–25.
[41] Yucel EK, Steinberg FL, Egglin TK, et al. Penetrating aortic ulcers: diagnosis with MR imaging. Radiology 1990;177:779–81.

[42] Bickerstaff LK, Pairolero PC, Hollier LH, et al. Tho racic aortic aneurysms: a population-based study. Surgery 1982;92:1103–8.
[43] Pressler V, McNamara JJ. Aneurysm of the thoracic aorta. J Thorac Cardiovasc Surg 1985;89:50–4.
[44] Mohiaddin RH, McCrohon J, Francis JM, et al. Contrast-enhanced magnetic resonance angiogram of penetrating aortic ulcer. Circulation 2001;103: 18–9.
[45] Pitt MP, Bonser RS. The natural history of thoracic aortic aneurysm disease: an overview. J Card Surg 1997;12:270–8.
[46] Schmidta M, Theissen P, Klempt G, et al. Long-term follow-up of 82 patients with chronic disease of the thoracic aorta using spin echo and cine gradient magnetic resonance imaging. Magn Reson Imaging 2000;18:795–806.
[47] Mohiaddin RH, Kilner PJ, Rees S, et al. Magnetic resonance volume flow and jet velocity mapping in aortic coarctation. J Am Coll Cardiol 1993;22: 1515–21.
[48] Roche KJ, Krinsky G, Lee VS, et al. Interrupted aortic arch: diagnosis with gadolinium-enhanced 3D MRA. J Comput Assist Tomogr 1999;23:197–202.
[49] Soler R, Rodriguez E, Requejo I, et al. Magnetic resonance imaging of congenital abnormalities of the thoracic aorta. Eur Radiol 1998;8:540–6.
[50] Desai MY, Stone JH, Foo TK, et al. Delayed contrast-enhanced MRI of the aortic wall in Takayasu's arthritis: initial experience. AJR Am J Roentgenol 2006;186:1197–8.
[51] Gotway MB, Araoz PA, Macedo TA, et al. Imaging findings in Takayasu's arthritis. AJR Am J Roentgenol 2005;184:1945–50.

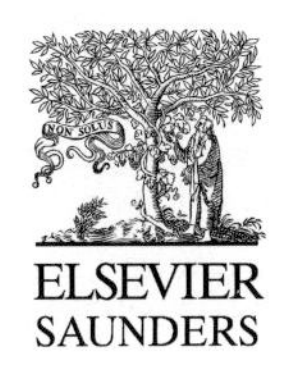

ELSEVIER
SAUNDERS

Cardiol Clin 25 (2007) 185–212

CARDIOLOGY
CLINICS

Magnetic Resonance Evaluation of Peripheral Arterial Disease

Dipan J. Shah, MD[a,*], Barbra Brown, NP[a], Raymond J. Kim, MD[c], John D. Grizzard, MD[b]

[a]*Nashville Cardiovascular MRI Institute, The Heart Group, PLLC, 1195 Old Hickory Boulevard, Suite 101, Brentwood, Nashville, TN 37027, USA*
[b]*Virginia Commonwealth University Health Systems, Department of Radiology, Richmond, VA, USA*
[c]*Duke Cardiovascular Magnetic Resonance Center, Duke University Medical Center, Durham, NC, USA*

Peripheral arterial disease (PAD) is a vascular disorder that results in progressive narrowing of arteries of the lower extremity because of atherosclerosis. This disease is common in the United States, with an estimated 5 million affected individuals over the age of 40 [1]. Although only 5% of these patients will suffer from symptoms (ie, intermittent claudication), and an even smaller percentage will experience limb threatening critical ischemia, the most common manifestation of PAD is a markedly increased risk of cardiovascular morbidity and mortality [2–4]. Although the initial evaluation for PAD is performed with basic physical examination, often supplemented by ankle brachial indices and segmental pressures, many patients will require imaging of the vasculature to definitively establish the presence of PAD, and to provide an anatomic roadmap to aid in performance of revascularization therapies for PAD.

Magnetic resonance angiography (MRA) has emerged over the last decade as the modality of choice in performing this imaging function. Although earlier time-of-flight techniques had significant limitations because of prolonged imaging times and image artifacts, currently available contrast-enhanced MRA using multistation bolus chase techniques is a rapid and robust technique that consistently allows comprehensive imaging from the level of the abdominal aorta to the proximal pedal vessels. Three-dimensional volumetric acquisitions are obtained at each station during the transit of gadolinium through the arterial system, and these are subtracted from a preliminary, noncontrast mask image to maximize vessel conspicuity. Maximum intensity projection (MIP) images then are prepared by means of post-processing, and are reviewed along with the source images. The acquisition of isotropic voxels (voxel size that is equal in all three dimensions) allows 360-degree rotation of the images into any obliquity, facilitating easy and accurate interpretation. Therefore, three-dimensional contrast-enhanced MRA combines the superior tissue contrast inherent in MRI with the improved vessel conspicuity resulting from digital subtraction technology and displays the results as a three-dimensional data set that can be rotated into any obliquity, a significant improvement over conventional two-dimensional projection angiography. Fig. 1 is an example of the coverage and image quality now possible with MRA.

In any magnetic resonance examination, there is virtually an unlimited number of permutations of selectable parameters (ie, scan duration, spatial resolution, slice thickness, and others), so the user can be easily overwhelmed by the variety of choices available. This article provides the reader with a clinically relevant practical approach to obtaining high-quality MRAs of the lower extremities. The physics underlying this imaging are discussed as they relate to practical matters such

* Corresponding author.
E-mail address: dshah@heartgroup.net (D.J. Shah).

0733-8651/07/$ - see front matter © 2007 Published by Elsevier Inc.
doi:10.1016/j.ccl.2007.02.006

Table 1
Siemens Avanto sequences

	Localizer		
Sequence	Coronal	Sagittal	Transverse
TR (ms)	3	3	3
TE (ms)	1.5	1.5	1.5
Flip angle (degrees)	64	64	64
Slice thickness (mm)	8	8	8
Number of slices	15	18	20
Field of view (mm)	500 × 500	500 × 500	500 × 500
Matrix (lines)	256 × 180	256 × 180	256 × 180
Averages	1	1	1
Acceleration factor	0	0	0
Bandwidth (Hz/pixel)	900	900	900
Scan duration (s)	23	23	23

as contrast timing schemes. Model protocols for various scanners are presented (Tables 1–5), and the rationale for the choices. In addition to the standard core protocol, alternative protocols are presented, so that the reader will have a sense of the full palette of options available, and be readily able to appreciate the relative advantages and disadvantages of each. Applications of these protocols in imaging various disorders then are discussed, with clinical exams presented. Pearls and pitfalls regarding imaging techniques and various tricks of the trade also are discussed.

Why use magnetic resonance angiography?

There are various imaging techniques available for imaging the aorta, iliac, and runoff vessels. To make an educated selection, it is helpful to consider what would constitute an ideal vascular imaging technique. An ideal technique would have the following characteristics:

- Easily performed (not require excessive operator skill)
- Rapidly performed (require only seconds to minutes of patient time)
- Easily interpretable (not require excessive time or expertise to accurately interpret)
- Risk-free and painless (not require arterial puncture, administration of ionizing contrast, or exposure to radiation)
- Applicable to, and accurate in a large range of patients
- Extensive anatomic coverage (because of the diffuse nature of atherosclerotic disease in the aorta, iliac, and runoff vessels).
- Three-dimensional in nature, allowing for an accurate vascular road map for percutaneous and surgical procedures

Catheter angiography

Although accurate, the technique is not risk-free (it requires a painful arterial puncture). It requires a 4- to 6-hour convalescent period after the procedure, involves exposure to iodinated contrast and radiation, has limitations in demonstrating small crural vessels, and is inherently not three-dimensional in nature.

CT angiography

CT angiography allows extensive anatomic coverage and is three-dimensional. Although it is noninvasive, it is not risk-free, as it requires ionizing radiation and the administration of iodinated contrast. Given that many patients with peripheral arterial disease also have

Table 2
Three-dimensional angio sequence

	Abdomen/pelvis	Thigh	Calf	Calf time resolved
TR (ms)	2.9	3.51	3.51	2.91
TE (ms)	1.1	1.25	1.25	1.07
Flip angle (degrees)	20	25	25	30
Slice thickness (mm)	1.4	1.4	1.2	1.3
Number of slices	88	80	104	60
Field of view (mm)	500 × 375	500 × 406	500 × 406	500 × 400
Matrix (lines)	384 × 245	512 × 291	512 × 291	448 × 186
Spatial resolution (mm)	1.4 × 1.3 × 1.4	1.4 × 1.0 × 1.4	1.4 × 1.0 × 1.2	1.9 × 1.1 × 1.3
Averages	1	1	1	1
Acceleration factor	2	2	2	2
Bandwidth (Hz/pixel)	500	360	360	470
Scan duration (s)	15	21	26	8.5
K space acquisition	Linear	Linear	Centric	Centric

Table 3
Siemens symphony (without parallel imaging) angio sequence

	Abdomen/pelvis	Thigh	Calf
TR (ms)	3.6	3.8	4.8
TE (ms)	1.5	1.7	1.8
Flip angle (degrees)	20	25	25
Slice thickness (mm)	1.5	1.4	1.1
Number of slices	64	56	80
Field of view (mm)	500 × 333	500 × 344	500 × 406
Matrix (lines)	384 × 182	512 × 194	512 × 291
Spatial resolution (mm)	1.8 × 1.3 × 1.5	1.7 × 1.0 × 1.4	1.4 × 1.0 × 1.2
Averages	1	1	1
Acceleration factor	NA	NA	Na
Bandwidth (Hz/pixel)	450	490	270
Scan duration (s)	19.8	19	43
K space acquisition	Linear	Linear	Centric

pre-existing renal compromise or are diabetic, this is obviously less than ideal. In addition, the presence of calcification and the need to subtract the adjacent bones make image interpretation more difficult, time-consuming, and possibly less accurate.

Magnetic resonance angiography

In many important respects, MRA fulfills the characteristics of an ideal imaging technique. It is quick to perform, with examination durations typically less then 30 minutes, and relatively easy of interpret. Multiplanar displays are performed easily, and three-dimensional imaging is standard. Most importantly, it does not require exposure to radiation or nephrotoxic contrast agents. Patients who have pacemakers and defibrillators traditionally have been excluded from undergoing MRA. All but the most severely claustrophobic patients are able to tolerate the procedure with administration of oral or intravenous anxiolytics. Although there may be limitations of availability in remote geographic regions, MRI scanners have becoming ubiquitous in most areas. As a result of the advantages outlined previously, MRA, where available, has assumed the role of diagnostic modality of choice.

Indications

The clinical indications for peripheral vascular MRI can be categorized into two groups. Most studies will be performed in the setting of chronic stable disease, while rarely the study will be requested for acute disease. Although special

Table 4
GE Signa 1.5T echospeed angio sequence

	Abdomen/pelvis	Thigh	Calf
TR (ms)	5	5	5
TE (ms)	MIN (2)	MIN (2)	MIN (1)
Flip angle (degrees)	30	30	30
Slice thickness (mm)	3.6	3.6	3
Number of slices	34	36	32
Field of view (mm)	440 × 296	440 × 296	440 × 296
Matrix (lines)	256 × 160	256 × 160	256 × 192
Spatial resolution (mm)	1.7 × 1.8 × 3.6 (interpolated to appear 1.8)	1.7 × 1.8 × 3.6 (interpolated to appear 1.8)	1.7 × 1.5 × 3.0 (interpolated to appear 1.5)
Averages	1	1	1
Acceleration factor	NA	NA	NA
Bandwidth	62.5	31.25	31.25
Scan duration (s)	20	19	29
-space acquisition	Centric	Centric	Elliptic centric
Interpolation	ZIP2	ZIP2	ZIP2

Table 5
Philips Intera 1.5T scanner

	Phillips Intera 1.5T	Software V11.1	
	Abdomen/ pelvis	Thigh	Calf
TR (ms)	5.7	SAME	SAME
TE (ms)	1.6		
Flip angle (degrees)	35		
Slice thickness (mm)	1.5		
Number of slices	70		
Field of view (mm)	430 × 302		
Matrix (lines)	512 × 512		
Spatial resolution (mm)	1.5 × .8		
Averages	1		
Acceleration factor	NA		
Bandwidth (Hz/pixel)			
Scan duration (s)	40		
K space acquisition	Linear		

considerations may need to employed in the evaluation of acute ischemic disease, peripheral vascular MRA can be used in both settings because of the rapid nature with which imaging can be performed.

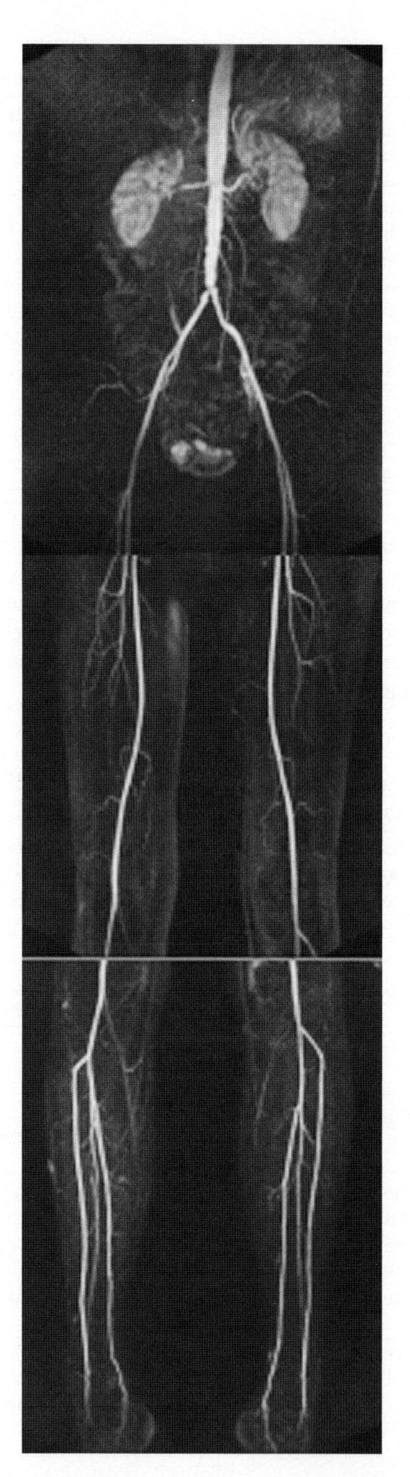

Fig. 1. Three-station magnetic resonance angiogram demonstrating the coverage and scan quality now available on a routine basis.

Chronic disease

Chronic forms of PAD include three general etiologies: atherosclerotic stenosis resulting in arterial insufficiency, aneurysmal dilation, or congenital diseases. Arterial insufficiency typically presents with classic claudication (pain induced by muscular activity such as walking that results in metabolic demands that exceed the delivery capacity of the supplying arterial circuit) but occasionally can present with claudication analogs such as leg cramping or fatigability. More severe forms of arterial insufficiency will present with rest pain or nonhealing ulcers. Aneurysmal dilation can occur in almost any arterial bed but most commonly will involve the aorta, iliac, or popliteal arteries. Congenital anomalies include persistent sciatic artery, popliteal entrapment syndrome, or Klippel-Trenaunay-Weber syndrome.

Acute diseases

Acute causes of vascular insufficiency may be imaged with MRA, provided that the patient is stable and capable of remaining motionless for this study. Pain control and coordination with the treating physician are important to allow optimal triage and treatment planning. Acute forms of PAD can be divided into three forms: cold leg syndrome, dissection, or blue toe syndrome:

Cold leg is the sudden, acute loss of perfusion to the lower extremity resulting in a pallor, coolness, and pain of the leg. This is most often caused by embolism, usually from the heart or the upstream aorta . Expeditious performance of the examination is necessary to minimize tissue loss if MRA is performed before intervention.

Dissection. MRA can be very useful to visualize the origination and extension of aortic dissection into the iliofemoral vessels. It also can be useful in discriminating between true and false lumens.

Blue-toe syndrome is an acute, but not emergent disorder resulting in a bluish appearance to one or more toes. It usually results from peripheral embolization from a more proximal source, such as an abdominal aortic aneurysm with mural thrombus, or an ulcerated plaque. It occasionally can occur from embolism from the heart.

Pulse sequences selection

Localization sequences

The selection of sequences used in peripheral MRA is based on their ability to fulfill a specific imaging purpose; localizers allow a global overview of the anatomy of the abdomen and lower extremities and facilitate easy localization of vascular structures within the imaged volume. Low-resolution steady-state free precession images (SSFP) images are ideal for this purpose and can be acquired in three planes in less than 30 seconds. These provide bright blood imaging of the vascular system. These usually suffice for vessel localization. In occasional circumstances, dark blood HASTE (Half-Fourier acquisition turbo spin echo) sequences can be obtained to improve vessel conspicuity, as can two-dimensional time-of-flight images, but these are not usually necessary.

Three-dimensional gradient echo angiographic sequences

The contrast-enhanced three-dimensional angiographic data set is acquired using a heavily T1 weighted spoiled gradient (SPGR) echo sequence obtained in the coronal plane (SPGR or turbo FLASH [fast low angle shot]). This sequence is the cornerstone of contrast-enhanced three-dimensional MRA, and is repeated at every imaging station. It is T1 weighted to visualize the intra-arterial contrast, which produces shortening of the T1 of blood from 1200 milliseconds to approximately 150 milliseconds. Spoiling is used to destroy any residual transverse magnetization and to accentuate the T1 weighting. The flip angle used is variable, but it is usually in the range of 20 to 35 degrees. The administration of repetitive radio frequency pulses to produce this flip angle every few milliseconds (typical repetition time 2.5 to 3.5 millieseconds) results in nearly complete suppression of background tissue, while still producing high signal in the arterial structures that are filled with gadolinium contrast. (Note: older texts may make reference to use of higher flip angles; however, this usually was done because older gradient systems were limited in the minimum TR achievable, and thus required higher flip angles for adequate tissue suppression. These are not necessary for most modern day scanners.) Subtraction of the postcontrast images from the precontrast mask images results in further suppression of soft tissue signal and an improvement in vessel conspicuity. In addition, use of fat suppression in the abdomen/pelvis and upper leg acquisitions will provide almost complete loss of soft tissue signal, with only a modest increase in imaging time.

As in any MR sequence, the user must weigh the relative advantages and trade-offs between improved spatial resolution and prolonged imaging time, but these issues take on special importance in imaging of the lower extremities. In the lower extremities, the need to image small structures with adequate resolution must be balanced with the need to image these arterial structures before venous filling contaminates the image. As a general rule, the resolution used and the slice thickness will vary such that the lower leg station is performed with the highest resolution and the thinnest slices.

Parallel imaging techniques (integrated parallel acquisition technique/sensitivity encoding/array spatial sensitivity encoding technique) have improved the ability to perform high-resolution imaging with fast image acquisition time significantly. This has resulted in a significant improvement in the robustness of peripheral runoff MRA, with fewer failed studies and markedly improved overall image quality. In its most common implementation, an acceleration factor of two is used, resulting in a decrease in imaging time (by nearly 50%) or an increase in spatial resolution (up to twofold). Most often, the improved efficiency is used to obtain some combination of both decreased time and improved resolution. The cost of this improvement relative to the nonaccelerated technique is a decrease in signal to noise by a factor of one divided by the square root of the acceleration factor (in this case two). That is, for a twofold increase in speed, the signal to noise drops to approximately 70% of the nonaccelerated technique, not 50%. Because gadolinium-enhanced MRA is a signal-rich technique, this trade-off is quite advantageous. At facilities having this capability, MRA almost always is performed using parallel imaging technology.

The parameters used for the coronal three-dimensional acquisition depend on various factors, and specific recommendations for various scanners are given in following sections. In general, the field of view should be maximized to obtain the greatest anatomic coverage possible for any given scanner, and to minimize the number of table movements required to encompass the desired anatomy. Newer scanners with a 500 mm field of view allow scanning from the diaphragm to the pedal vessels in three stations in virtually all patients, but on scanners with a 400 mm field of view, four stations often are needed in taller patients.

The three-dimensional slab thickness must be sufficient to cover the vessels of interest, and the slice thickness, number of slices, and the desired resolution are selectable parameters that can be varied to achieve the desired blend of spatial resolution, signal to noise, and imaging speed. As can be seen in Figs. 2 and 3, changes in imaging resolution, slice thickness, and number of slices all have an impact on scan duration. Imaging choices represent compromises between these competing priorities. Various other manipulations, including half-scanning techniques (useful if parallel imaging is not available, but not advisable in combination with parallel imaging), use of a rectangular field of view and zero filling interpolation are available in most modern scanners. These are considered in the protocol selection.

Automated table movement is now available on most scanners, along with dedicated peripheral phased-array coils. The table movement between stations should allow for overlap of the imaged anatomy, so that no gaps in coverage occur. For example, in a scanner with a 400 mm field of view, the table movement should be 300 to 350 mm between stations (therefore allowing 50 to100 mm of overlap at each station). In cases where a short patient is imaged on a large field-of-view scanner, the degree of overlap can be increased.

An additionally important parameter to be considered is the ordering of k space acquisition. Centrically ordered acquisitions are useful when the user wishes to acquire the central k space lines of

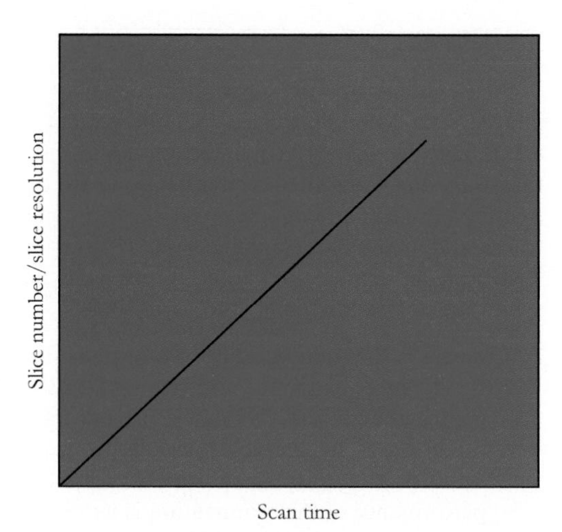

Fig. 2. For a given region of coverage, as the slice number or resolution increases, the scan duration increases.

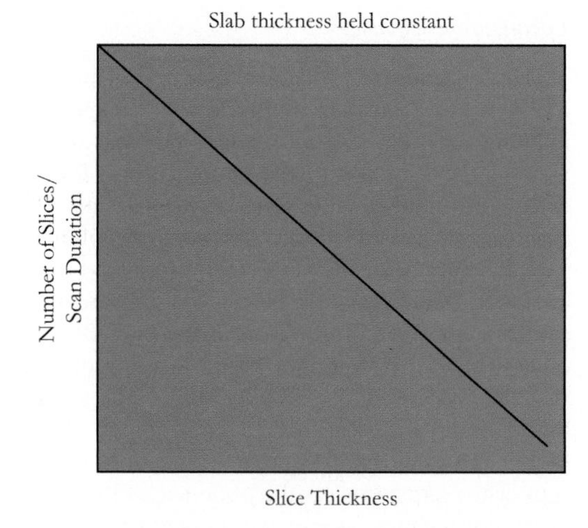

Fig. 3. For a given slab of coverage, as the slice thickness decreases (better spatial resolution), the number of slices and the imaging time increase.

data (which contain image contrast information) at the very beginning of the image acquisition. For example, when imaging the lower leg at the last station in a bolus chase acquisition, it is desirable to acquire the central k space lines immediately at the start of image acquisition, because there will be high arterial contrast concentration but minimal venous contrast concentration. If the central k spaces lines were acquired in the middle of the image acquisition (as with a linearly ordered sequence), there is greater likelihood of an increased venous contrast concentration, resulting in venous contamination of the image.

Supplementary sequences

Often, additional imaging to characterize the vessel wall may be desired, particularly in the abdomen, to better delineate the interface between thrombus, atheroma, and lumen. Sequences that may be chosen for this purpose include dark-blood HASTE, breath-held dark-blood T1 turbo-spin echo, breath-held T2 turbo-spin echo with fat-suppression, or a fat-suppressed volumetric T1 gradient echo sequence (VIBE). The addition of these sequences to the standard imaging protocol results in only a modest increase in total scan time, but can yield significant improvements in diagnostic ability. For example, these supplementary sequences are particularly useful in characterizing the extent of thrombus, atheroma, and vessel wall thickening in patients who have aneurysms. They should be performed in regions where aneurysms are prevalent such as the abdomen, inguinal regions, and popliteal fossae, to screen for aneurysms that could be missed on luminographic images alone. Additionally, these supplementary sequences are very useful in the accurate detection of peri-aortic hemorrhage, inflammation, or fluid collections. In addition to allowing improved characterization of the vascular structures, these sequences can be helpful in evaluating for associated abdominal and pelvic soft tissue pathology. (Please refer to the article on abdominal MRA elsewhere in this issue.)

Contrast and timing issues

Although timing is critical in all implementations of contrast-enhanced MRA, this is especially true in multistation bolus-chase MRA, where mistakes in timing may have a cumulative effect.

Two imperatives must be remembered regarding timing in runoff MRAs:

1. The acquisition of the central lines of k space must be synchronized to the presence of peak contrast in the arterial system being imaged.
2. The acquisitions of the central lines of k space must be completed before venous filling occurs, especially at the lower leg level.

Synchronization of the image acquisition with the arterial phase of contrast passage can be performed with use of a timing bolus or with a bolus-triggering technique.

Timing bolus

A timing bolus acquisition consists of a series of rapid (typically one per second) T1 weighted image acquisitions obtained in the axial plane through the region of the vessel of interest: in the present example the abdominal aorta. A 1 cm thick axial FLASH or SPGR acquisition is initiated simultaneously with the injection of 1 to 2 cc of contrast and 25 cc of flush, all administered at 2 cc/s. The image with maximal opacification (not the first image with contrast) can be determined visually or by using a region of interest (ROI) placed in the aorta with subsequent computer calculations. The appropriate time for the initiation of the scan is then calculated using the formula:

$$\begin{aligned}\text{Scan delay} = {} & \text{Circulation time} \\ & + (\text{the injection duration}/2) \\ & - (\text{the scan duration}/2)\end{aligned}$$

For example, an MRA of the abdominal aorta that takes 18 seconds to acquire might be performed using 20 cc of contrast administered at a rate of 2 cc/sec. The injection duration is 10 seconds, and the scan duration is 18 seconds. The circulation time obtained from visual evaluation of the axial images of a small test bolus is 19 seconds. Therefore, 19 + 5 - 9 equals 15 seconds is the appropriate time for the scan delay. Thus, the three-dimensional MRA sequence is initiated 15 seconds after the start of the contrast injection. This results in alignment of the midpoint of the arterial phase of the contrast bolus with the midpoint (time when the center of k space is acquired in a linear ordered sequence) of the image acquisition, with both occurring simultaneously at 24 seconds after the start of the contrast injection.

In actuality, it is desirable to have contrast present and at a relatively stable level throughout the scan. The foregoing formula represents conventional wisdom regarding the use of a timing bolus, and the dynamics of the bolus passage are not addressed, specifically, the degree to which the bolus disperses during its passage. One could argue that the reason this technique works is because of this prolongation of bolus duration, which allows for a greater contrast duration than is called for by the formula, and more nearly approximates the ideal. One also could argue that timing might be done most easily by simply choosing the start time of the scan to equal the circulation time (defined as the time of maximum opacification). No calculations are then necessary, and the scan will be obtained with contrast present in a steady state.

One advantage of the test bolus technique as outlined previously is that the scan will start simultaneous with the arrival of the maximum plateau phase of the contrast, with no time lost switching from scan monitoring to image acquisition, and the arterial phase of contrast passage will coincide with the center of k space acquisition. Therefore, this scan will finish, and the next position can be obtained more rapidly than when using a bolus triggering approach.

Bolus triggering

With bolus-triggering technique, the contrast is administered as intended for the scan, and multiple one per second images of the abdominal aorta are obtained in the coronal plane and displayed in real time on the scanner console. Then scan triggering usually is performed by the technologist based on the visualization of arterial contrast in the vessels of interest. Automated triggering also can be performed, by monitoring signal intensity within a region of interest, with scan initiation occurring when the specified region of interest exceeds a predetermined signal intensity threshold.

When using the bolus-triggering technique, because contrast is already present throughout the vasculature at the time of sequence initiation, centric ordering of k space acquisition is advised. The main advantage of the bolus-triggering technique is the ease of use; most technologists feel very comfortable with fluoroscopically monitored bolus- triggered techniques. Also, variation from the patient's baseline for any number of reasons is accounted for by the real-time nature of the scan initiation. For these reasons, the authors typically use this method in most cases. One caveat to keep in mind: although centric ordering is ideal with this methodology, some vendors do not have centric ordering available on three-dimensional MRA sequences with intrinsic fat suppression. In these instances, the three-dimensional MRA sequence will be linearly ordered, thus requiring the scan operator to trigger a few seconds before the expected peak arterial concentration in the vascular bed being imaged. Whenever the bolus-triggering technique is used, it is imperative for the operator to know whether the three-dimensional MRA sequence is centric or linearly ordered, so as to ascertain the optimal time for triggering.

Contrast administration

Various studies have evaluated bolus optimization strategies [5–7]. Given the prolonged scan times when viewed in aggregate, and the desire to minimize venous opacification, most often a biphasic contrast administration is chosen with an initial rate of approximately 1.2 to 1.5 cc/s for half the bolus administration followed by 0.4 to 0.5 cc/s for the remainder of the injection. This latter rate approximates the tissue extraction rate, which would allow arterial opacification with theoretically no venous filling. This results in a prolonged arterial phase of injection, with slow and delayed filling of the venous structures. For combined imaging of the abdomen, pelvis, and lower extremities, typically 40 cc of contrast are administered.

Minimizing venous contamination

The presence of venous contamination in runoff studies ranges in severity from the level of a nuisance that minimally complicates image interpretation (Fig. 4) to a complete disaster that renders interpretation impossible. In any case, the desire to minimize its presence drives much of the selection of imaging parameters and bolus administration techniques used. Venous contamination can be minimized by:

- Completing imaging within 60 seconds of study initiation
- Use of a biphasic administration of gadolinium, along with a slow prolonged infusion flush
- Use of venous compression devices at the level of the thighs (with pressures set to less than or equal to 50 mm Hg) to delay venous filling. Note: this technique should be used with caution in patients who have bypass

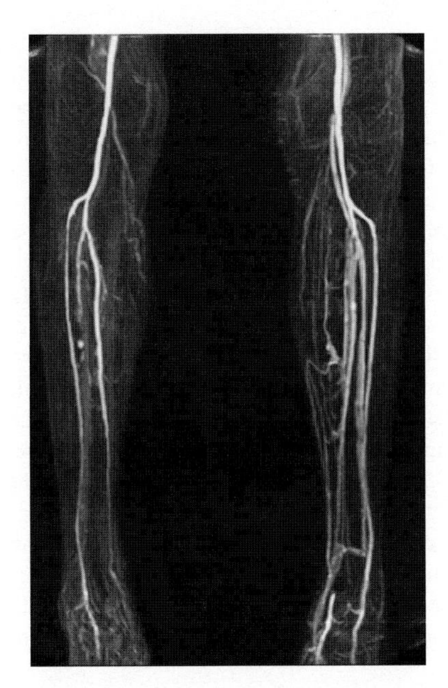

Fig. 4. Standard image at calf station showing venous contamination on the left, while timing on the right is appropriate.

grafts, as the grafts are often superficial in location and vulnerable to compromise by the compression device. Use of this technique has been reported recently in a series of 32 patients, and was demonstrated to slow down arterial transit times, increase arterial signal to noise, and reduce venous contamination [8].

Alternative techniques

Despite the optimization of imaging and contrast administration parameters, the frequent presence of venous contamination in the lower legs has stimulated the search for alternative techniques that can minimize this problem. In addition, although most patients tolerate the venous compression techniques well, some patients find them objectionable, and as mentioned previously, patients who have prior bypass grafts should probably not undergo thigh compression. Therefore, alternative techniques have been sought that can minimize the problem of venous contamination in the lower leg station. Hybrid imaging techniques, along with time-resolved angiographic techniques, have been used for this purpose.

Hybrid imaging

A newer strategy that may be used to solve the problem of venous contamination in the calf vasculature is the use of a dedicated high resolution imaging study at the lower leg level performed before imaging of the abdomen and pelvis. In this technique, initial mask images of the lower legs are obtained, followed by a timing bolus acquisition centered on the popliteal arteries. Using this timing bolus, appropriate imaging delay is instituted, and 15 cc of contrast administered at a rate of 1 cc/s with flush also administered at 1 cc/s for 25 cc. Two sequential three-dimensional high-resolution coronal image acquisitions then are obtained. Subsequently, the abdomen–pelvis and upper legs are imaged in the standard fashion as previously described using approximately 25 cc of contrast. Standard image-triggering techniques are used, and the table is moved one time. This technique was found to yield diagnostic images free of venous overlay in 95% of studies, and to demonstrate good agreement with selective digital subtraction angiography [9,10]. Other groups have reported similar findings, with a significant improvement in diagnostic accuracy at the calf level compared with standard bolus-chase methods [11].

Time-resolved hybrid imaging

An additional alternative involves the use of a time-resolved imaging sequence in the lower leg station. In this case, an initial scan with slightly lower resolution is performed repetitively in the lower legs, with a noncontrast image serving as the mask image. This acquisition only takes approximately 8 seconds, and typically is performed with the matrix size of 448 × 192. Sequential acquisitions are obtained during administration of 8 cc of contrast at 1 cc/s followed by 30 cc of flush, with up to15 sequential 8-second long acquisitions obtained. Each acquisition is a complete angiographic data set. Each one is subtracted from the mask, and only the resulting MIP image in the coronal plane is saved. The 15 MIP images generated subsequently are viewed as a movie loop. The study then is performed in the conventional fashion, with the lower leg high-resolution mask obtained followed by sequential table movement into the upper leg and abdomen–pelvis stations for the mask images. The antegrade bolus-chase technique then is used in the conventional fashion using the remainder of the contrast administration previously described. This technique has the advantage of being able to successfully image the arteries of the lower leg free of venous contamination, and also allows for visualization of discrepant flow if one leg is more severely diseased and has slower flow than the other. Figs. 4 and 5 show how this technique can be helpful in obtaining images free of venous contamination.

Although the previously described sequence was developed on a Siemens scanner, similar options are available on other scanners. Zhang and colleagues [12] reported on a series of patients where they used a two-dimensional projectional time-resolved angiographic technique with a temporal resolution of 2 seconds, and they demonstrated imaging free of venous contamination.

Suggested protocols are shown in Boxes 1 and 2.

Patient preparation and scan setup

Before scanning, the procedure should be explained to the patient, and emphasis should be placed on the need to remain still during the examination. This is particularly important given the multiple subtractions that will be required. If the patient has rest pain or skin ulceration, he or she should be reassured that appropriate care will be taken of the affected limb. There should be a thorough discussion regarding the characteristics of the scan, as this frequently will reduce the patient's anxiety and make the experience easier for the patient. An IV is required, and 20-gauge is preferred, although a 22 is acceptable given the low rate of contrast infusion. An antecubital vein is preferred. Hand veins may be used if necessary, although transit times will be prolonged. The patient should be placed on the table entering the gantry feet first, and the phased-array extremity coils placed, with attention to the patient's comfort. Additional body coils often will be placed over the lower abdomen, just above the extremity coil assembly. The patient should be notified that the table will move intermittently during the examination, and that compressive devices may be placed about the thighs to minimize venous contamination.

A dual-head power injector with the capability of multiphase bolus administration is preferred. Saline flush should be loaded along with the contrast in the injector before scan initiation.

Image acquisition

The scan protocol will vary somewhat depending on the protocol selected. In general, however, the scan sequence will be initiated with low-resolution scout SSFP images at the abdominal station, the upper leg station, and the lower leg station. Depending on user preference, additional localizers using either HASTE images or time- of-flight images can be used to localize the vessels of interest to ensure that they are enclosed in the

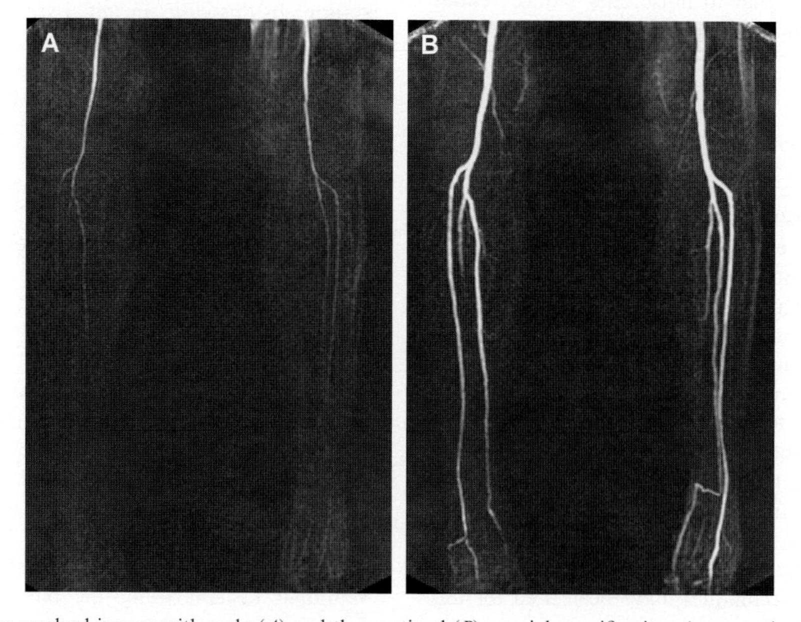

Fig. 5. Time-resolved images with early (*A*) and then optimal (*B*) arterial opacification, (same patient as Fig. 4.)

Box 1. Protocol steps: Siemens Avanto without time-resolved sequence:

Patient placed in magnet feet first, and centered at midabdomen
Abdomen True-FISP scout localizers (3 planes)—20 seconds
Table moves 375 mm (patient shorter than 5′10″) or 420 mm (patient taller than 5′10″)—2 seconds.
Upper leg three-plane scout—20 seconds
Table moves (see above)—2 seconds.
Lower leg three-plane scout—20 seconds
Three-dimensional standard angiogram noncontrast acquisition at lower leg (26 seconds)
Table moves to upper leg station—2 seconds.
Three-dimensional standard angiogram noncontrast acquisition—21 seconds
Table moves to abdomen/pelvis station—2 seconds.
Three-dimensional standard angiogram noncontrast acquisition—15 seconds
Contrast indicator clicked on (very important)
CARE-Bolus acquisition (in coronal plane centered on aorta) started
Contrast injected at 1.4 cc/s for 18 cc, then at .4 cc/s for remainder with flush at .4 cc/s
Three-dimensional angiogram dataset of abdomen/pelvis postcontrast acquisition triggered when contrast seen in abdominal aorta—s (in-line subtraction from precontrast mask preprogrammed, along with sagittal and coronal MIPs)
Table moves to upper leg level—2 seconds.
Upper leg Three-dimensional postcontrast angiogram dataset obtained—21 seconds (with in-line subtraction, MIPs preprogrammed)
Table moves to lower leg station—2 seconds.
Lower leg three-dimensional angiogram dataset acquired x 2—26 seconds each (sub/MIPs and others preprogrammed)
Additional VIBE postcontrast sequences at abdomen, femorals, popliteals as needed

Note: for venous studies following arterial studies, simply re-run the sequence in reverse order. Wait approximately 30 seconds and reacquire the lower leg, then the upper leg, then the abdomen/pelvis.

imaging volume. Subsequently, higher-resolution noncontrast images are obtained in all three stations, beginning at the lower leg and proceeding cephalad to the upper leg and the abdomen/pelvis station. Subsequently, the scan is initiated either following a timing bolus, or using fluoroscopic triggering. High-resolution angiographic images are obtained with the identical scan protocol used for the precontrast data set, and in-line subtraction can be preprogrammed, as can the creation of MIP images. The patient initiating a breath hold at the start of the scan improves image quality at the abdomen/pelvis station. The table then is moved sequentially such that the upper leg and lower leg stations are acquired sequentially. Two acquisitions at the lower leg level may be performed, to ensure that if there is significant disparity in flow, that both legs will be imaged adequately with arterial contrast present.

Post-processing and image interpretation

In-line subtraction of the postcontrast images from the precontrast mask image can be programmed in advance to be performed automatically, along with creation of MIP images in various imaging planes. Typically, postprocessing also will include a series of coronal MIP images that are rotated through 360 degrees.

The full-volume MIP images provide a quick review of the arterial structures, but review of the source images is required as well, as the MIP algorithm can result in obscuration of important findings. Because an MIP image is created by performing a ray tracing through the volume of tissue, it can miss lesions that are enclosed by high signal structures along the ray path. For example, in Fig. 6, the full-volume MIP image shows an irregularity of the proximal right common iliac artery that easily might be interpreted as

Box 2. Protocol steps: Siemens Avanto with time-resolved sequence

Patient placed in magnet feet first, and centered at midabdomen
Abdomen True-FISP scout localizers (three planes)—20 seconds
Table moves 375 mm (patient shorter than 5′10″) or 420 mm (patient taller than 5′10″)—2 seconds.
Upper leg three-plane scout—20 seconds
Table moves (see above)—2 seconds.
Lower leg three-plane scout—20 seconds
Lower leg noncontrast mask image for time-resolved sequence—8.5 seconds
Contrast indicator clicked on
Contrast injected at 1 cc/s for 8 cc total, with 25 cc flush at 1 cc/s
Time-resolved dynamic acquisition started at same time—programmed in advance for 10 to 15 repetitions, and for in-line subtraction and coronal MIPs—90 to 130 seconds
Contrast indicator clicked off (very important—later subtractions depend on this)
Three-dimensional standard angiogram noncontrast acquisition at lower leg (26 seconds)
Table moves to upper leg station—2 seconds
Three-dimensional standard angiogram noncontrast acquisition—21 seconds
Table moves to abdomen/pelvis station—2 seconds
Three-dimensional standard angiogram noncontrast acquisition—15 seconds
Contrast indicator clicked on (very important)
CARE-bolus acquisition (in coronal plane centered on aorta) started
Contrast injected at 1.4 cc/se for 18 cc, then at .4 cc/s for remainder with flush at .4 cc/s
Three-dimensional angiogram dataset of abdomen/pelvis postcontrast acquisition triggered when contrast seen in abdominal aorta—15 seconds (in-line subtraction from precontrast mask preprogrammed, along with SAG and COR MIPs)
Table moves to upper leg level—2 seconds.
Upper leg three-dimensional postcontrast angiogram dataset obtained—21 seconds (with in-line subtraction, MIPs preprogrammed)
Table moves to lower leg station—2 seconds.
Lower leg three-dimensional angiogram dataset acquired x2—26 sec each (sub/MIPs and others preprogrammed)
Additional VIBE postcontrast sequences at abdomen, femorals, popliteals as needed

Note: for venous studies following arterial studies, simply re-run the sequence in reverse order. Wait approximately 30 seconds and reacquire the lower leg, then the upper leg, then the abdomen/pelvis.

atherosclerotic plaque. Review of the source images in thin sections, however, clearly demonstrates the presence of clot.

Therefore, complete analysis of the angiographic datasets requires simultaneous interrogation of the axial, sagittal, and coronal imaging planes using the source data reviewed in multiplanar reformation mode on a commercially available workstation. Review of the unsubtracted dataset at the abdominal station is recommended, as it allows visualization of the vessel wall, and not just the lumen, as may be the case on subtracted images. In addition, other abdominal structures included in the study but poorly depicted by MIPs can be seen better. Fig. 7 demonstrates a renal cell carcinoma that is visualized better on thin MIPs and axial reformatted images than on standard MIP images. Sliding thin submaximal MIP images also allow visualization of the arteries without overlap of overlying structures, and are often useful as well. Multiplanar curved reformations can be performed as needed.

Modern workstations also can create images using the volume-rendering technique, and endoscopic views of the images. The volume-rendered three-dimensional images can be very dazzling in appearance, and are well-received by clinicians (Fig. 8). Although they can provide a unique

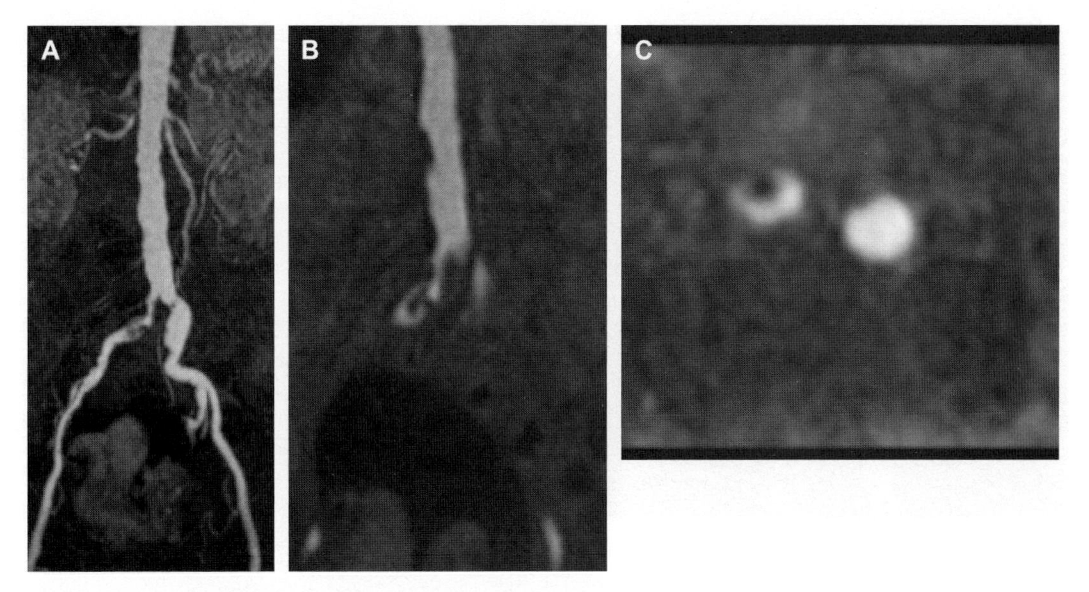

Fig. 6. Full-volume maximum intensity projection (MIP) (*A*) shows irregularity of the right iliac artery, which is noted to be caused by a focal filling defect on thin-section MIP (*B*), and is shown to be clot on axial image (*C*).

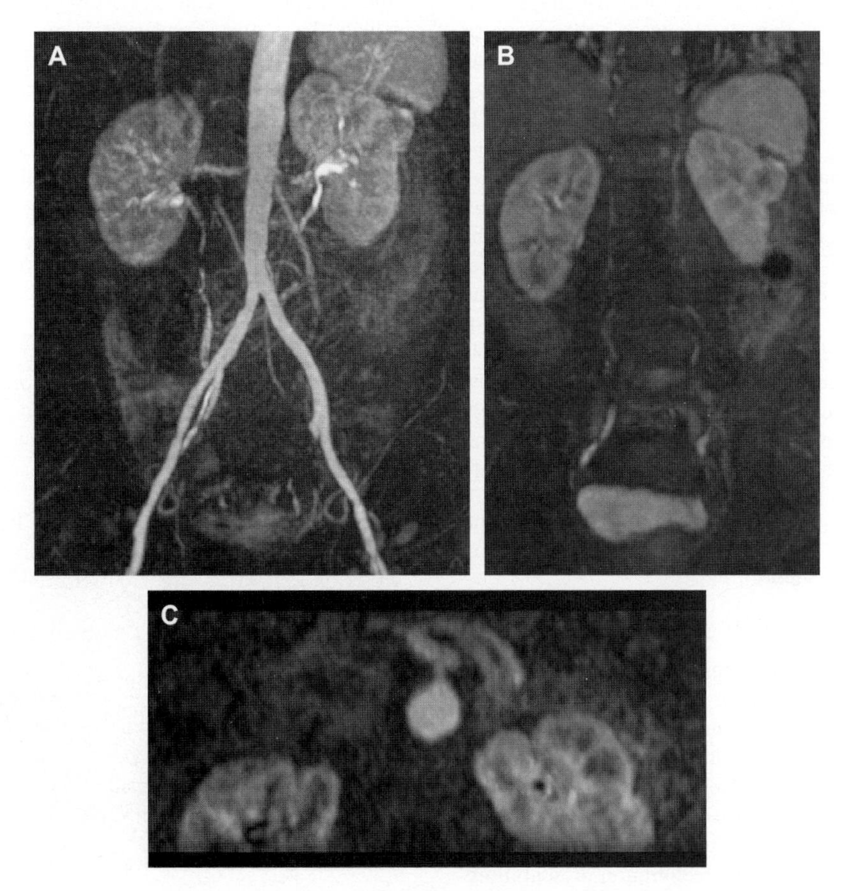

Fig. 7. Left renal carcinoma (*A*) better seen on subvolume maximum intensity projection (*B*) and axial reformation (*C*).

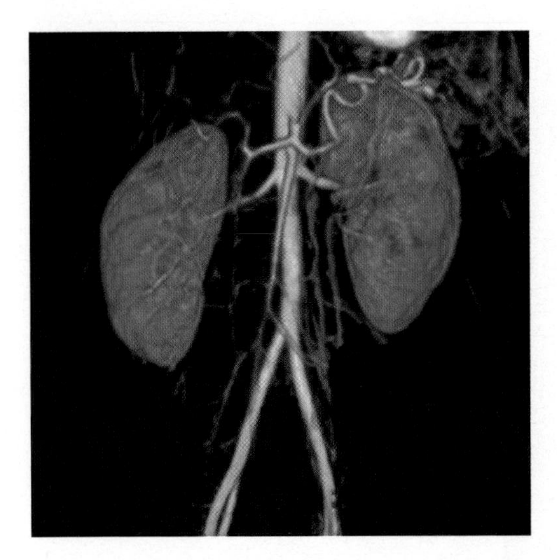

Fig. 8. Volume rendered magnetic resonance angiogram in color.

global overview of the relevant anatomy, they usually are not well suited to primary image analysis because of their tendency to either overestimate or underestimate lesions depending on the algorithm and thresholds used.

Automated evaluation of stenoses and MR angiographic data sets would simplify image interpretation, and potentially allow a more accurate, quantitative evaluation of the cross-sectional areas of stenosis. A study looking at the accuracy of semiautomated analysis of three-dimensional contrast-enhanced MR angiographic data sets for the detection and quantification of aortoiliac stenoses using commercially available software found that the overall sensitivity for the accurate detection of stenosis was approximately 89%, with specificity of 88%. Further studies are needed to validate this concept, but it certainly has intuitive appeal [13].

Clinical applications

Atherosclerotic peripheral vascular disease

As stated in the opening paragraph, this is the most common problem for which MRA of the aortofemoral circulation is requested. Because of its systemic nature, atherosclerosis tends to be a multisegmental disease, affecting various vascular territories. Nonetheless, recognized discrete syndromes often are found. Therefore, this next section addresses the more common presentations of atherosclerotic peripheral arterial disease, recognizing that significant overlap occurs. In addition, given that such imaging usually is performed preparatory to either surgical or percutaneous intervention, emphasis will be placed on a discussion of findings relevant to planned interventions. In short, it addresses what the surgeon or interventionalist needs to know.

Aortoiliac disease

High-grade occlusive disease of the terminal aorta or proximal iliac arteries often results in Leriche syndrome, a clinical entity characterized by the triad of diminished or absent femoral pulses, gluteal or thigh claudication, and impotence in males. Pallor and wasting of the lower extremities also may be seen in extreme cases. The aortic or proximal iliac occlusive disease may be total, as in the Fig. 9, or may be partial, as seen in Fig. 1. More distal manifestations often coexist.

In analyzing MRA in such patients, note should be made of the degree of occlusive change, and the status of collateral vessels. The point at which the native circulation is reconstituted is quite important, as it will determine the feasibility of percutaneous or surgical approaches. Specifically, the status of the more distal iliac and femoral arteries becomes extremely important [14]. For example, the length of iliac occlusion, if present, often determines whether the patient is a candidate for percutaneous treatment, or will require some open surgical therapy. In the treatment of

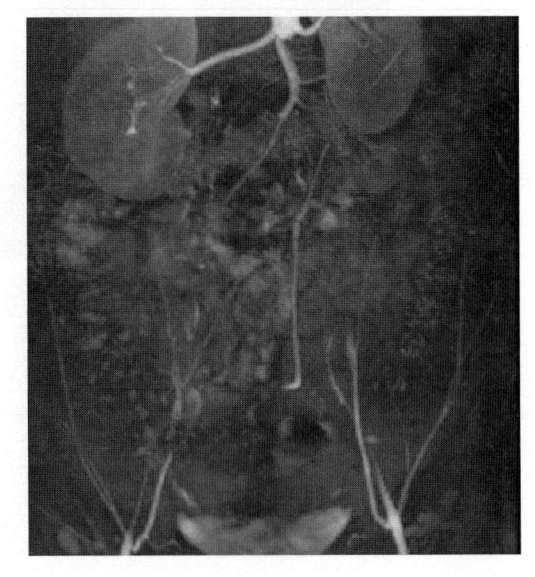

Fig. 9. Aortic occlusion just distal to the renal arteries.

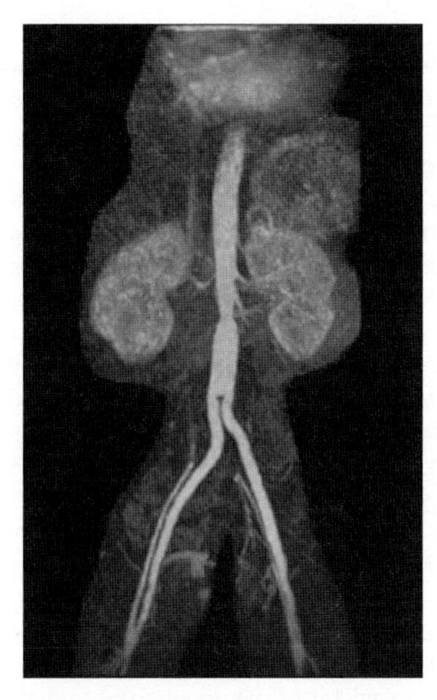

Fig. 10. Magnetic resonance angiogram demonstrating an aortobifemoral graft.

long-segment bilateral iliac occlusions, aortobifemoral open surgical repair often is preferred because of its superior patency. For short-segment iliac disease, even if bilateral, endovascular therapy often is preferred (Figs. 10 and 11).

Superficial femoral artery disease

Occlusive disease of the superficial femoral artery is often surprisingly symmetric bilaterally. High-grade occlusions often result in claudication of the calf musculature on walking, and if accompanied by severe runoff disease, may progress to rest pain (Fig. 12).

Analysis of MRA in this circumstance requires attention again to the length of the occluded or narrowed segment, as short segment occlusions are capable of percutaneous treatment, while longer segment occlusions more often require grafting. Particular attention should be paid to the level of reconstitution.

The level of resumption of a normal caliber vessel is quite important as it serves as the likely site of distal anastomosis [15]. Also, if the anastomosis can be made proximal to the articular portion of the popliteal artery, synthetic graft material remains a viable choice, sparing the patient's native veins for future use if necessary. If it is necessary to traverse the knee joint, however, synthetic material usually is not advised, and native veins are preferred.

Percutaneous treatment of infrainguinal atherosclerotic disease is an area of ongoing research, and the reader is referred to the recent literature [16,17]. Expansion of indications for percutaneous treatment in the infrainguinal region may prove to be quite helpful for patients who are poor operative candidates. For example, in patients who are poor operative candidates, subintimal recanalization techniques have been developed that often allow limb salvage [18]. Occasionally, stents are required in such patients also (Fig. 13).

Runoff disease

The usual patient with infra-articular runoff disease often presents with ischemic pain in the

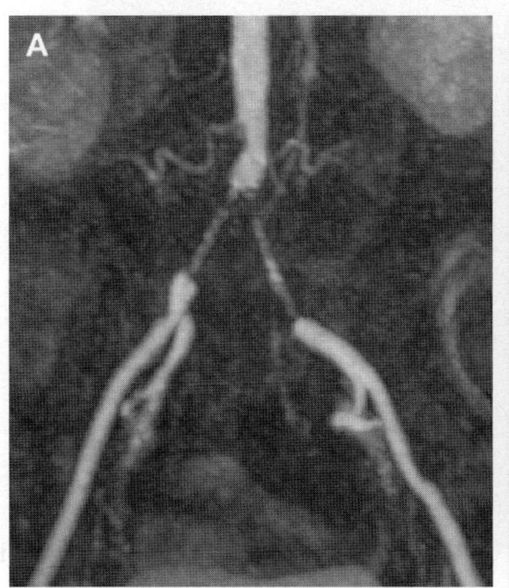

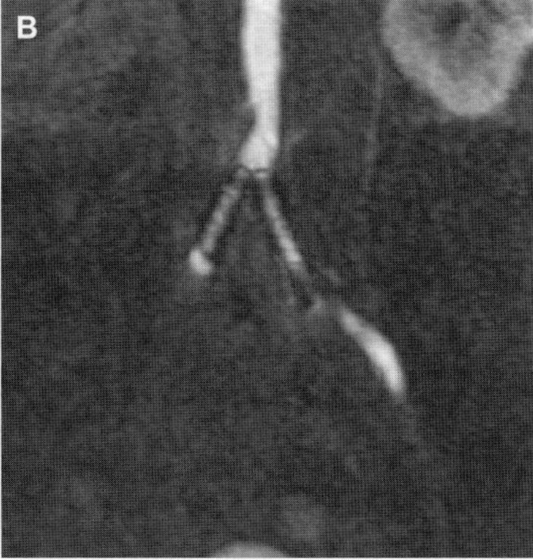

Fig. 11. Thick (*A*) and thin (*B*) maximum intensity projection images from a patient with bilateral iliac artery stents.

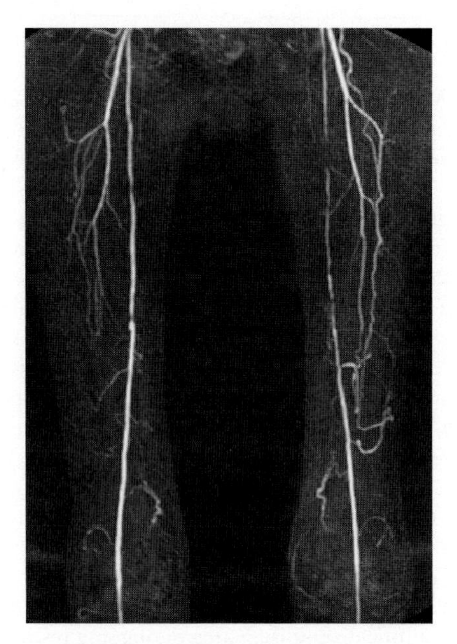

Fig. 12. Magnetic resonance angiogram showing mild superficial femoral artery plaques on right and multisegmental occlusive disease on the left.

foot, progressing to rest pain and even gangrene. Diabetics in particular are at risk for this more peripheral, small vessel involvement (Fig. 14) [19]. Early venous filling and arteriovenous shunting is not uncommon in patients who have severe runoff disease, particularly in those who have cellulitis and coexisting soft tissue infection, which may complicate image interpretation (Fig. 15). In fact, if the patient is known to have a foot or lower leg ulcer, steps to accelerate image acquisition are suggested. Alternatively, consideration should be given to the use of a time-resolved angiographic acquisition in this circumstance.

The status of the popliteal artery, the tibioperoneal trunk, and the vessels of the lower leg often determine whether the patient is a candidate for possible revascularization, or whether amputation is likely in the presence of rest pain. Given the multisegmental nature of atherosclerotic disease, it is sometimes possible by improving the inflow to restore limb viability in circumstances where the patient does not have anatomy favorable to intervention.

The status of the distal vasculature is important [20]. The study should demonstrate which, if any, vessels are patent in a continuous fashion from the knee to the ankle. In addition, likely sites of possible anastomosis should be identified, as should the caliber of the vessel distal to that point. It is often helpful to prepare unsubtracted images for demonstration of bony landmarks for the referring physician, to allow easy correlation of the angiographic images with the patient's anatomy.

Venous contamination if present can be minimized by using thin-section MIP images to eliminate venous overlap. In addition, rotating the imaging to various obliquities can help sometimes (Fig. 16).

Imaging of the pedal vessels sometimes may be required, and they may or may not be imaged

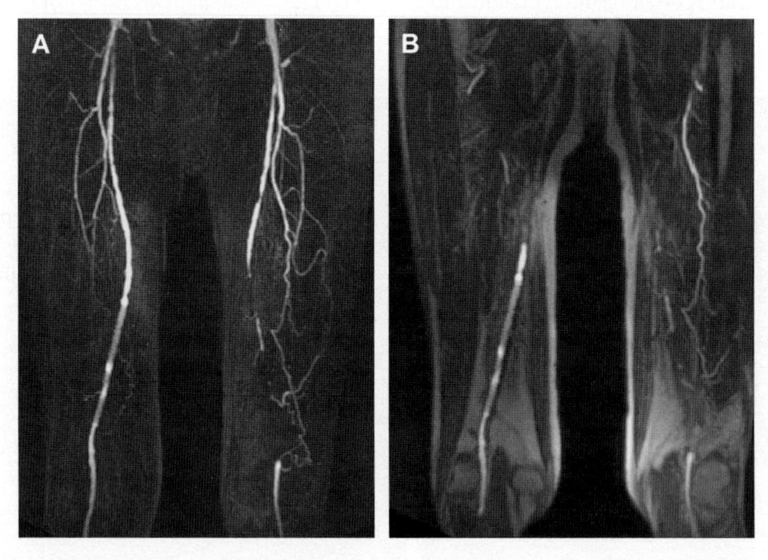

Fig. 13. Thick (*A*) and thin (*B*) maximum intensity projection images from a patient status after right superficial femoral artery (SFA) nitinol stent placement. Note also the left SFA occlusion.

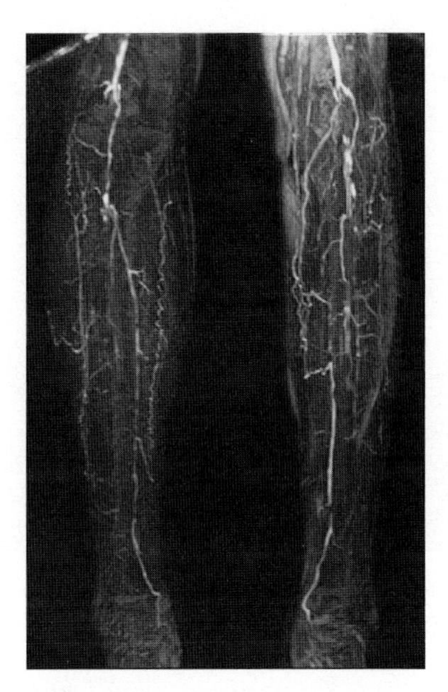

Fig. 14. Diabetic patient with severe bilateral run-off disease. Note that no single vessel extends in continuity from the knee to the ankle.

adequately on the standard multistation bolus chase angiography. In individual circumstances, two-dimensional time-of-flight images can be used at the time of the initial study if this is felt to be a clinical consideration. Alternatively, a dedicated high-resolution stationary examination of the pedal circulation can be performed at a separate time.

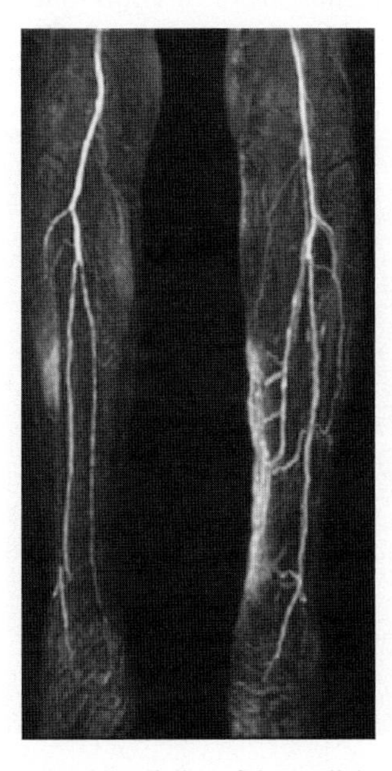

Fig. 15. Patient with cellulitis of the medial aspect of the left leg and the lateral aspect of the right leg.

Postoperative and postintervention imaging

Imaging of the postoperative patient seldom is performed simply as a surveillance procedure, but often for evaluation of suspected recurrence of occlusive disease, or more commonly, for progression of disease in the native vessels [21].

Aorto–bifemoral grafts (see Fig. 10) widely are used for treating long-segment iliac artery occlusions. Synthetic graft materials do not present a problem for MRI, but occasionally clips at the site of the surgical anastomosis may produce minimal artifact. Anastomotic complications including pseudoaneurysm formation can be visualized well. Fig. 17 A and B are images from the patient shown in Fig. 9 with aortic occlusion, now status post-aorto–bifemoral surgery, with a resultant pseudoaneurysm at the right femoral anastomosis.

In addition, because of the capability of reformatting the images into virtually any plane, rotation of the data set allows improved visualization of the surgical anastomosis. In Fig. 18, note that in this patient with a femoropopliteal bypass, that the straight anteriopostерior view of the anastomosis at the femoral site is poorly rendered because of overlap. Upon rotation, however, a mild-to-moderate stenosis is unmasked.

Stents

Endovascular stent placement frequently is performed to increase the long-term patency of percutaneous interventions. These are placed commonly in the iliac region, (see Fig. 11), but occasionally placement into the femoral vessels also is performed (See Fig. 13). As can be seen from these examples, visualization of luminal contrast in the presence of stents may be possible depending on the composition of the stent [22,23]. Specifically, nitinol-containing stents (as seen in Fig. 13) usually produce minimal if any artifact [24].

Stainless steel stents, however, particularly the Palmaz stent (Cordis Corporation, Miami Lakes, Florida), usually result in significant surrounding signal loss and as a result luminal visualization is not possible. If the presence of this stent is unknown, the reader may assume (incorrectly) that there is a short segmental occlusion (Fig. 19). The true nature of the abnormality, however, is easily clarified if radiographs are available. Even in the absence of radiographic or historical evidence of a stainless steel stent, an astute reader should be suspicious of this pseudo-stenosis based on the following: sharply marginated borders, the absence of collaterals, or the presence of stent artifact on

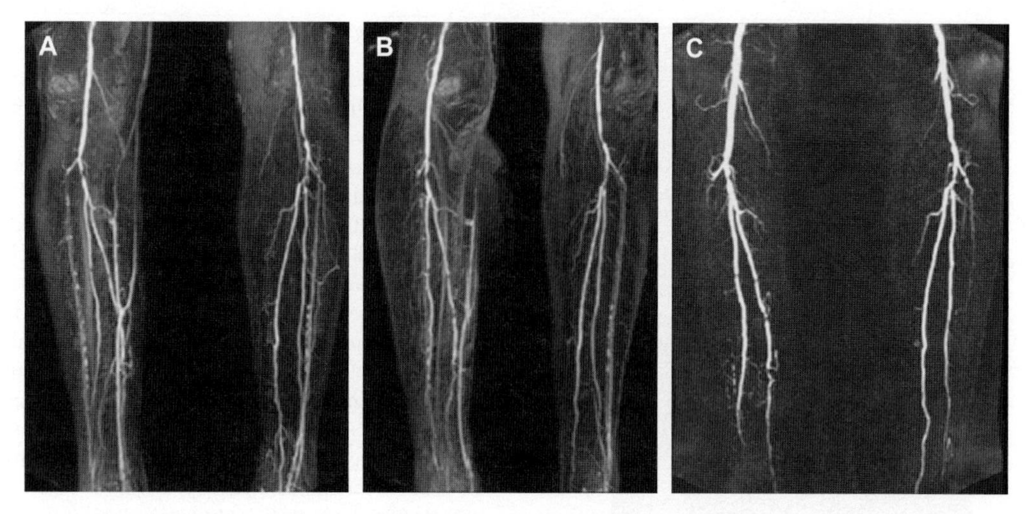

Fig. 16. In the anteroposterior image (*A*), the right posterior tibial artery is obscured by an overlying vein. Rotation of the image (*B*) offsets the vein, revealing significant posterior tibial artery disease, which is confirmed on the time-resolved image (*C*).

thin- section multiplanar images from the subtracted source images.

Patients who have undergone prior endovascular stent graft treatment of an abdominal aortic aneurysm may present subsequently for runoff imaging also. It should be noted that most of the current versions of the stent grafts produce minimal if any artifact [25]. MRA has been well-studied in evaluation of patients after covered stent graft repair of abdominal aortic aneurysm, and it has been found to be superior to CT for the detection of endoleak [26]. In this setting, delayed imaging through the aorta is necessary, and often is performed best with a VIBE technique. Fig. 20 represents a patient who had a prior endograft repair of an abdominal aortic aneurysm. Note the excellent depiction of the vessel lumen with minimal artifact. No evidence of delayed endoleak is seen on the accompanying three-dimensional volumetric acquisition (see Fig. 20B)

Buerger's disease

Buerger's disease, also known as thromboangiitis obliterans, is a disorder predominantly affecting young male smokers. The disorder, however, increasingly is being recognized in

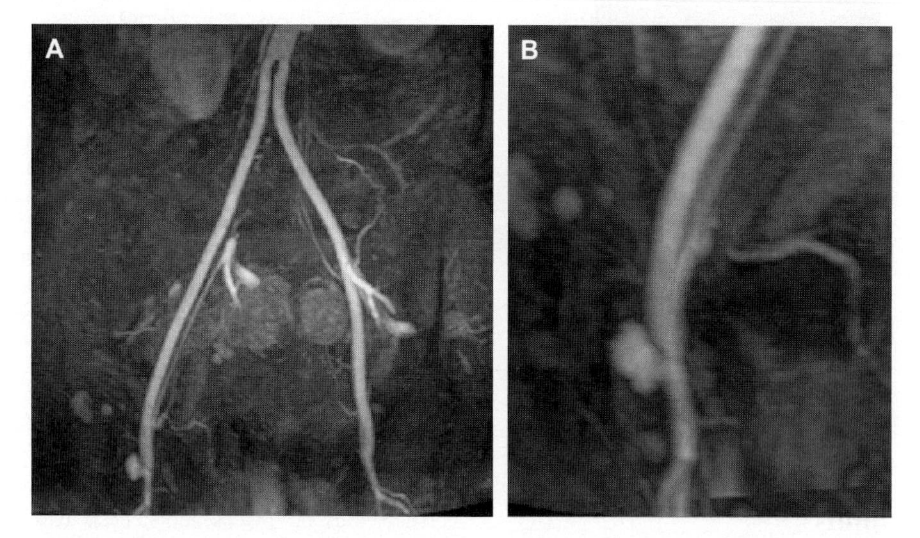

Fig. 17. Postoperative images on the patient seen in Fig. 9 with aortic occlusion status/post bypass grafting with a pseudoaneurysm at the anastomosis. Pelvic magnetic resonance angiogram (*A*) and magnified view (*B*) of the anastomosis.

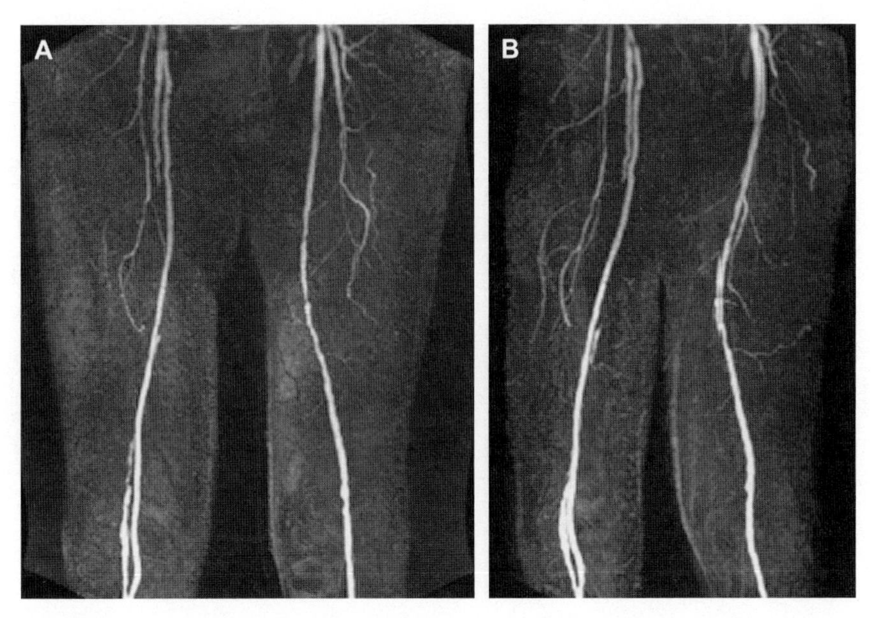

Fig. 18. Mild stenosis at origin of femoro-popliteal bypass graft better seen on oblique projection (*B*), than on antero-posterior image (*A*).

women smokers also. This disorder produces an obliterative arteritis of the medium and small vessels of the peripheral extremities, affecting both the upper and lower extremities. The characteristic angiographic hallmark is the presence of extensive distal occlusive disease accompanied by the development of corkscrew collaterals. In Fig. 21, an illustrative case is presented. Note the characteristic absence of distal runoff arteries, and the presence of multiple, irregular collaterals. It often can be differentiated from the more common atherosclerotic disease by the relative preservation of the inflow vessels.

Embolic disease

Peripheral arterial emboli affecting the lower extremity circulation typically originate either in

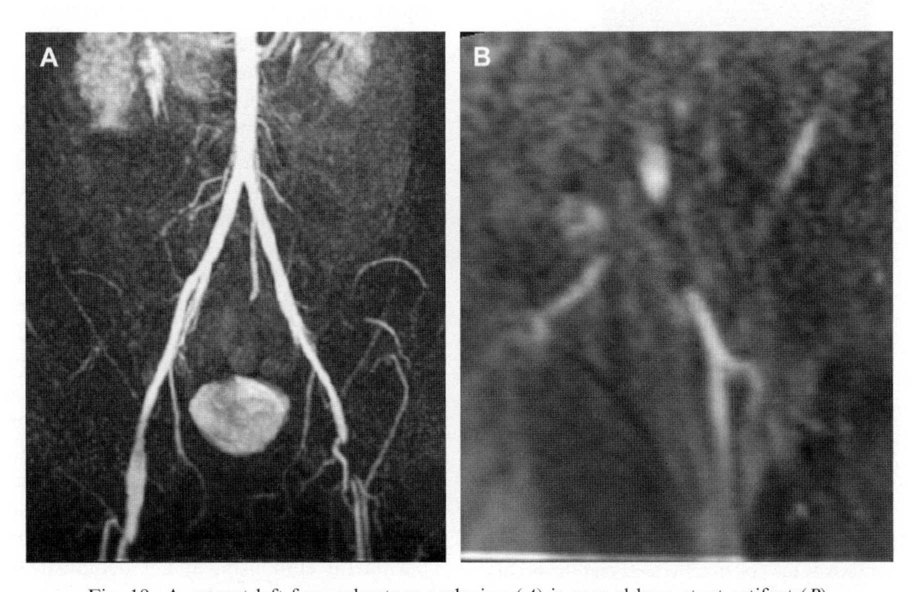

Fig. 19. Apparent left femoral artery occlusion (*A*) is caused by a stent artifact (*B*).

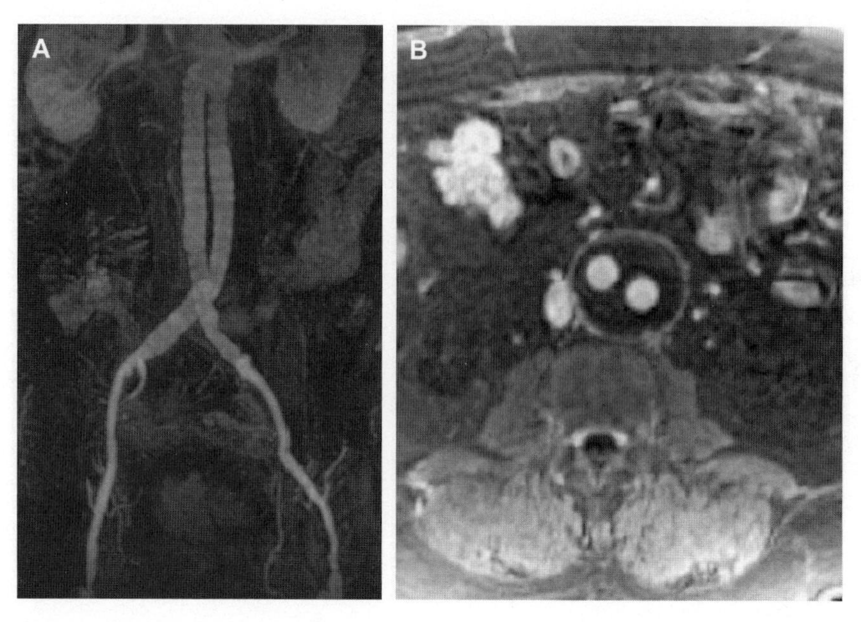

Fig. 20. Maximum intensity projection (*A*) and axial delayed volumetric T1 gradient echo sequence image (*B*) of aortic endograft.

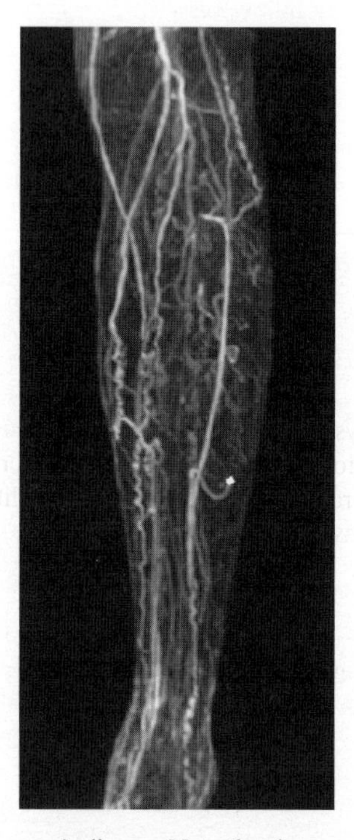

Fig. 21. Buerger's disease. Note the characteristic corkscrew appearance of the collateral vessels and the occlusive disease of the trifurcation vessels.

the heart or the thoracic or abdominal aorta. Emboli subsequently will lodge in the more peripheral vessels, when their size precludes further migration, or at sites of preexisting stenosis (see Fig. 6). Depending on the abundance of collaterals, the degree of ischemia that results can be quite profound, and MRA often needs to be performed in an urgent fashion [27]. Fig. 22 demonstrates the presence of a popliteal thrombus in a patient who presented with the acute onset of lower leg ischemia on the left. One can see from these images the excellent correlation between the MR appearance and the radiograph angiographic appearance. In this patient, thrombus lysis was performed with intra-arterial thrombolytics, and restoration of patency was achieved as can be seen in the accompanying figures.

When performing MRA for evaluation of acute ischemic syndromes, meticulous attention should be paid to the evaluation of the thoracic and abdominal aorta (for potential sites of embolism), and a cardiac imaging study should be considered to exclude ventricular or atrial thrombi, or a focus for intracardiac shunting (ie, patent foramen ovale or atria septal defect). Fig. 23 is a thin-section image reconstruction from an MRA of the thoracic aorta performed to evaluate for the source of recurrent peripheral embolism, and it demonstrates a left atrial thrombus. It should be noted that it has

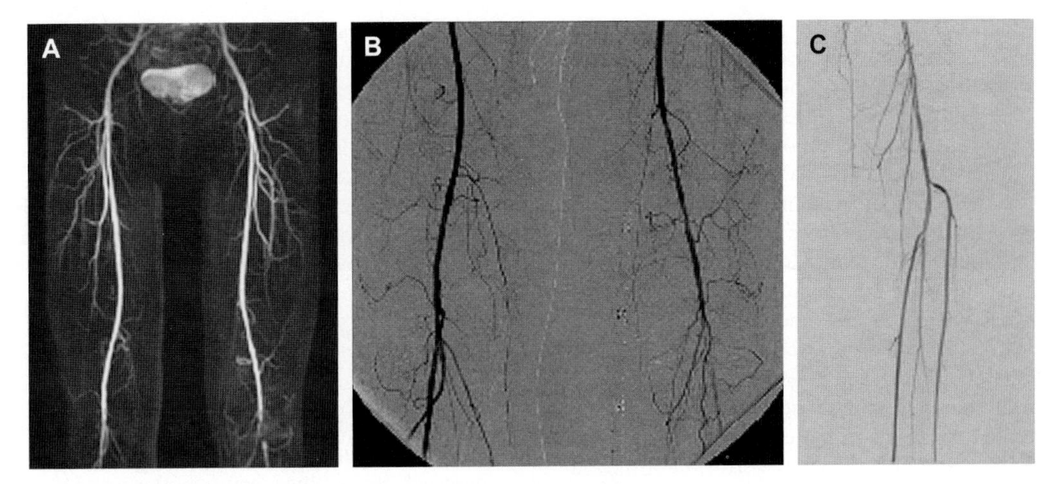

Fig. 22. Clot occludes the left popliteal artery on magnetic resonance angiogram (*A*), and is confirmed on digital subtraction angiogram (*B*). (*C*) After intra-arterial thrombolysis, restoration of patency is demonstrated.

been shown that cardiac MRI is superior to echocardiography for detecting ventricular thrombi, and dedicated cardiac MR evaluation should be considered in such patients [28].

Aneurysms and dissection

An aneurysm is a localized area of dilation within any blood vessel to more than 150% of the native reference vessel diameter (ie, a segment dilated to 1.5 cm or more in a vessel that has adjacent normal segment diameter of 1.0 cm would be considered an aneurysm). Areas of dilation that are less than 150% of the reference vessel diameter are referred to as ectasia (ie, a segment dilated to 1.3 cm in a vessel that has adjacent normal segment diameter of 1.0 cm would be considered an area of ectasia). Aneurysms can be the result of trauma, infections, or connective tissue abnormalities, but most frequently they are a consequence of atherosclerosis. Atherosclerotic aneurysms predominately involve the infrarenal abdominal aorta, and they are discussed in detail in the abdominal imaging section. Discussion also is referenced elsewhere in this article regarding endovascular stent graft treatment of such aneurysms. Aneurysms, however, can be present in any of the vessel in the pelvis and lower extremity arterial circulation.

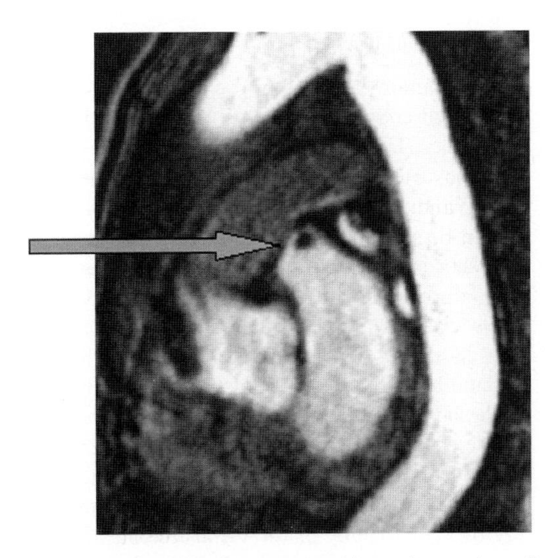

Fig. 23. Left atrial clot seen on thin-section review of thoracic magnetic resonance angiogram.

In occasional patients, generalized arteriomegaly may be evident, with extensive multisegmental aneurysm formation. In addition, multiplicity of aneurysms is seen frequently, and patients who have abdominal aneurysms are at increased risk for femoral aneurysms, and also popliteal artery aneurysms. These latter aneurysms are particularly prone to thrombosis and distal embolization. Evaluation requires recognition and study not only of the luminographic images, but also of the angiographic source images so as not to miss the vessel wall pathology. For this application, a VIBE sequence performed at the level of the popliteal artery is very useful to detect a small aneurysm with associated atheroma or thrombus resulting in a normal lumen caliber.

A dissection is a tear in the wall of a vessel separating the middle layer (media) from the outer layer (adventitia). Dissections in the abdominal, iliac, or femoral vessels are usually the result of propagation of a dissection originating in the thoracic aorta. Fig. 24 demonstrates the appearance of an aortic dissection extending from the thoracic aorta into the iliac vessels. Note the excellent depiction of the filling pattern of the various vascular structures on this volume-rendered MRA image. Which vessels fill from which lumen is the important information to be gleaned from an MRA study of dissection. Relative contributions of the true and false lumens to the supply of the abdominal and pelvic vasculature are important, and close attention should be paid to the relative perfusion patterns of the visceral organs. In particular, disparate perfusion of the kidneys often is evident in such patients and should be evaluated.

Although typically secondary to propagation from thoracic dissections, occasionally abdominal, iliac, or femoral dissections can be primary (ie, originate in and remain isolated to these vessels). Isolated lower extremity dissections can be a result of mechanical trauma (ie, a catheterization procedure), or can be truly spontaneous. Spontaneous dissections frequently are caused by an underlying connective tissue abnormality such as Ehlers-Danlos syndrome, as depicted in Fig. 25. This patient had a spontaneous right common iliac artery dissection, which extended into the right external iliac artery. This subsequently was treated with a covered stent graft, with exclusion of the false lumen, resulting in resolution. Note that the stent graft is made of nitinol and produces minimal artifact.

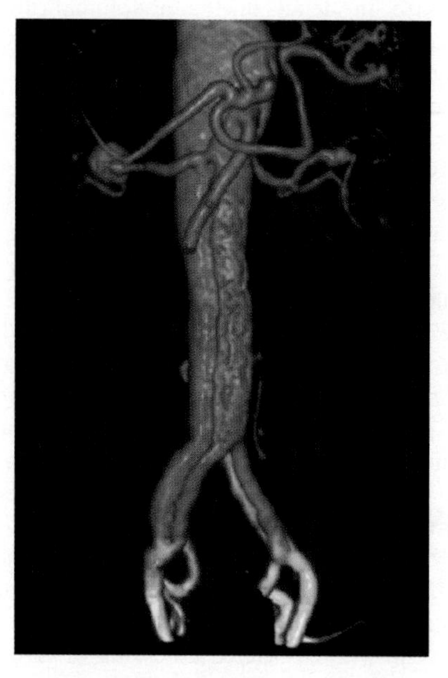

Fig. 24. Color volume-rendered image of aortic dissection extending into the iliac arteries. Note the incidental renal artery aneurysms.

Pseudoaneurysms most often are caused by prior trauma, or they may be a complication of surgical therapy. Fig. 10 shows an example of a postsurgical pseudoaneurysm.

Arteriovenous malformations and arteriovenous fistulas

Arteriovenous malformations (AVMs) are congenital malformations in which there are abnormal connections between the arterial and venous structures, without an intervening capillary bed, as in the patient represented in Fig. 26, who has an AVM of the midportion of the left foot. Both arteriovenous fistulas (AVF) and AVMs result in abnormal early opacification of venous structures. The AVM is recognized easily by the abnormal early venous filling during the arterial phase of imaging. Time-resolved imaging occasionally may be helpful in such instances, but a rapid frame rate is necessary for this purpose [29].

Arteriovenous fistulas are more commonly traumatic in origin, and they may result from iatrogenic intervention. Fig. 27 demonstrates a patient who has an arteriovenous fistula in the left femoral artery, resulting from a prior catheterization procedure.

Congenital disorders and miscellaneous

Uncommon causes of aortic narrowing include abdominal coarctation, also known as midaortic syndrome. This may be associated with other systemic arterial abnormalities as may be seen with Williams syndrome, or it may be seen occasionally in association with neurofibromatosis. In this disorder, an area of constriction is present in the midportion of the abdominal aorta, and often is associated with bilateral renal artery stenosis. Fig. 28 demonstrates a volume-rendered image and an angiographic image of such a patient.

Patients with Klippel-Trenaunay-Weber syndrome occasionally may present for angiographic imaging. In this disorder, abnormal arteriovenous connections may be present, and hemihypertrophy or hemiatrophy of the distal lower extremity often is seen. Abnormalities both of the arterial supply and of the draining veins may be present.

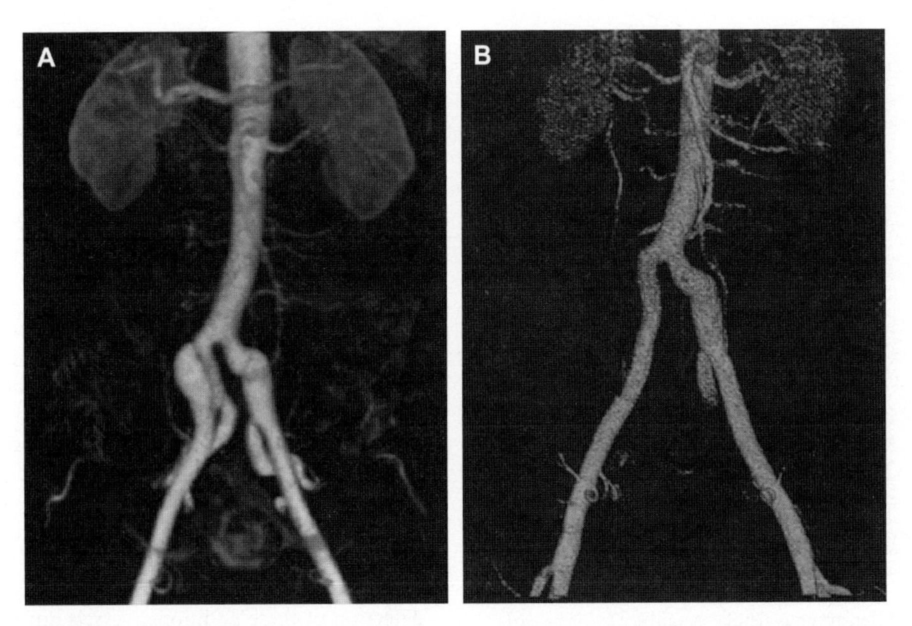

Fig. 25. Preintervention (*A*) and postintervention (*B*) images from a patient with right iliac artery dissection treated with a covered stent graft. Note the absence of stent artifact.

(Note: some authors separate Klippel-Trenaunay syndrome [KTS] from Parke-Weber syndrome [PWS], while others lump the two together as Klippel-Trenaunay-Weber syndrome. The distinction is that classic KTS has only anomalous venous structures and is a low-flow disorder, while patients who have PWS have arteriovenous fistlulae and high-flow lesions and have a worse prognosis.) Delayed imaging in the venous phase may be helpful in evaluating such patients.

Popliteal entrapment syndrome is a disorder that results from abnormal medial placement of the medial head of the gastrocnemius muscle, resulting in compression of the popliteal artery in the popliteal fossa during exercise. This disorder may go unrecognized if imaging is not performed with

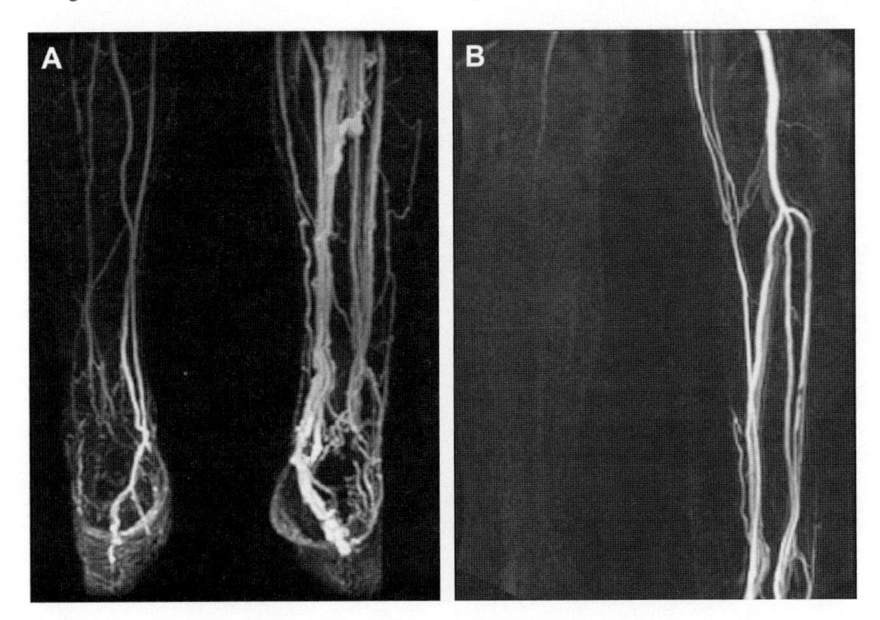

Fig. 26. Standard (*A*) and time-resolved (*B*) images of a patient with an arteriovenous malformation of the left foot. Note the early venous filling on the left that cannot be mitigated even with time-resolved imaging.

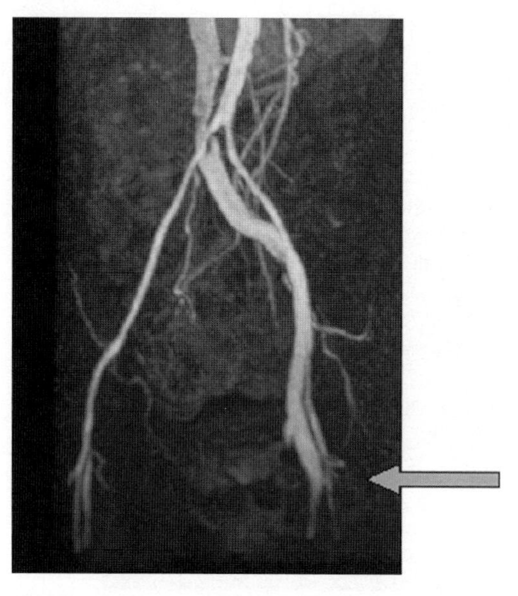

Fig. 27. Arteriovenous fistula secondary to prior catheterization procedure.

the patient attempting plantar flexion. In cases where this disorder is suspected, dedicated imaging at the level of the popliteal arteries is suggested, both at rest, and with provocative maneuvers [30].

Cystic adventitial disease is an uncommon disorder resulting in localized arterial narrowing that may progress to occlusion, often involving the popliteal arteries. It is characterized by the development of myxoid cystic changes of the adventitia, with resultant compression of the vessel lumen. Review of the axial source images is important in its recognition [31].

Comparison with alternative techniques

Comparison with DSA

MRA has been well-validated for the detecting and quantifying stenoses and occlusions in the aortoiliac and femoral vessels. Initial studies used two-dimensional time-of-flight imaging and demonstrated a high level of agreement with conventional angiography in the iliofemoral region [32]. In the lower legs, two-dimensional time-of-flight MRA detected all vessels identified by conventional angiography, and in addition demonstrated an additional 22% of runoff vessels that were not identified with conventional arteriography. The detection of these additional vessels not identified by conventional angiography altered the surgical management of the disorders in 17% cases [33].

Three dimensional contrast-enhanced MRA now has superseded two-dimensional time-of-flight imaging, and it shows an improved sensitivity and specificity. Several studies have demonstrated the superiority of contrast-enhanced MRA over two-dimensional time-of-flight angiography, with contrast-enhanced MRA demonstrating a significantly faster imaging time and a larger coverage area than

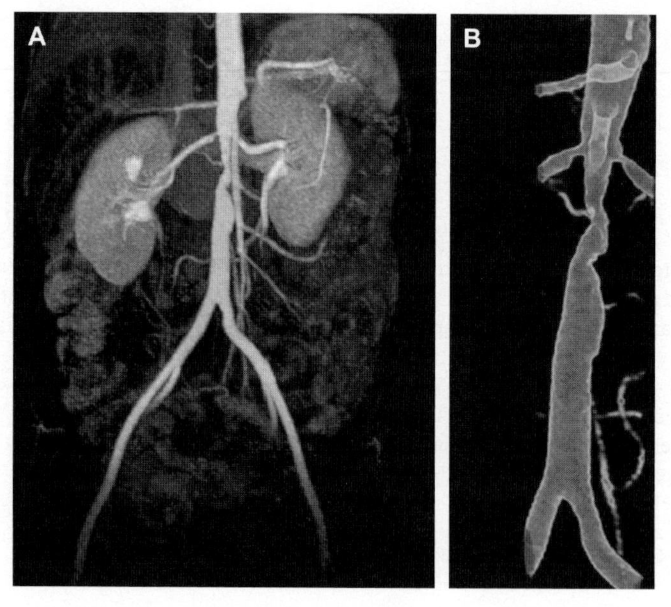

Fig. 28. Maximum intensity projection (*A*) and volume rendered technique (*B*) images of mid-aortic syndrome. Note the bilateral renal artery stenoses, which are frequent coexisting findings.

two-dimensional time-of-flight angiography [34,35]. The contrast-enhanced magnetic resonance angiogram also allows better visualization of the pedal vessels than two-dimensional time-of-flight imaging. As expected, the three-dimensional contrast-enhanced MRA images were found to be significantly less prone to artifact. In particular, three-dimensional contrast-enhanced MRA was able to visualize vessels with reversed diastolic flow, or if the flow extended in a retrograde fashion as is often the case with collateral vessels.

Multiple recent studies have demonstrated that contrast-enhanced MRA performed with a bolus-chase moving table technique has a sensitivity and specificity greater than 95% when compared with catheter angiography [36].

Magnetic resonance angiography versus CT angiography for runoff imaging

CT angiography using multislice spiral acquisitions has emerged recently as a noninvasive alternative to MRA [37]. In this technique, rapid thin-section imaging is performed in the axial plane from the level of the renal arteries to the feet during the prolonged administration of contrast material. Sixteen-slice scanners have made this technique feasible, and they are becoming widely available. In addition, newer 64-slice scanners are now available, and also allow thinner slice acquisitions and more rapid scanning. In fact, timing of the arterial bolus becomes important because of the ability of the scanner to outrun the contrast bolus.

Two recent studies have looked at the relative merits of MRA and multidetector CT angiography for evaluating peripheral arterial disease. A study of 157 consecutive patients randomized to either CT angiography using a 16-slice scanner, or bolus chase MRA using a high-performance gradient system demonstrated a minimal difference in observer diagnostic confidence favoring CT angiography, which was not statistically significant, and which diminished with increased observer experience. The patients in the MRA group required slightly more follow-up vascular imaging, likely related to the slightly decreased confidence [38]. The same researchers, however, subsequently also demonstrated that the interobserver agreement for MRA was higher than that for CT angiography for evaluating the degree of arterial stenosis or occlusion [39]. In particular, the presence of calcifications significantly decreased the interobserver agreement of multidetector CT angiography for the evaluation of stenosis. The small calf vessels with calcification present were the most problematic area. The authors did note that a high number of nondiagnostic segments were found on MRA, and speculated that performing an initial high-resolution sequence of the tibial vessels would reduce the number of nondiagnostic segments. Other studies have demonstrated that in the aortoiliac and renal arteries, the performance of MRA and CTA was essentially identical [40].

Anecdotally, the image interpretation time required for CT angiography is significantly higher than for MRA, largely because of the presence of calcification within the vessels of interest. Calcifications are not a problem in MRA, nor are the soft tissue and bony structures, which are suppressed with the acquisition technique itself or are subtracted from the mask images in the postprocessing steps.

At the present time, the choice of MRA or CT angiography for evaluation of peripheral vascular disease depends largely on scanner availability, with MRA preferred in general, and in particular in patients with pre-existing renal insufficiency or contrast allergy. CT angiography is an acceptable alternative, particularly in patients who have pacemakers, defibrillators, or other contraindications to MRA.

Artifacts and pitfalls

Artifacts always should be considered in the differential diagnosis of a suspected MRA abnormality. Stent artifact has been discussed previously as a potential cause of apparent localized vascular occlusion or stenosis. Stent artifact typically can be recognized on review of the source images, because of the characteristic MR appearance of metal. Indwelling metallic structures such as prosthetic joint replacements also may produce extensive artifact. These usually are recognized easily, but they may impair imaging significantly. They usually will result in extensive signal loss, with the resultant appearance of an occlusion, stenosis, or a missing segment of vessel. Fig. 29 shows the artifact produced by a total knee replacement on an MRA image of the popliteal region.

Additional artifacts may be seen as the result of poor timing of the arterial bolus. In particular, if triggering is performed too early, a ringing artifact frequently is seen. In unusual circumstances, this

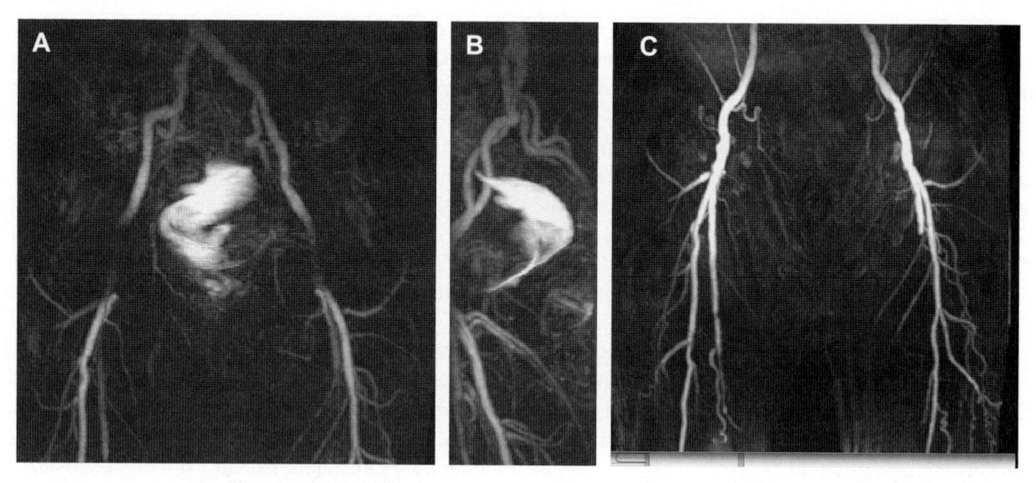

Fig. 29. Apparent bilateral femoral artery occlusions (*A*) produced by incorrect positioning of the imaging slab, as seen on a sagittal image (*B*). (*C*) Repeat examination with correct positioning.

appearance can mimic a dissection. Review of the source images and the characteristic appearance of this finding, however, usually allow the correct assessment to be made. In unusual circumstances, repetition of the acquisition with a second contrast bolus may be necessary [41].

Inappropriate positioning of the acquisition slices may result in exclusion of all or a portion of the vessel of interest from the imaging slab, resulting in apparent occlusion or stenosis. Fig. 29 demonstrates the appearance of an apparent area of occlusion in the femoral arteries. Review of the imaging slab positioning indicates that the vessels are not included in the image, explaining the resulting appearance. Repeat acquisition with appropriate positioning allows the proper evaluation to be made.

Image subtraction used in MRA demonstrably improves the contrast-to-noise ratio of the images, but can also lead to artifact. In particular, patient motion may result in such severe artifact as to limit the diagnostic value of the study.

Injection of undiluted contrast also may result in a pseudostenosis appearance, a finding most often seen during thoracic MRA, and this is noted most commonly in the subclavian region. This artifact results from the presence of undiluted contrast in the subclavian vein, which is in close proximity to the artery at its entry into the thorax, and which produces a resulting susceptibility artifact that results in apparent narrowing. Similar findings are possible in the abdomen, should a femoral venous catheter injection be performed.

New horizons

MRA imaging at 3 Tesla has been reported recently [42]. Given the increased signal to noise inherent in imaging at 3 Tesla, submillimeter image resolution is possible, with markedly accelerated imaging acquisitions using extensive parallel imaging protocols. This has the simultaneous benefit of decreasing scan time and diminishing the SAR impact of the higher field strength. Encouraging preliminary results have been reported [42].

A novel angiographic MRI technique is that of global coherent free precession imaging. In this technique, spins passing through a preselected region of interest acquire signal, while the background is suppressed, resulting in an angiographic appearance. The slab can be positioned freely, resulting in dynamic image acquisitions [43]. This manipulation can be performed in real-time from the scanner console. Possible future applications include real-time evaluation of the coronary arterial flow and guidance of interventional procedures.

Summary

It can be seen from the foregoing that MRA of the abdomen, pelvis, and lower extremities can be performed easily and rapidly for various clinical indications. The technique is robust and reproducible, and results in images that are the diagnostic equivalent of digital subtraction angiographic images, without radiation or an arterial puncture.

Certain inherent advantages present in three-dimensional imaging make it preferable in most circumstances. Continued improvements in scan hardware and software will allow more rapid acquisitions, further minimizing the potential for venous contamination, and allowing simultaneous improvement in spatial resolution.

Pearls

Positioning the three-dimensional angiographic slab is critically important. Knowledge of the underlying anatomy is key. The smaller the slab, the shorter the scan time and the quicker imaging is accomplished. One must be certain to include all relevant vessels, however.

In the upper leg, the arteries course posteriorly as they descend toward the knee. Therefore, the slab should be tilted in the sagittal plane such that the front of the slab encompasses the skin along the anterior aspect of the thigh at the top and extends posterior to the back of the knee at the bottom.

At the abdomen/pelvis level, remember that the iliac arteries can dip quite far posteriorly, and should be the marker for the most posterior aspect of the slab. The anterior margin of the slab must include the skin anterior to the femoral heads, which can serve as the marker for the front of the slab. If these regions are not included in the slab, the slab needs to be made thicker (increase slice number or thickness).

If a vessel possibly is occluded, remember to look for a stent on thin section images.

MIPs are not enough. Multiplanar thin section review of the images is essential to avoid missing significant lesions.

If the timing is off, or in case of technical glitches, consider rapidly repeating the acquisition and using subtraction and thin-section imaging review to salvage the study.

If information about the venous structures also is desired, the series of imaging sequences can be re-run in reverse order (from lower leg to abdominal station) after the arterial acquisition, with a 30-second pause in between.

References

[1] Selvin E, TP Erlinger. Prevalence of and risk factors for peripheral arterial disease in the United States: results from the National Health and Nutrition Examination Survey, 1999-2000. Circulation, 2004. 110(6): 738–743.

[2] Murabito JM, Evans JC, Larson MG, et al. The ankle–brachial index in the elderly and risk of stroke, coronary disease, and death: the Framingham Study. Arch Intern Med 2003;163(16):1939–42.

[3] Criqui MH, Langer RD, Fronek A, et al. Mortality over a period of 10 years in patients with peripheral arterial disease. N Engl J Med 1992;326(6):381–6.

[4] Newman AB, Shemanski L, Manolio TA, et al. Ankle–arm index as a predictor of cardiovascular disease and mortality in the Cardiovascular Health Study. The Cardiovascular Health Study Group. Arterioscler Thromb Vasc Biol 1999;19(3): 538–45.

[5] Hany TF, McKinnon GC, Leung DA, et al. Optimization of contrast timing for breath hold three-dimensional MR angiography. J Magn Reson Imaging 1997;7(3):551–6.

[6] Prince MR, Chabra SG, Watts R, et al. Contrast material travel times in patients undergoing peripheral MR angiography. Radiology 2002;224(1):55–61.

[7] Wang Y, Chen CZ, Chabra SG, et al. Bolus arterial–venous transit in the lower extremity and venous contamination in bolus chase three-dimensional magnetic resonance angiography. Invest Radiol 2002;37(8):458–63.

[8] Zhang HL, Ho BY, Chao M, et al. Decreased venous contamination on 3D gadolinium-enhanced bolus chase peripheral MR angiography using thigh compression. AJR Am J Roentgenol 2004;183(4): 1041–7.

[9] Morasch MD, Collins J, Pereles FS, et al. Lower extremity stepping-table magnetic resonance angiography with multilevel contrast timing and segmented contrast infusion. J Vasc Surg 2003;37(1): 62–71.

[10] Meissner OA, Rieger J, Weber C, et al. Critical limb ischemia: hybrid MR angiography compared with DSA. Radiology 2005;235(1):308–18.

[11] Binkert CA, Baker PD, Petersen BD, et al. Peripheral vascular disease: blinded study of dedicated calf MR angiography versus standard bolus chase MR angiography and film hard copy angiography. Radiology 2004;232(3):860–6.

[12] Zhang HL, Khilnani NM, Prince MR, et al. Diagnostic accuracy of time-resolved 2D projection MR angiography for symptomatic infrapopliteal arterial occlusive disease. AJR Am J Roentgenol 2005; 184(3):938–47.

[13] de Vries M, de Koning PJ, de Haan MW, et al. Accuracy of semiautomated analysis of 3D contrast-enhanced magnetic resonance angiography for detection and quantification of aortoiliac stenoses. Invest Radiol 2005;40(8):495–503.

[14] Brothers TE, Greenfield LJ. Long-term results of aortoiliac reconstruction. J Vasc Interv Radiol 1990;1(1):49–55.

[15] Leng GC, Davis M, Baker D. Bypass surgery for chronic lower limb ischaemia. Cochrane Database Syst Rev 2000;3:CD002000.

[16] Muhs BE, Gagne P, Sheehan P. Peripheral arterial disease: clinical assessment and indications for

revascularization in the patient with diabetes. Curr Diab Rep 2005;5(1):24–9.

[17] Ramdev P, Rayan SS, Sheahan M, et al. A decade experience with infrainguinal revascularization in a dialysis-dependent patient population. J Vasc Surg 2002;36(5):969–74.

[18] Lipsitz EC, Ohki T, Veith FJ, et al. Does subintimal angioplasty have a role in the treatment of severe lower extremity ischemia? J Vasc Surg 2003;37(2): 386–91.

[19] Lapeyre M, Kobeiter H, Desgranges P, et al. Assessment of critical limb ischemia in patients with diabetes: comparison of MR angiography and digital subtraction angiography. AJR Am J Roentgenol 2005;185(6):1641–50.

[20] Raffetto JD, Chen MN, LaMorte WW, et al. Factors that predict site of outflow target artery anastomosis in infrainguinal revascularization. J Vasc Surg 2002;35(6):1093–9.

[21] Bertschinger K, Cassina PC, Debatin JF, Ruehm SG, et al. Surveillance of peripheral arterial bypass grafts with three-dimensional MR angiography: comparison with digital subtraction angiography. AJR Am J Roentgenol 2001;176(1): 215–20.

[22] Klemm T, Duda S, Machann J, et al. MR imaging in the presence of vascular stents: a systematic assessment of artifacts for various stent orientations, sequence types, and field strengths. J Magn Reson Imaging 2000;12(4):606–15.

[23] Lenhart M, Volk M, Manke C, et al. Stent appearance at contrast-enhanced MR angiography: in vitro examination with 14 stents. Radiology 2000;217(1): 173–8.

[24] Letourneau-Guillon L, Soulez G, Beaudoin G, et al. CT and MR imaging of nitinol stents with radiopaque distal markers. J Vasc Interv Radiol 2004; 15(6):615–24.

[25] Ayuso JR, de Caralt TM, Pages M, et al. MRA is useful as a follow-up technique after endovascular repair of aortic aneurysms with nitinol endoprostheses. J Magn Reson Imaging 2004;20(5):803–10.

[26] Cejna M, Loewe C, Schoder M, et al. MR angiography vs CT angiography in the follow-up of nitinol stent grafts in endoluminally treated aortic aneurysms. Eur Radiol 2002;12(10):2443–50.

[27] Costantini V, Lenti M. Treatment of acute occlusion of peripheral arteries. Thromb Res 2002;106(6): V285–94.

[28] Barkhausen J, Hunold P, Eggebrecht H, et al. Detection and characterization of intracardiac thrombi on MR imaging. AJR Am J Roentgenol 2002;179(6): 1539–44.

[29] Herborn CU, Goyen M, Lauenstein TC, et al. Comprehensive time-resolved MRI of peripheral vascular malformations. AJR Am J Roentgenol 2003; 181(3):729–35.

[30] Elias DA, White LM, Rubenstein JD, et al. Clinical evaluation and MR imaging features of popliteal artery entrapment and cystic adventitial disease. AJR Am J Roentgenol 2003;180(3):627–32.

[31] Wright LB, Matchett WJ, Cruz CP, et al. Popliteal artery disease: diagnosis and treatment. Radiographics 2004;24(2):467–79.

[32] Quinn SF, Sheley RC, Semonsen KG, et al. Aortic and lower-extremity arterial disease: evaluation with MR angiography versus conventional angiography. Radiology 1998;206(3):693–701.

[33] Owen RS, Carpenter JP, Baum RA, et al. Magnetic resonance imaging of angiographically occult runoff vessels in peripheral arterial occlusive disease. N Engl J Med 1992;326(24):1577–81.

[34] Sharafuddin MJ, Stolpen AH, Sun S, et al. High-resolution multiphase contrast-enhanced three-dimensional MR angiography compared with two-dimensional time-of-flight MR angiography for the identification of pedal vessels. J Vasc Interv Radiol 2002;13(7):695–702.

[35] Vosshenrich R, Kopka L, Castillo E, et al. Electrocardiograph-triggered two-dimensional time-of-flight versus optimized contrast-enhanced three-dimensional MR angiography of the peripheral arteries. Magn Reson Imaging 1998;16(8): 887–92.

[36] Steffens JC, Schafer FK, Oberscheid B, et al. Bolus-chasing contrast-enhanced 3D MRA of the lower extremity. Comparison with intra-arterial DSA. Acta Radiol 2003;44(2):185–92.

[37] Willmann JK, Baumert B, Schertler T, et al. Aortoiliac and lower extremity arteries assessed with 16-detector row CT angiography: prospective comparison with digital subtraction angiography. Radiology 2005;236(3):1083–93.

[38] Ouwendijk R, de Vries M, Pattynama PM, et al. Imaging peripheral arterial disease: a randomized controlled trial comparing contrast-enhanced MR angiography and multidetector row CT angiography. Radiology 2005;236(3):1094–103.

[39] Ouwendijk R, Kock MC, Visser K, et al. Interobserver agreement for the interpretation of contrast-enhanced 3D MR angiography and MDCT angiography in peripheral arterial disease. AJR Am J Roentgenol 2005; 185(5):1261–7.

[40] Willmann JK, Wildermuth S, Pfammatter T, et al. Aortoiliac and renal arteries: prospective intraindividual comparison of contrast-enhanced three-dimensional MR angiography and multidetector row CT angiography. Radiology 2003;226(3):798–811.

[41] Lee VS, Martin DJ, Krinsky GA, et al. Gadolinium-enhanced MR angiography: artifacts and pitfalls. AJR Am J Roentgenol 2000;175(1):197–205.

[42] Huber ME, Kozerke S, Pruessmann KP, et al. Sensitivity-encoded coronary MRA at 3T. Magn Reson Med 2004;52(2):221–7.

[43] Klem I, Rehwald WG, Heitner JF, et al. Noninvasive assessment of blood flow based on magnetic resonance global coherent free precession. Circulation 2005;111(8):1033–9.

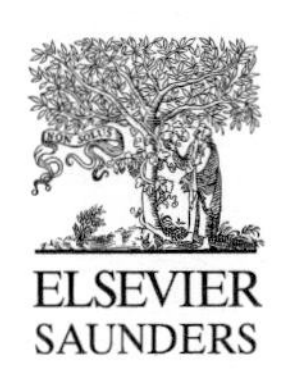

ELSEVIER
SAUNDERS

Cardiol Clin 25 (2007) 213–220

CARDIOLOGY
CLINICS

Index

Note: Page numbers of article titles are in **boldface** type.

doi:10.1016/S0733-8651(07)00019-7

D

R

S

T

U